Supportive Care in Respiratory Disease

Supportive Care Series

Volumes in the series

Surgical Palliative Care
Edited by Geoffrey P. Dunn and Alan G. Johnson

Supportive Care in Respiratory Disease, Second Edition
Edited by Sam H. Ahmedzai, David R. Baldwin, and David C. Currow

Supportive Care for the Renal Patient, Second Edition
Edited by E. Joanna Chambers, Edwina A. Brown, and Michael J. Germain

Supportive Care for the Urology Patient
Edited by Richard W. Norman and David C. Currow

Supportive Care in Heart Failure
Edited by James Beattie and Sarah Goodlin

Supportive Care for the Person with Dementia
Edited by Julian Hughes, Mari Lloyd-Williams, and Greg Sachs

Supportive Care in Respiratory Disease

SECOND EDITION

Edited by

Sam H. Ahmedzai

David R. Baldwin

David C. Currow

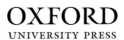

OXFORD
UNIVERSITY PRESS

OXFORD

UNIVERSITY PRESS

Great Clarendon Street, Oxford ox2 6DP

Oxford University Press is a department of the University of Oxford.
It furthers the University's objective of excellence in research, scholarship,
and education by publishing worldwide in

Oxford New York

Auckland Cape Town Dar es Salaam Hong Kong Karachi
Kuala Lumpur Madrid Melbourne Mexico City Nairobi
New Delhi Shanghai Taipei Toronto

With offices in

Argentina Austria Brazil Chile Czech Republic France Greece
Guatemala Hungary Italy Japan Poland Portugal Singapore
South Korea Switzerland Thailand Turkey Ukraine Vietnam

Oxford is a registered trade mark of Oxford University Press
in the UK and in certain other countries

Published in the United States
by Oxford University Press Inc., New York

British Library Cataloguing in Publication Data
Data available

Library of Congress Cataloging in Publication Data
Supportive care in respiratory disease / edited by Sam H. Ahmedzai, David R.
Baldwin, David C. Currow. — 2nd ed.
     p. ; cm. — (Supportive care series)
  Includes bibliographical references and index.
  ISBN 978-0-19-959176-3 (alk. paper)
  I. Ahmedzai, Sam, 1950- II. Baldwin, David R. III. Currow, David. IV. Series: Supportive care series.
  [DNLM: 1. Respiration Disorders—therapy. 2. Chronic Disease—therapy. 3.
Palliative Care—methods. WF 145]
  LC classification not assigned
  616.200429—dc23   2011032794

Typeset in Minion by Cenveo, Bangalore, India
Printed and bound by
CPI Group (UK) Ltd, Croydon, CR0 4YY

ISBN 978–0–19–959176–3

10 9 8 7 6 5 4 3 2 1

Preface to the Supportive Care Series

Supportive care is the multidisciplinary holistic care of patients with chronic and life-limiting illnesses and their families—from the time around diagnosis, through treatments aimed at cure or prolonging life, and into the phase currently acknowledged as palliative care. It involves recognizing and caring for the side-effects of active therapies as well as patients' symptoms, co-morbidities, psychological, social, and spiritual concerns. It also values the role of family carers and helps them in supporting the patient, as well as attending to their own special needs. Supportive care is a domain of health and social care that utilizes a network of professionals and voluntary carers in a 'virtual team'. It is increasingly recognized by healthcare providers and governments as a modern response to complex disease management, but so far it can lay claim to little dedicated literature.

This is therefore one volume in a unique new series of textbooks on supportive care published by Oxford University Press, which has already established itself as a leading publisher for palliative care. Unlike 'traditional' palliative care, which grew from the terminal care of cancer patients, supportive care is not restricted to dying patients and neither to cancer. Thus, this series covers the support of patients with a variety of long-term conditions, who are currently largely managed by specialist and general teams in hospitals and by primary care teams in community settings. It will, therefore, provide a practical guide to the supportive care of the patient at all stages of the illness, providing up-to-date knowledge of the scientific basis of palliation and also practical guidance on delivering high-quality multidisciplinary care across healthcare sectors. The volumes—edited by acknowledged leaders in the specific fields discussed in each volume—will bring together research, healthcare management, economics, and ethics through contributions from an international panel of experts of all disciplines. The underlying theme of all the books is the application of the latest evidence-based knowledge, in a humane way, for patients with advancing disease.

As Series Editor, I bring decades of research and clinical experience of acute medicine and palliative care. My work has spanned St Christopher's Hospice and the Leicestershire Hospice in England—both of which have been inspirational leaders of traditional palliative care; and the Academic Unit of Supportive Care at the University of Sheffield, England. I have advocated the supportive care approach to cancer and other chronic disease management and I am delighted to be collaborating on this series. I am committed to delivering high quality of end-of-life care when it is necessary, but constantly seeking to influence colleagues in all relevant healthcare disciplines to adopt the principles of modern supportive care to benefit a wider range of patients at earlier stages of illness.

I aim, through this series, to inform and inspire other doctors, nurses, allied health professionals, pharmacists, social and spiritual care providers, and students, to improve the quality of living for all patients and families in their care.

Sam Hjelmeland Ahmedzai
Professor of Palliative Medicine
Academic Unit of Supportive Care
The University of Sheffield
Royal Hallamshire Hospital
Sheffield, UK

Foreword to First Edition

The starting point to support patients with any long-standing medical condition is to listen to them and understand those things which are compromising the quality of *their* lives. For one individual, it may be the burden of a particular symptom such as breathlessness; for another it may be the consequential limitation on some particular activity such as their inability to get upstairs or to get out and about. Different problems have different solutions. This is a very timely book because it demonstrates the importance of the art as well as the science of medicine and brings the two together. In recent years there have been magnificent advances in the treatment of many lung conditions. Some of the world's most common diseases such as tuberculosis can be cured before there is irreparable damage to the lungs, and immunization and antibiotics can prevent other forms of long-standing disabilities such as bronchiectasis following measles or whooping cough. Removal of damaging environmental agents including tobacco can reduce the burden of chronic obstructive pulmonary disease, many occupational lung diseases, and lung cancer. Likewise anti-inflammatory medication can now transform other common and less common lung diseases if administered early enough. Advances in surgery can eliminate areas of localized disease, greatly improving symptoms and prolonging life. Indeed, flushed with the success of so many advances, made possible through modern scientific medicine in the pathogenesis and treatment of lung diseases, it is easy to overlook the burden of persisting symptoms and the compromise to normal life that a large number of patients are still compelled to endure.

The fact is that in spite of modern advances there remain a large number of patients with persisting conditions such as asthma which require continuing support, those with irreversible airways obstruction, destruction of alveolar units (eg emphysema) or lung scarring from a variety of causes, which result in loss of lung reserve and limit exercise through breathlessness and other pathophysiological mechanisms. Some patients have other bothersome symptoms such as chronic cough and sputum. In turn these often compromise sleep and lead to general debility. Such continuing symptoms often lead to social isolation, anxiety and depression, and a general lack of self-esteem and confidence. All undermine the quality of life. Only too often, especially when doctors are under severe pressure of time, these patients are regarded as untreatable and simply left to their own devices without support until, often after years of unnecessary suffering and deteriorating health, the need for palliative care to ease their terminal distress is recognized. The importance of the distinction between supportive and palliative care cannot be overemphasized. Of course many good doctors are well aware of the physical and psychological burden of chronic lung disease and over the years have tried their best to relieve their patients' symptoms. More recently there has been much more focused attention on the basic mechanisms underlying respiratory symptoms and this has led to the evaluation of a wide variety of techniques to improve respiratory performance as well as the development of scientific measurements to validate and quantify the improvements obtained in terms of quality of life, as well as the cost effectiveness of doing so. What has been lacking is a comprehensive and fully-referenced book where all these advances in supportive medicine in respiratory disease are brought together.

This substantial book, with contributions from many international specialists, reviews systematically the advances in this field across the whole range of lung diseases and sets new standards in both primary and secondary care to support patients with continuing respiratory disabilities. Indeed it goes much further because the principles of supportive medicine outlined here and the ways in which therapies may be evaluated are often equally applicable to those with non-respiratory disorders. In this way, this book makes a major contribution to the field of medical care of patients with chronic disease and emphasizes the responsibilities that doctors, other healthcare workers and society in general have for those who we are currently unable to cure, but for whom so much can still be done to lighten their burden.

Margaret Turner Warwick
November 2004

Preface

In the years since the first edition of this volume, supportive care has become an increasingly important concept in most fields of healthcare but despite this, its implementation is still often an afterthought or not thought of at all. This is even the case where supportive care is arguably the most important part of care. For example, most people with lung cancer are offered 'best supportive care' with or without disease modifying treatment. However, in reality such patients receive very variable levels of supportive care, all under this one umbrella term.

In this, the second edition of *Supportive Care in Respiratory Disease*, we re-emphasize how important supportive care is in respiratory disease by updating the sections on generic aspects, mechanisms, and treatment of the more common symptoms, and show how supportive care applies in specific settings and diseases. Part one gives, by way of introduction, a discussion of the meaning of terms associated with supportive care and examines some important concepts. Anatomy and physiology is covered to assist in interpretation of later chapters and the concepts associated with quality of life and economic evaluations are explored. Part 2 deals specifically with the science of the generation of dyspnoea and its measurement. Part 3 reviews several aspects of supportive interventions which apply to many diseases. Parts 4–6 deal more specifically with conditions and other common symptoms, and finally Part 7 deals with specific diseases where supportive care should play a particularly dominant role.

We are greatly indebted to all the authors who have given their expert appraisal of the literature and their valuable opinions, and hope that the reader will gain new insight, as we indeed have during the course of producing this book, into this essential topic. We are also grateful to our secretaries for assisting us in our editing, and of course to the editorial team at Oxford University Press for their administrative help and constant support.

Contents

Contributors *xiii*

Part 1 **Supportive care in respiratory medicine**

1 Palliation and supportive care *3*
Sam H. Ahmedzai

2 Anatomy and physiology *37*
Martin F. Muers

3 Quality of life: models and measurement *53*
Michael E. Hyland and Samantha C. Sodergren

4 Principles of economic evaluation *61*
Sarah Willis

Part 2 **Mechanisms and assessment of dyspnoea**

5 The genesis of breathlessness: what do we understand? *71*
Jeremy B. Richards and Richard M. Schwartzstein

6 Multidimensional assessment of dyspnoea *91*
Ingrid Harle and Deborah Dudgeon

Part 3 **General supportive interventions**

7 Pharmacological treatment of respiratory symptoms *111*
David C. Currow and Amy P. Abernethy

8 Oxygen and airflow *123*
Christine McDonald and James Ward

9 Occupational therapy, environmental modifications, and pulmonary
rehabilitation *145*
Sally Singh and Louise Sewell

10 Non-pharmacological strategies for dyspnoea *163*
Virginia Carrieri-Kohlman and DorAnne Donesky-Cuenco

11 Nutrition and cachexia *185*
Josep M. Argilés, Sílvia Busquets, Mireia Olivan, and Francisco J. López-Soriano

Part 4 **Dyspnoea in special situations**

12 Diffuse airflow obstruction and 'restrictive' lung disease *197*
Mary McGregor and David R. Baldwin

13 Neuromuscular and skeletal diseases, and obstructive sleep apnoea   *215*
John Shneerson

14 Hyperventilation syndrome   *233*
Julie Moore and Sally Singh

Part 5 **Cough and expectoration**

15 Physiology and pathophysiology of cough   *253*
Ian D. Pavord

16 Expectoration: pathophysiology, measurement, and therapy   *271*
Alyn H. Morice

Part 6 **Pain**

17 Pain assessment in respiratory disease   *281*
Elaine Cachia, Jason Boland, and Sam H. Ahmedzai

18 Pain in respiratory disease: mechanisms and management   *289*
Jason Boland, Elaine Cachia, Russell K. Portenoy, and Sam H. Ahmedzai

Part 7 **Specific diseases**

19 Supportive care in cystic fibrosis   *309*
Andrew Clayton

20 Assessment and management of respiratory symptoms
of malignant disease   *319*
Jennifer Chard, Peter Hoskin, and Sam H. Ahmedzai

21 Comprehensive supportive care for chronic pulmonary infections   *347*
Gary T. Buckholz and Charles F. von Gunten

Index   *369*

Contributors

Amy P. Abernethy
Associate Professor of Medicine,
Discipline of Palliative and Supportive
Services, Flinders University, Australia;
Duke Comprehensive Cancer Center; and
Department of Medicine,
Division of Medical Oncology, Duke
University Medical Center (DUMC),
Durham, NC, USA

Sam H. Ahmedzai
Head of Academic Unit of Supportive
Care and Honorary Consultant Physician,
University of Sheffield, UK

Josep M. Argilés
Cancer Research Group, Biochemistry
and Molecular Biology of Cancer, Faculty
of Biology, University of Barcelona, Spain

David R. Baldwin
Consultant Respiratory Physician,
Respiratory Medicine Unit, Nottingham
University Hospitals, UK

Jason Boland
Academic Unit of Supportive Care,
The University of Sheffield, UK

Gary T. Buckholz
Director, Palliative Medicine Fellowship
Program, The Institute for Palliative
Medicine at San Diego Hospice, CA, USA

Sílvia Busquets
Cancer Research Group, Biochemistry
and Molecular Biology of Cancer, Faculty
of Biology, University of Barcelona, Spain

Elaine Cachia
Specialist Registrar in Palliative Medicine,
Sheffield Teaching Hospitals NHS
Foundation Trust,
University of Sheffield, UK

Virginia Carrieri-Kohlman
Professor, Department of Physiological
Nursing, University of California,
San Francisco, CA, USA

Jennifer Chard
Andrew Clayton
Department of Respiratory Medicine,
David Evans Centre, Nottingham City
Campus, Nottingham University
Hospitals, UK

David C. Currow
Professor, Discipline of Palliative and
Supportive Services, Flinders University,
Australia

DorAnne Donesky-Cuenco
Assistant Adjunct Professor, Dyspnea
Research Group, Department of
Physiological Nursing, University of
California, San Francisco, CA, USA

Deborah Dudgeon
Queen's Palliative Care Medicine
Program, Kingston, Ontario, Canada

Fabio Fulfaro
Medical Oncology Operative Unit,
University of Palmero, Palmero, Italy

Ingrid Harle
Queen's Palliative Care Medicine
Program, Kingston, Ontario, Canada

Peter Hoskin
Consultant Clinical Oncologist, Mount
Vernon Hospital, Northwood, Middlesex,
and Professor of Oncology, University
College London, UK

Michael E. Hyland
Professor of Health Psychology, School Of
Psychology, University of Plymouth, UK

Francisco J. López-Soriano
Cancer Research Group, Biochemistry
and Molecular Biology of Cancer, Faculty
of Biology, University of Barcelona, Spain

Christine McDonald
Professor and Director, Department of
Respiratory and Sleep Medicine, Austin
Health and Melbourne University,
Victoria, Australia

Mary McGregor
CT2 Medicine, Pilgrim Hospital,
Boston, UK

Julie Moore
Pulmonary Rehabilitation Department,
Respiratory Medicine, University
Hospitals of Leicester, UK

Alyn H. Morice
Professor, Hull York Medical School,
University of Hull, Cardiovascular &
Respiratory Studies, Castle Hill Hospital,
Cottingham, UK

Martin F. Muers
Consultant Physician, Leeds Chest Clinic,
Leeds General Infirmary, UK

Mireia Olivan
Cancer Research Group,
Biochemistry and Molecular Biology of
Cancer, Faculty of Biology,
University of Barcelona, Spain

Ian D. Pavord
Consultant Physician and Honorary
Professor of Medicine, Institute for Lung
Health, Department of Respiratory
Medicine, Glenfield Hospital, University
Hospitals of Leicester NHS Trust, UK

Russell K. Portenoy
Chairman and Gerald J. Friedman
Chair in Pain Medicine and Palliative
Care, Department of Pain Medicine and
Palliative Care, Beth Israel Medical
Center; Chief Medical Officer,
MJHS Hospice and Palliative Care; and
Professor of Neurology and
Anesthesiology, Albert Einstein College
of Medicine, New York, NY, USA

Jeremy B. Richards
Division of Pulmonary and Critical Care
Medicine and Department of Medicine,
Beth Israel Deaconess Medical Center and
Harvard Medical School, Boston,
MA, USA

Carla Ripamonti
Pain Therapy and Palliative Care Division,
National Cancer Institute, Milan, Italy

Richard M. Schwartzstein
Division of Pulmonary and Critical Care
Medicine and Department of Medicine,
Beth Israel Deaconess Medical Center and
Harvard Medical School, Boston,
MA, USA

Louise Sewell
Senior Pulmonary Rehabilitation
Specialist, Glenfield Hospital, University
Hospitals of Leicester NHS Trust, UK

John Shneerson
Consultant Physician, Respiratory
Support and Sleep Centre, Papworth
Hospital, UK

Sally Singh
Pulmonary Rehabilitation Department,
Respiratory Medicine, University
Hospitals of Leicester, UK

Samantha C. Sodergren
School of Psychology, University of
Plymouth, UK

Charles F. von Gunten
Provost, Center for Palliative Studies, San
Diego Hospice & Palliative Care,
University of California, San Diego,
CA, USA

James Ward
Department of Respiratory and Sleep
Medicine, Austin Health, Victoria,
Australia

Sarah Willis
Research fellow in Health Economics,
London School of Hygiene and Tropical
Medicine, UK

Part 1

Supportive care in respiratory medicine

Chapter 1

Palliation and supportive care

Sam H. Ahmedzai

Changing aims of medicine

Medicine has undergone significant changes many times in history, but perhaps none so dramatic as those in the latter part of the 20th and beginning of the 21st centuries. Particularly in the last 50 years, there has been a shift in focus from the restricted view of the physician at the bedside, in the clinic, or at the operating table, to the broader vision of community and social networks. Public health medicine has become a major force in planning and delivering healthcare, whereas previously this was determined by the interests of individual practitioners, who worked largely in independent settings with little accountability or need to cooperate with other colleagues. The birth of the World Health Organization (WHO) and its subsequent influence on the public health policies of most countries can be seen as both a reflection and a driving force of this global change.

At the same time, paradoxically, other contemporary influences have made patients' views more powerful, which has led healthcare practitioners to think more carefully about the psychological and social implications of their actions. These influences include the rise of consumerism, at least in the Western world, and the growing disenchantment many people have felt with the unchallenged authority of medicine and nursing. In some countries, there has also been an increasing role of non-governmental organizations, or charities, which have become significant agencies for stimulating social reform, funding research, influencing policy, and even competing with, or at least supplementing, state healthcare systems for providing direct medical care to the public. (The rise of charities in the latter part of the 20th century is rather different from their role in the 19th century, when they were dominated by religious principles and were largely concerned with relieving the pitiful conditions of the very poorest people in society.) Examples of the modern organizations are the many national cancer leagues and international bodies such as the International Union Against Cancer (UICC) and the international hospice movement.

A central theme with all the diverse charitable organizations has been the recognition of the importance of the individual patient and his or her family, and their needs at different stages of illness and the road to recovery. Parallel to the development of the charitable organizations has been the growing role for volunteers in health and especially social care. In many cases this aspect has been crucial to the charities' outreach work. Volunteers have been particularly important, for instance, in the implementation of palliative care principles in Europe, Australia, India, Africa, Southeast Asia, and the Americas.

These shifts in healthcare thinking can be seen reflected in the changing aims of medicine. Table 1.1 shows how the originally simple purpose of medicine has moved from making a diagnosis, followed by attempting a cure and if that were not possible, then trying to palliate the consequences, into broader and more humanistic objectives. The first of these modern objectives is the increasing investment into prevention and earlier detection of disease, reflecting the current view that earlier intervention with many diseases may result in a better chance of disease eradication. Other key elements of the new aims of medicine include: recognizing the value of prolonging life, even if the patient cannot be 'cured'; rehabilitation to enable people whose lives have been changed by disease (or treatment), to restore better function and reclaim personal and social roles; and the value placed on care at the end of life.

There is perhaps now greater honesty among physicians about the true chances of 'curability', with recognition that prolonging life is itself a worthy aim of medicine, even if the disease cannot be cured. In a similar vein, oncologists have realized that 'response rates' to anticancer therapies by themselves do not always translate into benefit for patients, and are therefore increasingly incorporating subjective endpoints such as symptom relief and quality of life as markers of their interventions (1, 2).

MacDonald has stated this as a challenge to his fellow oncologists to see cancer management as more than curing cancer, or prolonging life, but also from the point of view of improving the *quality* of life of the patients (3). Of course, in chronic disease management, notions of 'cure' are often meaningless. In the respiratory field, chronic obstructive pulmonary disease (COPD), pulmonary fibrosis, industrial lung diseases, neuromuscular disorders, and even some chronic infections such as tuberculosis cannot be thought of as curable, and so a different attitude to their management has emerged.

Rehabilitation is becoming integral to the plan of disease management, both in acute and chronic conditions. Some rehabilitation is required because many treatment interventions themselves compromise the independence of the patient, e.g. surgery. Other motivations for rehabilitation come partly justified by humane reasons of improving

Table 1.1 Changing aims of medicine

Older aims	Newer aims
	Prevention
Diagnosis	Early and accurate diagnosis
Cure	Cure
	Prolonging life
	Rehabilitation
Palliation	Palliation
Terminal care	End of life care
(Death seen as a failure and dying as usually terrible)	(Death seen as inevitable and dying as potentially tolerable)

health, and partly by socioeconomic arguments about restoring the patient to a former occupation, or allowing a family carer to resume work or being less reliant on outside help. Pulmonary rehabilitation in COPD is a good example of these phenomena and programmes are becoming widespread within respiratory disease services (see Chapter 9 and 12).

According to the *Compact Oxford English Dictionary*, the definition of 'to palliate' is: 'to alleviate the symptoms of a disease without curing it; to relieve superficially or temporarily; to mitigate the sufferings of; to ease'.

Deriving from the Latin word '*palliare*', to cloak, the dictionary definition given above is not particularly helpful in the fuller clinical context that this volume will be considering. For this purpose, a more comprehensive definition is proposed: medical palliation is the relief of a symptom or a problem associated with an illness, without necessarily curing the underlying disease process; and in the case of a life-threatening illness, without primarily attempting to prolong life.

The terms 'necessarily' and 'primarily' are important parts of this definition, but frequently in clinical practice they may be overruled. As will be seen throughout this volume, in many areas of medicine the best palliation may well be achieved through measures which are in fact designed to cure or to prolong life, by being directed against the underlying primary disease process. Examples are the impressive relief of physical symptoms of lung cancer through the use of life-prolonging cytotoxic chemotherapy; and the resolution of fever, cough, and haemoptysis with the use of combination antibiotics in pulmonary tuberculosis.

In many other cases, however, symptoms may be better controlled by interventions which act directly on them, by mitigating the pathological processes caused by the primary disease which give rise to symptoms remote from the primary disease site. An example of this is the management of nausea and vomiting which arises in some patients with squamous cell cancer of the lung. The mechanism of the emetic stimulus is hypercalcaemia, which is caused by the production of a parathormone-like substance from the tumour. Treating the hypercalcaemia systemically by means of intravenous bisphosphonates is dramatically helpful for reducing emesis (and other hypercalcaemia-related symptoms such as confusion), without any need directly to treat the primary cancer (4).

A further mechanism of medical palliation is the relief of symptoms and other problems by interventions which are not targeted at the causative disease *nor* at its pathophysiological consequences, but by tackling directly the subjective perception of the symptom/problem. The use of opioids such as morphine for pain control is an example of this mechanism. In the case of pain during angina, the distress is caused by ischaemia in the cardiac muscle. Morphine promptly relieves the pain, not by restoring blood supply (as would glyceryl trinitrate), nor by intervening in the pathology of coronary artery disease (as would cholesterol-reducing agents), but by its direct effect on the brain's perception of pain originating in visceral tissues. It does this by interacting with mu-opioid receptors in the brain and spinal cord, far from the site of the pathology.

Another way of relieving the nausea in the patient with hypercalcaemia could be the administration of a butyrophenone drug such as haloperidol. This works without having any impact on the underlying malignancy or the elevated serum calcium, but by modulating dopaminergic D2 receptors in the chemoreceptor trigger zone in the brainstem. There are examples of this type of palliation in the field of psychological care: the relief of anxiety by the use of anxiolytic drugs, or by explanation and information. Thus it is not always strictly 'medical' palliation that may be helpful, but also the contributions from other healthcare disciplines such as nursing or psychology.

In order to improve the clarity in describing and attributing the palliative actions of healthcare interventions, a classification of palliative interventions is shown in Table 1.2. This table shows that to the three types of palliation described above, a fourth has been added—called type 1 or preventive palliation. This type of palliation is included for completeness, because it emphasizes that appropriate preventive measures can also relieve symptoms, even if they cannot stop the onset or progress of a disease. An example of this is the improvement in delirium in elderly people by attention to good ambient light and noise reduction at night (rather than the use of neuroleptic agents, which in this classification, would represent type 3 palliation) (5). The purpose of introducing this taxonomy is to clarify the aims of palliation, so that we can better understand how to use different approaches to maximum advantage. The classification may also be useful in guiding us to use appropriate outcome measures to evaluate the potential benefit of different palliation techniques.

Figure 1.1 shows how we can develop these types of medical palliation into a generic algorithm, which attempts to explain how and when palliation works.

The generic model could be used in several ways: first, as an educational tool for teaching healthcare professionals about the impact of disease on patients' lives and how other

Table 1.2 A proposed classification of palliative interventions based on intention

Type of palliation	Intention	Example—cancer	Example—COPD
Type 1	Prevention/prophylaxis	◆ Smoking prevention/ cessation ◆ Cranial irradiation to prevent brain metastases	◆ Smoking prevention/ cessation ◆ Exercise programmes to prevent de-conditioning
Type 2	Direct targeting of the primary disease process	◆ Lobectomy ◆ RT for bone metastases	◆ α-1 antitrypsin replacement ◆ Corticosteroid
Type 3	Manipulation of the pathophysiological consequences of the primary disease process	◆ Bisphosphonate for symptoms of hypercalcaemia, e.g. nausea, confusion	◆ Broncho-dilator for airflow obstruction
Type 4	Alteration of the perception or secondary effects of the symptom	◆ Drug treatments for symptoms of hypercalcaemia, e.g. emetic, neuroleptic	◆ Therapies to reduce perception of dyspnoea, e.g. oxygen, opioid

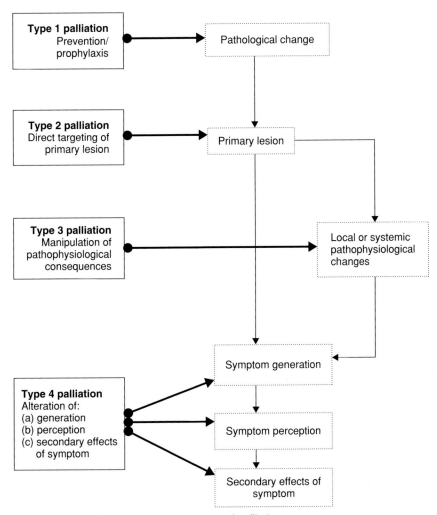

Fig. 1.1 Generic model of symptom perception and palliation.

intrinsic and extrinsic factors modify that impact. Second, as an information tool for explaining to patients themselves and their family carers, why and how specific palliative interventions are hoped to work, and to help them understand why some treatments may fail. Third, the model can be used to expose key aspects of the disease or patient's psychological condition which could be further researched to lead to more effective interventions for the future.

Factors determining symptom perception and the success of palliation

So far we have considered how a palliative intervention may bring about its effect. There is another important aspect to this discussion, and that is the role of the individual's own psychic traits and state, and how that may affect the success or failure of an intervention. It is a commonplace observation in healthcare that no two patients respond with the same degree of pain to an injury, and even the same person may report different levels of pain with the same pathology at different times, depending on other conscious or subconscious processes. Increasing age is thought to be accompanied by reducing tendency to complain of some physical symptoms such as pain; and at the same time older people appear to require lower doses of analgesic drugs to achieve pain control. Recent studies have shown that not only do men and women report some symptoms to different extents, but they also react differently to some classes of drugs (6, 7). The reasons for these findings are no doubt complex, and could include true differences in end-organ subjectivity, changes in metabolism of drugs, social conditioning, and biases of observers.

Care of dying patients

The final layer in Table 1.1 is the introduction of a new objective for medicine, that of 'end of life care'. It could be said that care of the dying has always been central to medicine, but it is fair to comment that it had to be included in medical care during the centuries before curative treatments were available. In the 16th century an anonymous author defined the role of a physician as: 'To cure sometimes, to relieve often, to comfort always'.

The medical establishment subsequently adopted an increasingly distant position from patients with diseases which could not be cured. Only in the last two centuries has the care of a dying person been recognized by the body of physicians as a worthy end in itself. The origins of terminal or 'end of life' care go back many hundreds of years, but it became an organizational reality only in the latter half of the 19th century in the first Christian hospice-like institutions of Ireland, France, and England. A discussion of the hospice movement is beyond the scope of this volume, but its relevance and contribution to modern supportive care should never be underestimated (8).

Why have end of life care and the recognition of comfort as a valid goal of healthcare become more widely recognized recently? Part of the explanation derives from the secular trends described earlier, and sociologists have commented on the public's concern with the increasing 'medicalization' of life and death, and the perceived 'sanitization' of the dying process (9). Over the last 50 years, the tendency has been for most deaths in developed countries to occur in hospital, rather than at home. One reason for this is that the notion of 'home' and who resides there has itself changed because of demographic shifts, including increased mobility of populations and the break-down of nuclear families in many Westernized societies.

Non-industrialized societies may not have the same opportunities for admitting terminally ill patients to hospital or hospice, but in other ways have embraced the concept of providing high-quality specialized end of life care. In India, for example, Rajagopal and Kumar have argued that the Western hospice model cannot be widely implemented partly because of the sheer size of the terminally ill population (one million cancer patients who mostly present with advanced incurable disease), but also because the hospice concept is not suited to Indians culturally (10). In response, they describe the 'Calicut model', in which families are mobilized to assist the dying patient, aided by existing cancer services and boosted by non-governmental charitable organizations. In 1998 nine Central and Eastern European countries joined to make the 'Poznan Declaration', which emphasized the desire to pursue palliative care but stressed the need for national policies, education, and awareness programmes and improved drug availability (11). Building more hospices was not a viable option here, as in many other parts of the world.

The unifying principle behind these international developments is the recognition that terminally ill patients (usually identified as having incurable cancer, but increasingly embracing life-limiting non-malignant diseases) have a need to receive good quality care at the end of life. In the words of the preamble of the Poznan Declaration: 'It is a human right to receive effective cancer pain relief and palliative care. It is unethical to tolerate unnecessary and unacceptable suffering'.

Clearly this statement could equally apply to a patient with a potentially curable cancer, or to one with a progressive non-malignant chronic disease such as severe COPD or fibrosing alveolitis—or even to one with an acute and self-limiting condition which produces pain and suffering. However, the spirit which has captured the world in the past 30 years, since the establishment of St Christopher's Hospice in London and the Royal Victoria Hospital palliative care unit in Montreal—the two pioneers of hospice, home, and hospital-based care—is the care of people dying from cancer. In the following discussion we will explore the nature of this concentration of emotion, energy, and resources for end of life care, and an argument will be proposed that life—*before it comes to the end*—with either chronic or curable distressing illnesses, is also worthy of equally energetic dedication from the healthcare professions. This is the basis of the concept of 'supportive care'.

In summary, rehabilitation, palliation, and end of life care—together with the underlying principle of always giving comfort—are important in the field of respiratory disease. To justify this one needs only to look at the 'curability' of pulmonary diseases, or even when they cannot be cured, at the realistic prospect of prolonging life. Naturally the possibilities of cure or increased survival depend not only on our current knowledge and treatments, but on social and economic variations in the general health of a nation, as well as on the physiological and psychosocial resistance of the individual patient. Table 1.3 shows how powerless medicine really is in halting the deadly progress of so many pulmonary diseases, which highlights the enormous possibilities for relieving suffering!

Models of palliative care

Let us now consider a healthcare approach which incorporates elements from the preceding discussions about symptom perception, medical palliation, and the need to consider incurable and fatal diseases. This approach has come to be known as 'palliative care'. The historical explanation for this new use of 'palliative' is because of the reluctance of the newly developing terminal care services in French-speaking Canada in the 1970s to use the term 'hospice', which had already been accepted in Britain. To the francophones in

Table 1.3 Curability, possibility of prolonging life and ability to palliate in various pulmonary diseases

Condition	Cure?	Prolong life?	Palliate?
Infections			
Acute bronchitis	++	++	++
Pneumonia	+	++	+
TB	+/−	++	+
HIV		++	++
Chronic disorders			
COPD	−	++	+
Cystic fibrosis	−/+	+	+
Pneumoconiosis and industrial lung diseases	−	−/+	−/+
Malignancy			
Primary lung cancer	−/+	++	++
Mesothelioma	−	−/+	+
Metastatic cancer	−	−/+	+

Key: − = never; −/+ = sometimes; + = frequently; ++ = always.

Montreal, the word 'hospice' implied a residential system for elderly people, with strongly negative connotations. It is said that Balfour Mount, a surgeon working in the Royal Victoria Hospital and who had been inspired by Dame Cicely Saunders to establish the first terminal care service in Canada, started to use the term 'palliative care' as an alternative to both hospice and terminal care. This new usage rapidly gained currency on both sides of the Atlantic and is the favoured expression worldwide today to describe what are essentially end of life healthcare services. It is, however, somewhat regrettable that the same term 'palliative' has been used to describe the *healthcare system* as is used for the *relief of symptoms*, since this has only added to the confusion about what the former is.

What actually *is* palliative care? A common starting point for understanding this is the WHO view which was first published in its landmark 1986 *Cancer pain relief and palliative care* booklet. The second edition (1990), gives the following definition (12):

> Palliative care is the active total care of patients whose disease is not responsive to curative treatment. Control of pain, of other symptoms and of psychological, social and spiritual problems is paramount. The goal of palliative care is achievement of the best possible quality of life for patients and their families.

This definition has been extremely influential, just as the pain relief programme, which accompanied it in the *Cancer pain relief and palliative care* booklet, has been. But has this definition stood the test of time? In one way it clearly has, as so many other organizations and publications refer to and borrow from it. Also these sentences have clearly been powerful in opening the minds of clinicians, and perhaps more importantly, of policymakers to release the resources needed to improve the care of cancer patients at the end of life.

Who could argue with the need to control pain, breathlessness, and other symptoms, to achieve the 'best quality of life' for patients and families, and to offer a support system to help patients live as actively as possible?

But the premise on which all these statements were based is that the patient has to have an incurable and fatal cancer. How can we reconcile that with the humane need to offer care to people who have potentially curable cancer; or those with cancer whose life may be still extended; and to all those whose primary disease is *not* cancer? The WHO definition makes reference to 'many aspects of palliative care' being applicable to earlier stages of disease. However, this only underlines the perception that palliative care itself is confined to terminally ill patients. In response to these limitations, the WHO issued a revised definition in 2002 (13):

> Palliative care is an approach that improves the quality of life of patients and their families facing the problems associated with life-threatening illness, through the prevention and relief of suffering by means of early identification and impeccable assessment and treatment of pain and other problems, physical, psychosocial and spiritual.

This addresses some of the concerns expressed above, namely that relief of suffering and the improvement of quality of life need not be confined to those who are deemed to be dying. However, the diagrammatic representation of palliative care initiated in the 1980s, represented in Figure 1.2, still heavily implies that palliative care should be associated with the end of life. This model has been influential in advising policy-makers on allocating resources for palliative care for cancer patients who are incurable. Unfortunately, it has also unavoidably been seen as a *clinical* model, encouraging surgeons and oncologists to practice their interventions in *separate compartments* of the healthcare system from the palliative care services. This may be efficient and convenient for the services, but it leads to discontinuity from the point of view of the recipients. The WHO model also imposes an additional, unnecessary trauma for patients who need to be transferred at a vulnerable time from what is often loosely called 'active' to palliative care. Furthermore, a too literal reading of the WHO resource model implies that curative treatment is superior to, and has to *take precedence* over, palliative care. Leaving aside the question of how 'curable' many cancers really are at the outset, this view gives individual clinicians involved in curative treatments (and also in primary care) the discretion to withhold referral to palliative care until it is thought that the 'time is right'.

In 1987 a group of doctors in the UK convened a new association for those working in the newly emerging field of medical practice in hospices and community- or hospital-based

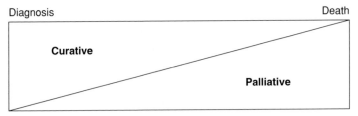

Fig. 1.2 The WHO model of resource allocation in cancer care.

palliative care services. Forming what is now called the Association for Palliative Medicine of Great Britain and Ireland, they adopted a new definition of what shortly afterwards became recognized by the Royal Colleges of Physicians in the UK as the specialty of palliative medicine. The definition is: 'Palliative medicine is the study and management of patients with active, progressive, far-advanced disease for whom the prognosis is limited and the focus of care is the quality of life'.

This definition has no doubt helped medical colleagues in other established specialties to understand and accept what palliative medicine is trying to do. But again, we can see that there is an unmistakable emphasis on the end of life. The definition also uses terms which are not themselves clear. To take the elements separately:

◆ *Active, progressive*—how does one determine this, even in malignant disease? We may know when a cancer is actively progressing, from biochemical markers, radiological and perhaps clinical signs, but how can we be sure when it is *not* active, but stable? Are symptoms and other problems from stable disease not worthy of attention? Patients who have come through devastating disease and invasive treatments may be medically 'stable', but they may well have major need for rehabilitation: whose task is to provide that? And how much 'progression' needs to occur before palliative medicine becomes relevant? Should cancer patients be referred at the time when the first metastasis is detected; or should they wait until the oncologist or surgeon has exhausted second-, or third-line therapies?

◆ *Far-advanced disease*—what does this evocative term actually mean? Does 'far' imply distance, in other words, metastatic disease in the case of cancer? But if a disease is only locally advanced, e.g. lung cancer which is causing pain through intercostal nerve infiltration or breathlessness through bronchial obstruction, then does palliative medicine have no part to play? If, on the other hand, 'far-advanced' is another way of saying 'end-stage' regardless of metastatic status, perhaps it would be better to use plainer language. If we consider non-malignant diseases, does the concept of 'far-advanced' still have currency and a measurable threshold—e.g. when does it start in COPD, musculoskeletal disorders, or tuberculosis? Furthermore, if the specialty of palliative medicine does not consider that it should study and manage symptoms and problems in disease which are *not* 'far-advanced', whose responsibility should this be?

◆ *The prognosis is limited*—this is more helpful than the original WHO statement 'not responsive to curative treatment', because it implies that some patients may be eligible for palliative medicine right from the time of diagnosis, regardless of how successful 'curative' treatment may be for them. It would be helpful if there were consensus about what constitutes 'limited prognosis'—commonsense suggests that it should apply if the probability of cure (i.e. not dying from this disease) is less than 50%. Seen this way, the large majority of solid malignancies at diagnosis, with the exception of basal cell carcinomas of skin, carry a 'limited prognosis'. How limited does the prognosis need to be in order for palliative medicine to be involved? Should it be measured in terms of chance of survival, e.g. less than 10%; or does 'limited' mean that the actual survival time is now estimated to be short, e.g. months rather than years? These are not facile questions, because they have everyday implications for the referral criteria to palliative medicine used by doctors and hospice services in general. All too often one hears regret that a patient was referred 'too late'. Paradoxically, the public's observation that services such as hospices and specialist palliative care nurses and doctors are usually activated when the prognosis *is* poor, often turns into a reason for them to resist referral for themselves or a relative, until 'it is really necessary'. The definition therefore both requires a limited prognosis and ensures it.

◆ *The focus of care is quality of life*—it is hard to disagree with this element of the definition. In practice, quality of life is not routinely measured from the patient's point of view, and so it is difficult to verify if this goal is actually being achieved. Several studies have shown that physicians and also nurses do not reliably estimate patients' quality of life, or even the symptoms and other concerns which contribute to it (14, 15). There is also increasing evidence that improved symptom control by itself does not necessarily lead to a measurable improvement in quality of life, even when validated quality of life instruments are employed (16). Even when quality of life is measured in clinical trials, there are numerous weaknesses in study design and the statistical analysis (17). This is in contrast to, say, increased survival being the 'focus' of oncology or improved pulmonary function being the 'focus' of pulmonary rehabilitation—i.e. routinely measured and objectively auditable goals.

The purpose of dissecting and challenging these definitions is to show that palliative care (if it wishes to retain this convenient but euphemistic name) has a duty to be crystal clear in its objectives and its sphere of influence. If palliative medicine is not only concerned with incurable, malignant disease and with care at the end of life, then these references should be stripped from the definition.

From this discussion of the meaning and scope of palliative care, three strands emerge. First, there is the question of the purpose and importance of the definition of palliative care. Does it really matter exactly what is meant by this term? What harm does it do if different countries and different professional disciplines hold the words to mean different types of healthcare? The answer to these questions has two parts, semantic and organizational. It seems to be a retrograde step to allow ambiguity and contradictions into the very words which we use to describe a clinical discipline or healthcare policy. It would not be helpful if 'oncology' meant to some people a discipline covering all neoplastic disease and its consequences, but other people restricted it to only the metastatic stage of cancer, whilst others chose to include some benign growths which did not display malignant changes. At the organizational level, would it be considered reasonable if a country's professional association for pulmonary medicine declared that it would henceforth only concentrate on diseases which ultimately cause death, but not on acute or chronic conditions which would need to be picked up by other healthcare agencies?

The second issue is regarding the ability of countries to seek consensus on definitions of palliative care. One promising compromise (rather than true consensus) emerged from a working group of 24 palliative care, cancer, and pain specialists which was convened by the European School of Oncology in late 2000 (18). The purpose of this workshop was to propose a new European programme of activities and priorities for harmonizing and improving palliative care across the European Union. The workshop proposed the following new definition which builds on the previous ones and tries to clarify the problems noted above (18):

> Palliative care is the person-centred attention to physical symptoms, psychological, social and existential[1] distress and cultural needs in patients with limited prognosis, in order to optimise the quality of life for the patients and their families or friends.

The workshop also agreed that it is essential to separate palliative care interventions which can and should be undertaken by *any healthcare professional*, and those which should fall within the responsibility of *specialists with postgraduate training*. This view gave rise to the following further definitions of how palliative care could be implemented:

> *Basic palliative care* is palliative care which should be provided by all healthcare professionals, in primary or secondary care, within their duties to patients with life-limiting disease.
>
> *Specialized palliative care* is palliative care provided at the expert level, by a trained multiprofessional team, who must continually update their skills and knowledge, in order to manage persisting and more severe or complex problems and to provide specialized educational and practical resources to other non-specialized members of the primary or secondary care teams.

It is immediately apparent that these definitions, which were submitted in early 2001 to the Council of Healthcare Ministers of the European Union, are not 'water-tight'. That is, they still allow some ambiguity about how seriously ill and near to death a patient needs to be before he or she is considered to fall within the purview of palliative care. The term 'specialized' was used in preference to 'specialist', as in most European countries palliative care is not yet recognized as a specialty within medicine or nursing. However, given the history of the field and the existing large variations between the 12 countries contributing to these statements, these definitions represent useful starting points for further work.

An updating of this pan-European approach came with the recently completed 'EuroPall' project, which sought to move beyond the definitions, by documenting the actual implementation of palliative care, through a Delphi technique followed by data collection in 21 European countries (19).

The last issue is that if there should be uniformity in how palliative care is defined, across both geographical and professional boundaries, then how should that standardization be reached? Does it need international ratification, like the definition of 'pain' which has been adopted by the International Association for the Study of Pain, and serves as a reference point for studies and policies? It would seem appropriate that the WHO, which launched the first helpful but now outdated definition, should take on the responsibility of coordinating a new universal statement of what palliative care is. A good starting point would be the joint European statements presented above, together with the current

---

[1] *Existential* here includes 'spiritual' and 'religious', but is not confined to people with established faiths.

definitions used by governments and the national palliative care organizations which have chosen to develop their own definitions. It would also be wise to agree that a review of any new definition should be made within at least 5 years, so that it is updated in the light of further global changes in theory and practice.

Palliative medicine as a specialty

The specialty of palliative medicine has been mentioned above, but it is worth emphasizing that it is still recognized in only very few countries of the world. In the UK, entry is based on general professional training resulting in the postgraduate membership of either a Royal College of Physicians or of General Practice, and there is then a 4-year training programme leading to accreditation as a consultant physician in palliative medicine. Even in the UK, where the specialty has been officially recognized since 1987, there is not universal clarity of its place alongside other hospital-based specialities, or vis-à-vis general practice.

MacDonald, a Canadian haematology oncologist, has asserted that colleagues in his discipline, even with training in symptom control, will never reach the level of knowledge and skills as those of a palliative medicine doctor. He has further stated that (20):

> Palliative medicine should be recognised as an integral component of an overall cancer programme. The benefits of liaison are obvious: continuity of care, ready access for patients to all therapies, better coordination between cancer centres, the home, and community institutions, and increased emphasis on symptom control research and education.'

The scope of this volume goes far beyond cancer, and the question which arises is: how could the emergence of a specialty of palliative medicine help improve the medical care of patients with non-malignant diseases, as it is believed to have done for cancer? The answer is not clear—most palliative care services still concentrate their efforts on cancer patients. In the UK, the 4-year postgraduate training programme for doctors includes compulsory time in chronic (i.e. non-malignant) pain clinics and in HIV/AIDS services, and requires trainees to keep informed of palliative care issues in other disciplines. However, there is no corresponding compulsory time for palliative medicine trainees to learn in respiratory medicine or cardiology units, even though it is increasingly recognized that palliative care could usefully be extended to patients with advanced respiratory and cardiac disease (21, 22). This could make specialists in these latter subjects understandably nervous and even sceptical about the competence and usefulness of the palliative contribution that 'specialists' in palliative medicine can offer to them.

The comments above have referred to palliative medicine. So far other professions have been lagging behind in declaring specialisms in palliative care, except that nursing appears to have embraced the concept and often has sections of palliative care nursing within national associations or international oncology societies. In the UK, nurses may train as specialist practitioners in palliative care, and practise their skills in hospices, home care, or hospital teams, alongside—and often out-numbering—specialist doctors. Other members of multidisciplinary palliative care (which will be discussed below) are typically 'borrowed' from generic services and are not currently required to undergo postgraduate training in their fields.

Why do we need a new concept of supportive care?

From the preceding section, it should be clear that the scope of palliative care—and the goals of medical and nursing specialties which practise it—are based on an uncertain premise. This is the notion of incurable and soon to be fatal disease, which is usually but not always cancer. The emphasis of palliative care on symptom control and quality of life is admirable, but it seems to promote these to the exclusion of prolonging life. Is this in the best interests of patients and their families? What of the large numbers of patients who are hovering between being potentially curable and having frankly incurable disease? Who should look after the symptoms, psychological concerns, and quality of life of patients who are undergoing curative or life-prolonging therapies, both with cancer or any other life-threatening disease? What of the needs of patients who have been through 'curative' treatment and are now, at least temporarily, regarded as 'survivors'? Clearly the specialists who work with these groups of patients cannot be expected also to be experts in all aspects of palliation, as their technical knowledge and practical skills need to encompass prevention, accurate diagnosis, and attempts to cure or prolong life. To whom can they turn for help? This is where the concept of supportive care has to be invoked.

For many years, supportive care has been spoken of within oncology as a set of specific interventions and manoeuvres aimed at reducing the toxicity of anticancer treatments. For example, anti-emetic therapy for cytotoxic and radiation therapy-induce nausea and vomiting took a great stride forward with the introduction of the serotonin (5HT-3) antagonist drugs, and this also gave a boost to supportive care in oncology services. Similarly, the more recent introduction of bone marrow growth factors, which enable faster recovery of white blood counts after cytotoxic drugs, and erythropoietin which protects against anaemia, have been important elements of support for some cancer patients undergoing aggressive chemotherapy. Antifungal therapies and improved antibiotic regimens, nutritional advice, and supplementation—sometimes with parenteral feeding—are further examples of advances in the last two decades of cancer supportive care.

Undoubtedly these forms of support are helpful and reassuring to the patients, who benefit from reduced morbidity and mortality from anticancer treatments. Their oncologists also naturally feel relieved that the interventions can be both less toxic and more-over, because anticancer treatments can be maximized, often more effective. But supportive care can be more comprehensive and inclusive, in terms of the benefits to patients and professionals, and also in terms of the diseases and the stages of disease that it covers.

First, supportive care need not be restricted to the end of life. Indeed, cancer supportive interventions were originally *not* deployed at the end, but rather in the earlier stages of disease, to allow patients to tolerate more aggressive curative treatments. Similar technologies and interventions can be useful in patients with more advanced cancer, and in some cases they can be transferred to other diseases. Supportive care interventions which are directed at symptom control may be palliative by virtue of using type 1 (preventive), type 2 (primary disease-directed), type 3 (distant effects-directed), or type 4 (symptom perception) palliation, as described above. As such, they are therefore not confined to use only in early stage disease. If we broaden our view of what constitutes a supportive care intervention, then the possibility of a truly humane, holistic and respectful system of care becomes possible for patients at any stage of disease, with any serious illness.

Talking of supportive care rather than palliative care may also avoid the situation that has now arisen, in that the word 'palliative' (which was introduced as a euphemism for 'terminal' or 'hospice' care) has been 'found out' by patients, who are suspicious when it is mentioned. It is unlikely that 'supportive care', even if it were only used cynically as a new euphemism for 'palliative care', would ever in turn be regarded with the same suspicion for two reasons. First, the terms 'support' and 'supportive' are commonplace words with a real vernacular meaning, as opposed to 'palliative'. Second, if supportive care is deployed from the outset at the beginning of illness as well as at later stages, then the public (and healthcare professionals) should not categorize it as an end of life intervention.

How can supportive care be elevated to this new role? Klastersky, one of the pioneers of supportive care in oncology, believes that the process has already begun and that supportive care is a real entity in modern cancer services (23):

> Basic supportive care is part of any general practitioner's (GP's), and at least practising oncologist's, medical armamentarium . . . Supportive care consists of many subspecialties of the traditional medical and nursing care system and encompasses a broad and highly interesting variety of facets.

He feels that supportive care is a *generic set of skills and knowledge*, rather than being a distinct *specialty*, such as palliative medicine (23):

> Such a definition carries many practical difficulties because it brings under a 'common hat' many different subspecialties that differ considerably in approach, technique and healthcare personnel . . . A common – interdisciplinary and multiprofessional – forum is thus necessary to bridge these various aspects, all of which have one common aim: comprehensive supportive care in cancer.

The driving force behind this concept lies in its emphasis on multidisciplinary team-working, which is fundamental to many branches of healthcare today. But this type of teamwork goes beyond the scope of the typical groupings which operate in cancer and respiratory medicine. Typically, multidisciplinary (or interdisciplinary, or multiprofessional) teams operating in cancer, rehabilitation, or similar services arrange to meet physically in a room on a regular—usually weekly—basis, to discuss patients and plan their investigations or care. In contrast, comprehensive supportive care invokes the concept of a *virtual* team, composed of collaborating professionals (and in some circumstances, volunteers) from different disciplines, and representatives from relevant discrete multidisciplinary teams, making complementary contributions at all stages of illness—without their all having to be present in the same room, building, or even healthcare sector. Thus, comprehensive supportive care is in reality delivered by a *network* of individuals, teams, and resources.

Implementing a comprehensive supportive care network

How can this idea be implemented? A model has been proposed which describes how supportive care fits in with other aspects of healthcare during a serious illness, and which also gives a legitimate place to palliative care in cancer and other diseases (24).

The 'Sheffield model' is composed of two components: a reductive step and an integrative step. The former (Figure 1.3) dissects and separates the elements of care into three streams: those interventions which are directed at modifying or eradicating the disease process (e.g. COPD, cancer, HIV); care directed towards helping the person who has that disease; and thirdly support for the family (or other significant carers) of the person who is experiencing the disease. The model uses the term 'therapy' for these elements, as they are more than just medical treatments—they should include holistic assessments of the aims of interventions at each stage in the disease progression, and contributions for care can come from a variety of clinical non-clinical sources.

Note that this model allows for the patient's and family's needs to be recognized and met *even before a formal diagnosis is made*, i.e. during the screening and investigation phases. This will be increasingly important in the future, as genetic screening programmes and other forms of early disease detection, e.g. by imaging or biochemical markers screening campaigns, become more widely applied. Potential 'patients' in these programmes often have special fears and information needs, which can lead to anxiety and other consequences within the family. Moreover many patients, especially if they are elderly, have comorbidity with a variety of other longstanding or intercurrent illnesses or mental concerns, and these also need support and practical help. In the acute phases of investigation and diagnosis-making, it is easy for hard-pressed professionals to miss or disregard these concerns. If ignored, comorbidity may become the reason for some patients to refuse or withdraw prematurely from potentially helpful or life-prolonging treatments. In their turn, family members also need support to ease their concerns and—if patients have to give up work or household duties—financial worries. Note also in Figure 1.3, that the family's support needs go on after the patient may die, as some family members (or close friends) could have abnormally disturbed grief reactions.

Note that the reductive model in Figure 1.3 does not show a temporal relationship between the stream of disease-directed therapies, and the therapies aimed at supporting the patient and family. This is because supportive care needs may arise at any point in the disease trajectory: they certainly do not only surface when 'the disease is no longer curable'. Providing supportive care for patients' and families' needs at the earliest possible stage should be just as desirable as starting disease-directed therapies as early as possible.

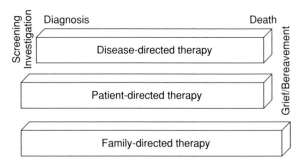

Fig. 1.3 The Sheffield model of comprehensive supportive care: Part 1—the reductive model.

In cancer, an earlier start with anticancer treatments may mean the difference between cure or life-prolongation; in COPD, early education and lifestyle modifications may have a better impact on functioning and quality of life. Similarly many supportive care therapies, whether they are directed at symptoms, psychological concerns, socio-economic difficulties, or existential fears probably are more useful if they are started early.

Until recently, the evidence for this model was lacking, as no formal trials have been conducted with comprehensive supportive care starting at the onset of a life-threatening disease. A US randomized trial of early introduction of 'palliative care' in patients with advanced non-small cell lung cancer (NSCLC) has, probably for the first time, shown that such a step led to improved physical and psychosocial outcomes for patients many months later (25). Surprisingly, the study also showed a significant (3-month) survival advantage for patients who were randomized to early palliative care. The most likely explanation (apart from a chance finding) is that patients who received 'palliative care' were less likely to accept the more aggressive forms of anticancer treatments which, paradoxically, could have shortened their lives. Although the study described their intervention as 'palliative care', in fact it involved at least monthly contacts with a service that essentially provided supportive care from the beginning of the disease.

Another example of the benefits of early initiation of supportive treatment comes from preoperative or perioperative anaesthetic or analgesic interventions, which can lead to significant reduction in pain experience in the short and medium term (26). Similarly, prevention of psychological distress and conditioning could also be a legitimate target. Earlier psychological intervention with cancer patients and their relatives may help to prevent or mitigate later family stresses (27). With COPD, it has been shown that physical restrictions induced by dyspnoea and reduced exercise tolerance induces a vicious circle of reducing physical and social functioning, which then lead to physical muscle de-conditioning that aggravates the dyspnoea (28). The logical response to this finding is educational and motivational exercise training programmes for COPD patients, offering type I palliation of dyspnoea.

The second part of Sheffield model aims to clarify the integrative approach to delivering care to the patient and family. It does this by aggregating the three elements of care from the reductive model (Figure 1.3) into an integrated clinical and organizational scenario, represented in Figure 1.4. It is immediately apparent that this diagram is based on the highly influential WHO resource model for organizing cancer services, which has been discussed above (Figure 1.2). However, a major problem with the WHO diagram was that in practice the resource model became seen as a clinical guideline, suggesting that 'curative' therapies should be tried and seen to fail, before palliative care could be introduced. This has led to the common situation of patients with cancer being initially cared for by mostly surgeons and oncologists, who rightly offer and try disease-directed therapies. Often in this phase the presenting symptoms and psychological needs of the patient are overlooked, or managed ineffectively by clinicians who are not trained in palliation and who have rudimentary communication skills. (Primary care teams, which may have both to offer, are frequently unable to help the patient at this stage because the

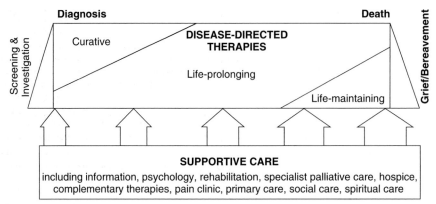

Fig. 1.4 The Sheffield model of comprehensive supportive care: Part 2—the integrative model.

focus of care is at the hospital, and they may receive little information about the patient's status.) Comorbidity issues and family needs are also frequently ignored. On the day when the patient attends the clinic and is told that the disease has 'failed to respond (or has progressed/recurred)' and that 'there is nothing more that the oncologist can do', they receive two severe psychological blows. First they are devastated at the news itself, and second by being referred to another service—the primary care team or the local palliative care team (if indeed, one exists). Patients and families find this period of sudden transition very traumatic, and many of them initially turn down the offer of palliative care at this time because of the 'shell-shock' and because of the previously mentioned fears that palliative care is synonymous with terminal care (29).

The Sheffield model handles this area somewhat differently. Whereas the WHO approach was designed to advise governments and oncologists on how to allocate resources in cancer control programmes, the Sheffield integrative model is primarily aimed at *advising clinicians and local services planners* on how to make the support of patients with chronic disease and their family carers as comprehensive, integrated and 'shock-free' as humanely possible. It encourages the involvement of some supportive services even during the screening and diagnostic stages. In genetic screening for certain cancers, for example, whole families may need information and reassurance. During lung cancer diagnostic work-up, presenting symptoms of cough, haemoptysis, pain, and dyspnoea have to be palliated. In lung cancer it is not unusual for a patient to die from metastatic disease even before a tissue diagnosis is confirmed. If the WHO model is applied too literally, he or she may not be offered palliative care. Should such patients be denied the benefits of good support, just because they do not possess the requisite clinical label?

The Sheffield integrative model (Figure 1.4) identifies two main sectors of healthcare—those which are directed at the primary disease process ('disease-directed therapies') and those which are aimed at patient's and families' needs ('supportive therapies'). It can be seen that the upper block which represents 'disease-directed therapies' looks superficially like the block of cancer therapies in the WHO resource allocation model. There are three main differences: first and foremost, the Sheffield model has dissociated the patient- and family-directed needs and therapies from the management of the primary disease. Put another way, palliative care does not need to follow after curative treatments (30). Second, the disease-directed therapies now can be focused on any chronic life-threatening disease, not just cancer. Indeed, the concept of separating out 'disease-modifying therapies' is well established in fields of other chronic disease management, e.g. rheumatoid arthritis (31). Third, the sequence of treatments within the block of disease-directed therapies are more realistically (one could say more honestly) represented. *'Curative'* therapies should of course be applied first. With many chronic inflammatory, degenerative and also neoplastic diseases, this part of the sequence may be very limited. For them a larger part of the time may be spent with offering the patient *'life-prolonging'* treatments. In small cell cancer, these include chemotherapy which can usefully provide years of extra survival; in non-small cell disease, the benefit may be measured in months. In HIV/AIDS, modern combination antiviral therapies fall into this category. It is not helpful for clinicians to talk to the patient and family about this phase of treatment in terms of 'chances of cure'; rather, there should be honest discussion about how many extra years, months, or possibly weeks may be gained. Most patients would feel less disillusioned and cheated by their professional advisers if they were aware at the outset, that the disease will not be cured—i.e. they will eventually succumb to the disease or its effects, regardless of how dramatically successful the initial treatment may be.

The final part of the sequence within disease-directed therapies is a relatively new concept, that of *'life-maintaining'* therapies. By this is meant those interventions which are required to keep a patient alive and functioning to a level that is acceptable to him or her. The period of time that life may be maintained can vary from days to months. The interventions include regular blood transfusions in a patient with widespread malignancy and bone marrow replacement, as occurs in myeloma or advanced breast cancer. Other examples are assisted ventilation for patients with motor neuron disease/amyotrophic lateral sclerosis (MND/ALS) who have total respiratory muscle paralysis; or artificial hydration in a patient with malignant oesophageal obstruction and who would otherwise die within days of dehydration. Note that in these examples patients will inevitably die anyway even with the life-maintaining therapies, from the systemic complications of advanced disease—the situation being discussed here is *not* analogous to long-term artificial ventilation and total nutrition in a patient with coma after head injury. Life-maintaining therapies are respectful and humane if they reflect the wishes of the patient (and ideally also the family, although there are often conflicts at this stage of illness). They are disrespectful and become unethical if they are imposed by medical teams to keep a patient living who would otherwise die, and who has not sought for longer survival.

Who could benefit from comprehensive supportive care?

Clearly not all supportive interventions are necessary for patients or family members at each stage of the disease. Early in a serious illness, information and psychological counselling may be more important than symptom control. Before there is a confirmed histological or radiological diagnosis, symptom palliation will be predominantly of types 3 and 4, i.e. modifying the distant effects of a disease or relieving the subjective distress arising from it, without tackling the primary cause. Once the diagnosis is made, it is important that alongside initial disease-directed therapies aimed at cure or prolonging life, patients are honestly and realistically informed about the goals of treatment. Their symptoms, comorbidity, and treatment-related toxicities can then be managed using all of the appropriate types of palliation. As discussed above, this is the phase when 'traditional' oncology-based supportive care, using anti-emetics, antimicrobials, and, latterly, growth factors and have become a routine part of cancer management using chemotherapy. Currently at this stage however, patients in most settings are *not* routinely offered the broader elements of the Sheffield model of supportive care which are directed to the patient's and family's wellbeing.

If the patient does fail to respond to disease-directed therapy, then the responsibility of care should pass *gradually*—rather than at present, *suddenly* on the day of 'bad news'—to the supportive care virtual team. In some centres, this will involve the patient being discharged to the coordinating umbrella of the primary care team, which will in turn negotiate and obtain specialist help from palliative medicine and nursing, and other relevant services such as dietetics, physiotherapy, social work, and perhaps a member of the clergy, depending on the patient's and family's needs. In order to do this effectively, primary care teams need education and training. In some cases, the specialist palliative care team may, for a variable period, have to 'take over' the care of a difficult problem, and occasionally the patient may never return to the primary care team if the problem warrants long-term admission. In many cases staff within primary care team do not have the requisite skills for giving more than generic palliative care. Patients have a right to access specialists either in the community or in centres such as hospices or hospital-based teams, who can then make a trained assessment, initiate appropriate treatment, and refer back to the general practitioner or family doctor and community nursing services for continuity.

It must be stressed that it is not only palliative care services which have expertise in the broader interdisciplinary network of supportive care. Some patients may benefit more from the attention of an occupational therapist, dietician, or art therapist than from any medical or nursing professional. In many places, these professionals will not be found in the local palliative care service. Information resources are becoming more widely available, both through an actual presence in hospitals and hospices, but also via booklets and telephone advice from national help lines, and increasingly, via the Internet. Cancer has been well served in this respect: for example, in the UK, the major information resources for cancer include Macmillan Cancer Support and Cancer Research UK. However, non-cancer patients are also now being served by support groups and national organizations such as the British Lung Foundation, which offers the 'Breathe Easy' programme for patients with COPD and other chronic non-malignant chest diseases. Just as oncologists have come to realize and accept that palliative care can have a positive contribution for their patients, so must palliative care professionals open up their minds to the possibility that, for certain patients with specific needs, other disciplines may have an even more important role than they do.

What is a supportive care network composed of?

We have seen that the modern supportive care 'virtual team' operates as a network of different individuals, teams and resources. What are the constituents of this network? Table 1.4 shows one concept of how existing services can be configured to form the network. In this diagram, there are three groups of professionals operating. Group A is recognizable as having the typical composition of a specialist palliative care service, at least within the UK and many other Western countries. The key members of this group are: physicians (preferably trained to a specialist level in this subject); nurses (also with post-basic training); social workers; chaplains or religious advisers; pharmacists; and physiotherapists. In many countries and services, volunteers assist these professionals, e.g. in providing diversional and social activities in hospices and at day centres. Within these settings, and increasingly in hospitals, Group A staff physically meet on a regular basis to discuss individual patients and overall strategy.

Group A could be regarded as a core element of the supportive care service, at least where palliative care services are well established. It has already been acknowledged that these staff are most familiar with caring for cancer patients and their families, towards the end of life. They are frequently supplemented by a second group which is composed of professionals who are usually based in other departments and who do not have specific palliative care training. Group B includes: psychologists, dieticians, occupational therapists, speech and language therapists, and complementary therapists. Many of these will be known as the core elements of a rehabilitation programme. A newly emerging discipline within this group is the creative arts therapists, who may bring painting, other practical arts, writing, or music into the clinical setting. (In many UK palliative care services, especially the independent hospices, arts therapy and complementary therapies are provided, but they cannot be regarded as 'essential' to Group A.)

A third group of disciplines shown in Table 1.4 consists of teams from other settings which have an impact on the patient's and family's care. For cancer patients these would include the oncology team, which is naturally focused on providing disease-modifying therapies. For chronic respiratory disease patients, the pulmonary service is included in Group C. The key point is that Group C services are included not for their investigative

Table 1.4 Composition of comprehensive supportive care network

Group	Professionals	Health or social care sector
A	Palliative care physicians and nurses; social workers; chaplains/priests; physiotherapists; volunteers	Hospice; day care; hospital-based team; community-based team
B	Psychologists; dieticians; occupational therapists; speech and language therapists; complementary therapists; art therapists; volunteers	Hospital services; community services; some hospices; free-standing agencies; private services
C	Respiratory department; oncology service; pain clinic; breathlessness clinic; lymphoedema service; primary care team; information resource	Hospital services; community; some hospices; telephone or Internet-based resource

and 'disease-directed' activities, but for their supportive care interventions. Thus, these services may include nurses who specialize in respiratory care; or psychologists, dieticians, and physiotherapists of their own. Moreover, individual physicians working in group services may also be interested and have received training in aspects of specialist palliation and psychological support. During the times when the patient is receiving active input from the oncology or respiratory unit, these staff may be the main source of supportive care. A useful function of an oncology unit or respiratory unit is to be the hub of coordination where Group A and Group B members can telephone for liaison or physically attend meetings to discuss shared patients.

Other Group C elements include hospital-based pain clinics, which may provide both ward and out-patient (ambulatory) support for chronic pain management. Often their main workload consists of chronic non-malignant pain, but they work closely with palliative care teams to provide specialist advice and practical procedures for certain types of pain (see Chapter 18, this volume). Teams and clinics specializing in other symptoms are less common, but a recent development has been the hospital-based breathlessness clinics. These were initially entirely staffed by nurses, which seems contradictory to the current trend towards multidisciplinary team-working. As their skills mature and other practitioners recognize their value, which has been demonstrated in at least one randomized clinical trial (32), ideally they will become multiprofessional resources like pain clinics and will offer help to patients who have diagnoses other than cancer. Another example of a specialist supportive care service which has already made significant impact in non-malignant disease is the lymphoedema clinic (33). Some palliative care services offer a lymphoedema service for patients with breast or pelvic or genital cancers that cause limb swelling. The specialized clinics are increasingly supporting patients with chronic 'benign' lymphoedema—often still within a palliative care setting.

It is relevant to include the primary care team in Group C, as many GPs and community nurses have undergone postgraduate training in aspects of palliation and can provide the bulk of symptom control and psychological support for their patients. Until now, however, the training has been very much modelled on palliative care, i.e. advanced stage, cancer-focused, programmes. Finally, resources such as information centres which guide patients towards better understanding of their predicament and help them make more informed choices, will increasingly figure within Group C supportive care. Some of these resources are simply racks of leaflets in a clinic, whilst others are fully established as staffed information points in hospital departments. Increasingly, patients are turning to the Internet for information and guidance and specific resources are being set up: the monitoring of their quality is vital for patients' choices to be rational (34).

Table 1.5 demonstrates the crucial times in the illness process, from screening to possible death, where different elements of the new supportive care virtual teams or networks could have an input. Although this table has been based on the author's experience primarily with cancer, it should be possible for other specialties to adapt this skeleton of a supportive care framework. Thus Table 1.5 shows how staff from all three supportive care groups could also be involved in the stages of diagnosis and progress of COPD and

Table 1.5 Opportunities for supportive care interventions

	Cancer	COPD	MND/ALS
Screening and investigation	C, B	C	C, B
Breaking bad news	C, B	C, B	C, B
Initial disease-directed treatment	C, B	C, B	N/A
Recurrence	C, B, A	N/A	N/A
Progression	A, B, C	C, B, A	B, A, C
Terminal care	A, B, C	C, B, A	A, C, B
Bereavement support	A, C	C	A, C
Information at all stages	C, B, A + Internet	C, B + Internet	A, C + Internet

Key: the resources for offering patients and families supportive at each stage in the three diseases are summarized using the taxonomy of health and social care sectors presented in Table 1.4. The order in which they are presented here is in decreasing likelihood of the sector being relevant for each need.

A = typical palliative care team; hospice; B = other supportive care services; C = hospital-based specialties; pain clinic; information resources; primary care; N/A = not applicable

of MND/ALS. For the future of respiratory supportive care, it will be important for experts from within respiratory medicine itself and supportive care professionals within Group A and B to develop these strategies together.

In the early stages of a chronic disease, it is reasonable for Group C services to take the lead and coordinate other services as needed. With advanced disease, in countries where palliative care is recognized and well resourced, it is customary for the specialist palliative care teams of Group A to form the nucleus and hub of the network. One problem with this is that even in the UK, where hospice units have flourished for 40 years, there is still great variation between different services, often in the same city or region. Surveys of European palliative care services over the past 20 years show that they are far from homogeneous in terms of their staffing structures and what they can offer patients and families (19, 35). In non-malignant disease services, it is quite reasonable—and probably desirable—for teams operating outside of palliative care structures to take the leading role for individual patients. For example, physiotherapy and nursing teams, ideally operating from a pulmonary disease service, may be the lead agencies for COPD or MND/ALS.

Towards the end of life, for some patients the key input will come again from the acute hospital-based services or from the primary care teams within Group C. Within the field of cancer, oncologists in Western countries have learnt to be accommodating so that patients gradually shift their reliance from themselves to the palliative care team. Once there has been greater collaboration between pulmonary services and other supportive care professionals, the same could follow for chronic respiratory disease.

It is crucial, as discussed above, that patients are not 'handed over' suddenly and without warning from the primary hospital unit to the local palliative care unit, or back to the primary care team, on the day that the news of failure to respond to curative therapy, or of recurrence, has been broken. This is more likely to happen with cancer patients, because of how recurrence or progression is diagnosed. It should theoretically be less likely to occur with chronic lung disease, as the decision to move over to a palliative care programme could be discussed over several admissions for acute respiratory failure (36). However, the problem here is that respiratory units do not have the years of experience of working along-side group A or B services. On the other hand with MND/ALS, at least in the UK, there has been longstanding collaboration between Group C and palliative care services, so that as the patient progresses, respite admissions to a hospice may be seen as routine intervention, and final admission for terminal care could be at the hospice or respiratory unit. (See Chapter 13, this volume, for discussion of management of neuromuscular disorders.)

Relationship between supportive care and palliative care

It may be helpful at this point to emphasize the differences and overlaps between traditional palliative care and the new model of supportive care. In essence, the Sheffield model attempts to provide a *comprehensive framework*, so that palliative care (and the special setting of hospice care) should be seen as components of supportive care. In some diseases such as lung cancer, and for individual patients, palliative care could be the most important element of supportive care. For other diseases such as COPD or HIV/AIDS, present day palliative care may have little practical to offer. However, it may still help by sharing its knowledge base with clinicians attending to these diseases. The management of pain, for example, is essentially the same in cancer, COPD or MND/ALS, so long as logical means of palliation (of types 3 or 4) are employed according to their known or putative modes of action. The differences in approach arise in the implications for, say, respiratory depression, if opioids are used in these three situations. The use of cytotoxic chemotherapy is obviously one example of a type 2 treatment which is only relevant for oncology. Ventilatory support is used in both COPD and MND/ALS but is not useful in cancer. There are few other areas of symptom control—and probably even less in psychological, social, or spiritual support—which are unique to a disease.

Several possible problems may arise if a palliative care philosophy dominates in the setting up of comprehensive supportive care networks. First, it may bring 'traditional' models and ways of working, which have been largely tested and refined in hospices, into situations where such methods are inappropriate or even unhelpful. An example was the early response of the UK hospice movement to incorporate HIV/AIDS patients: often these patients were much younger, and from a different social background from the usual older hospice cancer patients, and this hospice model was rejected and gradually super-seded by separate units being established for AIDS (37). Because COPD and some other chronic lung disease patients are demographically more similar to cancer patients (especially lung cancer), then perhaps this particular problem may be less acute with these illnesses. Indeed, more palliative care units in the UK are reporting that they admit COPD as well as heart failure patients, and although no series have been published, it appears that this approach could be feasible.

However, another problem arises, which is that cancer-based palliative care services are equipped to deal with patients whose prognosis is relatively short and fairly certain. A frequently voiced concern in palliative care circles themselves is how they can then cope with diagnostic groups in which there is far greater uncertainty. Respiratory physicians could also feel ambiguous about referring patients to hospice-based care, where facilities for radiography and even percutaneous oximetry are limited or absent. These physicians and also the patients could understandably feel nervous about palliative care policies which might deny patients intravenous antibiotics and other interventions which can be useful to maintain life, and even for symptom control. Patients being admitted to many palliative care units are commonly not offered the choice of cardiopulmonary resuscitation (CPR) in the event of a respiratory or cardiac arrest. Many have argued that CPR is anyway futile for many patients with advanced disease and terminal disease, but could hospices which may in future take patients at an *earlier* stage, have the skills to determine whether resuscitation or other forms of life support (e.g. temporary assisted ventilation) could be appropriate? (36, 38). It is clear that if palliative care services are to incorporate more patients with non-malignant illnesses like COPD or interstitial lung diseases, then there would have to be a large educational programme for staff in those units, ideally led from acute respiratory care services.

A perceived 'risk' to patients is the cancer-oriented palliative care teams' attitudes to the use of opioids in symptom control, which could be seen by untrained respiratory or cardiological specialists as being 'too casual'. There generally are no doubts about the benefits of morphine or its newer analogues for pain control in *cancer* patients. There is now convincing evidence for opioids in the relief of dyspnoea, in both cancer and COPD (see Chapter 7, this volume). However, in reality many patients with advanced non-malignant diseases who are very distressed by breathlessness are denied the benefits of opioids by respiratory physicians, neurologists, and GPs. The problem here is actually a tension between the knowledge base and expertise of palliative care, and the doubts over opioids of other clinicians. The usual reasons expressed for the latter are: fear of respiratory depression (which need not happen if the opioid is titrated carefully upwards) (39, 40); fear of addiction in patients with a relatively uncertain prognosis (although *physical dependence* may occur temporarily when opioids are withdrawn, *anti-social addictive behaviour* is hardly ever seen in palliative care); and general reluctance to use the newer opioids if the physician is not familiar with them. The point about including these issues here as potential 'problems' of instilling a palliative care culture within supportive care, is that they represent more of a educational challenge than a true organizational one.

Supportive care needs at earlier stages of illness

If comprehensive supportive care is meant to be more than a new euphemism for palliative care, then what elements of it are distinctive? It is difficult to be very precise about this, because both supportive care and palliative care are implemented so variably in different places. However, a good example of what supportive care can offer, beyond the *normal* scope of palliative care services, lies in the support that is needed by patients and families in the earlier stages of disease. As the diagram of the Sheffield integrative model (Figure 1.4) shows, such elements include information services and rehabilitation.

Considerable research has been conducted in recent years on the information needs of patients with serious life-threatening illnesses, particularly cancer (41). It is acknowledged that patients and families need information as early as possible in the illness, and many specialized services for cancer, HIV and conditions such as MND/ALS have developed written, audio, video, and latterly Internet-based information packs. The informational needs of patients with cancer are known to change during the first weeks and months of illness: they shift from a desire for information about the disease process and its causes, to information about support services (42). It should be remembered that the need for information can start even before the illness is formally 'diagnosed', e.g. during the work-up for cancer or interstitial or industrial lung disease.

Rehabilitation is now so much established in many services aimed at COPD and cancer patients following surgery that it may be regarded by those teams to be integral to their package of care. That is how supportive care should of course be seen, but rehabilitation is essentially person- and family-directed, rather than disease-directed. Seen this way, it does not need to be provided by the same service which is making the diagnosis and arranging disease-directed therapy. The packages of rehabilitation in such centres attend to physical, psychological, and social needs. In Europe, cancer rehabilitation is very well developed in Germany and Scandinavian countries, e.g. patients in Germany can expect to receive up to 3 weeks of in-patient rehabilitation in a specialist hospital after the completion of cancer treatment (43, 44). In the UK, most cancer patients do not receive such a formal programme of rehabilitation, even after curative but debilitating surgery for lung cancer. By contrast, many UK respiratory units are developing pulmonary rehabilitation programmes for COPD and other lung diseases, as have been successfully established in the USA.

Complementary therapies are another form of supportive care, to which patients are increasingly turning *in addition to* conventional disease-directed treatments from healthcare services. Clinical care providers need to know how to direct patients towards reputable and preferably validated therapies and local therapists, rather than leaving them to learn by trial and error. There needs to be a clear distinction between complementary therapies which are taken up by the patients *alongside* conventional care—sometimes provided in the same unit, and which many help them to complete disease-directed therapies—and alternative therapies, which in a disease like cancer can lead to patients *opting out* of potentially beneficial conventional treatments, often at great personal expense. However, it could be a problem for some patients if they access alternative therapies when evidence-based interventions can change the course of the illness.

Supportive care for cancer survivors

In the past decade, there has been a growth of interest in the issues surrounding cancer 'survivorship' (45). Like some of the other medical concepts described in this chapter, there is no hard and universally recognized definition of makes a cancer 'survivor'. In the

UK, it is now taken to be someone who has completed primary treatment, whether it is surgery, chemotherapy, or radiotherapy. The term includes patients who have entered complete remission, those who have continuing but stable disease, and even those who have advancing disease (though patients at the 'end of life' are not, for obvious reasons, called survivors). One of the practical benefits of recognizing the phase of survivorship is that patients—and their families—who have continuing supportive care needs are not forgotten when they are discharged from hospital-based care. Many patients have the physical or psychological scars of surgical and medical interventions. Long-term post-surgical pain is increasingly recognized, e.g. after thoracotomy for lung cancer (46, 47). The sequelae of chemotherapy include painful neuropathy, endocrine suppression, cardiac damage, pulmonary fibrosis, etc.—collectively, these are known as 'late effects'. Until recently, these problems were not even recognized in individual patients. Now there are starting to be services set up specifically for managing late effects, or else supportive care teams are taking on such patients.

Examples of support for survivors include occupational therapy, which is often included within a full rehabilitation programme; nutritional support; exercise programmes; psychosexual counselling; financial and welfare benefits advice. Palliative care services usually have access to these professionals, but it is unnecessary to refer a patient to palliative care just for this advice.

End of life care

An exploration of the management of supportive and palliative care would be incomplete without a discussion of end of life care. This is often also called 'terminal care', although many patients and also professionals feel uncomfortable with the harshness of the word 'terminal', at least in English. In UK palliative care circles, the expression 'terminal care' is indeed used, but it then refers to comfort measures which dominate in the last few hours, days or possibly weeks of life. Because these phrases will continue to be used more or less idiosyncratically by different people in different countries, it is difficult to make rigid definitions. In terms of the Sheffield model of supportive care (Figure 1.4), it may be helpful to conceive of *end of life care as beginning for a particular individual, when the aims of disease-directed therapy move from life-prolonging to life-maintaining; and of terminal care starting when the decision is made to withdraw even life-maintaining treatments.* Unfortunately, these movements across phases are not always easy to distinguish, especially if one is the professional who is very close to the day-to-day decision-making for that individual. (The corollary of this is that it is often easy to see, in retrospect, when the changing aims of management failed to keep step with the actual deterioration in the patient's condition.)

What is special about this phase of chronic disease management? One answer to this is that for many, how a society takes care of its dying members is a good judge of its civilization. Another response is that dying is still seen as one of the greatest spiritual challenges for humanity, both in religious and in the increasingly secular cultures. A third, pragmatic response is that there is only one chance to get it right with the dying—the dead do not complain! Finally, there is the pedagogic view that if we 'get it right' with one patient's end of life care, this may have an educational effect on other members of that patient's family, who may thus develop a more positive attitude to death and dying. The opposite of this is frequently seen when a bad experience in watching a loved one die in physical, psychological, and spiritual distress, can heighten a relative's anxieties and mistrust of the medical profession.

There are numerous excellent textbooks and journals devoted to improving end of life care, that only a few points need to be made here, to add to the specific aspects of symptom control covered in other chapters in this volume (48–50). These points will mainly relate to how supportive care needs to be different at the end of life, if indeed it needs to differ from other stages of disease management:

Physical symptom management

- The pharmacology of some drugs requires more careful monitoring of doses and their timing, e.g. if the patient is developing liver or renal failure.

- As patients become physically weaker and also slip into unconsciousness, the oral route for medication becomes less reliable and even impossible—in this situation, the common alternatives include rectal and parenteral routes.

- With parenteral medication, subcutaneous injections are usually preferred by patients to intravenous or deep intramuscular injections, and many of the drugs used in the terminal stage are suitable for this route.

- In the terminal stage, some patients may become distressed, severely and constantly, by refractory symptoms (pain, dyspnoea, agitation). There is a growing literature on the use of planned and controlled 'palliative sedation' for the relief of this situation, which also distresses those watching and caring for the patient (51).

- The drugs which can be used to achieve reversible sedation include benzodiazepines (e.g. midozalam); opioids; and neuroleptics (e.g. haloperidol or levomepromazine). It is important that the sedation is openly declared to have the goal of palliating symptoms or terminal agitation rather than being a form of unofficial euthanasia (see discussion of assisted dying, below).

Psychological aspects of management

- As patients deteriorate they frequently become cognitively impaired or lapse into unconsciousness, which means that opportunities for discussing details of management with patients are reduced and so more reliance must be placed on communication with relatives or other carers.

- The implication of this is clearly that discussions are better held earlier, when patients are mentally clear and participating in decision-making, about their wishes for specific interventions. Older people and patients with life-threatening illnesses are being encouraged to prepare advanced directives or 'living wills' in which their preferences for more or less active interventions at the end of life are explicitly stated.

◆ Because experience has shown that patients' views about these interventions change as disease progresses, they should be advised to review and update these directives, preferably in discussion with family carers.

Social aspects of the patients' and families' lives

Whereas in western countries it is normal and desirable for patients to try to retain social independence for as long as possible, in some cultures it is accepted for dying people to play a 'sick role' and become dependent on family and healthcare staff. However many individuals vary from these societal norms and it is important for the multidisciplinary care team to be as accommodating as possible to allow patients their dignity in performing as many activities of daily living as their condition permits.

Spiritual and cultural aspects of care

◆ Existential (also called spiritual) fears may dominate some individuals, not only at the end of life but throughout a life-threatening illness. However, these may certainly become more acute in the terminal stage, especially if the patient becomes aware of impending death and has not had the chance to prepare in advance. This is an argument for earlier and open discussion of existential doubts—not for the denial of prognosis to patients!

◆ In many cultures and for specific patients, the answer to existential doubts will be found in spiritual/religious doctrines. Such patients should be allowed full access to their religious advisers in the latter stages of disease, when being admitted to a hospital could prevent them from attending their own place of worship.

◆ Even for 'non-religious' people or those who have weaker faiths, access should exist to staff members who have special training in discussing existential issues.

◆ Attention must be paid, when a person is dying in hospital or in a hospice, to cultural imperatives with respect to the preparation of the body after death and means of disposal. This may mean that family members, rather than staff from other religions, should be allowed to take over these tasks.

Needs of the family and other carers

Caring for a patient who is approaching death imposes special difficulties for relatives and close friends. The supportive care teams should be aware of the needs of those who are involved with the care:

◆ There may be, apart from the expected 'anticipatory grieving' for any terminally ill person, a disproportionate fear of impending loss and future helplessness, especially for those who have been dependent on the dying person. Such individuals may need extra support from social workers and nurses to help them prepare for life alone, and for elderly people this may mean facing the possibility of receiving formal care themselves, perhaps by admission to a care institution.

◆ At the time of death and for some weeks or months afterwards, some individuals may need extra bereavement counselling. The supportive care team may possess such skills, or it may need to refer the relative to a psychological service, if the primary care team or community nursing services are unable to respond to this.

◆ Some carers may need financial advice and support from the state, especially if the patient had been the wage-earner and the illness had been relatively short. For this reason, it is advisable that all people who have a life-threatening illness diagnosed should be assessed for future financial needs at an early stage, by a social worker or specialist nurse trained in social benefits.

Needs of healthcare professionals

Healthcare professionals themselves have special needs with respect to the care of patients approaching the end of life, which may not have been covered in the basic education or postgraduate training in their specialty. This is more likely to be a problem for medical staff in, say, oncology or respiratory medicine and surgery, than for specialist nurses or physicians in palliative medicine where these issues are part of the training. Some areas which cause most concern for staff, when dealing with terminally ill patients, include:

◆ Lack of confidence in communicating openly with dying people about prognosis and the changing aims of treatment. This is particularly likely to cause distress for patients and/or families who can see that the disease is progressing but the physician cannot or prefers not to acknowledge this.

◆ As a result of this, the physician may strive—beyond what is 'reasonable'—to prolong life with inappropriate disease-directed therapies, or to maintain it with artificial nutrition and hydration, blood transfusions, and other supportive measures. Even if the physician acknowledges that the patient is deteriorating, he or she may still be so concerned with pursuing disease-directed investigations and therapy that the person- and family-directed therapies are overlooked or even over-ruled. In some cultures where the decision of the attending physician is paramount and cannot be questioned, this may be socially condoned. Increasingly in the West, this attitude is actively challenged, even by other professional team members. The adage that 'death should not be seen as a failure' is most helpful to those who can see the limitations of modern medicine, or who can recognize their own their own fallibility. Of course there will be times when death comes unexpectedly soon, or as a result of an adverse effect of a therapy, or because some potentially preventable complication was not anticipated—in these cases, the circumstances and timing of the death may indeed be seen as technically a 'failure' of medicine and its current resources. But it is pointless and harmful for the physician to see it as a personal failure or—unconsciously—to blame the patient or family, or even professional colleagues, for 'giving up'.

◆ Repeated exposure to witnessing deaths which are inexpertly managed from the point of view of physical symptoms and psychological or spiritual distress, can lead to professionals themselves becoming worn down. In some cases, this can lead to 'burn-out', when the job is made into a routine and there is little personal engagement and no satisfaction (30). The best prevention for this is to work in a supportive team—giving support to fellow professionals as well as patients. This can only work, however, if professionals admit to their fallibility and their need to share their distress at witnessing patients and families suffering.

◆ There are special dilemmas for staff who work in acute healthcare settings where diseases *can* be cured or at least where patients' lives may be substantially prolonged. Compared to this setting, working in a hospice where all patients have a uniformly terminal prognosis is relatively straightforward. One solution for this is for patients' progress to be monitored and discussed in a multidisciplinary team, so that it is easier to acknowledge when the chances of cure are receding and later, when it becomes clear that life can no longer be prolonged. Sometimes if the patient is very well known to the hospital unit over a long time, it may be difficult for the team members to confront the fact that the patient is deteriorating. Where there is a well established and trusted palliative care service, it may be helpful to call in a member from this to see the patient and family separately. This colleague can then act as the patient's advocate, tactfully advising the respiratory or oncology team that the goal of therapy needs to be changed.

Assisted dying and euthanasia

This chapter would be incomplete without reference to the growing worldwide debate on assisted dying and euthanasia. The debate is relevant to supportive care in respiratory disease, because the chapters in this volume demonstrate that the potential for suffering and for premature death from pulmonary diseases is great. As these illnesses come towards their terminal stage, is there a place for hastening death in a positive way to ease the patient out of extreme distress?

The traditional response of palliative care—and especially of the hospice movement—worldwide has been to totally reject these interventions on grounds of clinical need as well as morality. It is often said that if palliative care were to be more widely available, then people would ask less for assistance with death. Recently these views have been increasingly challenged. It is argued that some patients are still left in an unacceptable physical, psychological, and existential distress even after receiving the best that palliation can offer. Others may live in countries where high-quality palliative care just cannot be offered. It is also argued that it is a fundamental human right to have control over ones death as it is over most aspects of life. The changes in legislation in the Netherlands and Belgium to decriminalize euthanasia, and the law in Oregon, USA which allows physicians to assist patients to commit suicide are quoted as examples of a seemingly inexorable secular global trend towards the acceptance of these views.

This has to be countered with the following arguments. First, it is the duty of healthcare systems constantly to find ways of preventing and curing disease, and if that is not possible, then to prolong and maintain life when it is humane to do so, and always to relieve distress. It has never been a recognized function of healthcare to hasten deaths, even if popular opinion wishes for this facility. Some express fears that in a culture that openly condones assisted dying, older and vulnerable individuals may feel under some pressure to end their lives for the good of their families. Carefully conducted surveys have shown that many physicians, e.g. geriatricians who are in regular contact with frail and terminally ill people, feel on the whole uncomfortable with the notion that they may be called upon to assist in hastening death (52, 53).

Occasionally clinicians are faced with a terrible situation, e.g. massive haemoptysis or stridor when no disease-modifying treatments are available. To give sedation in order to stop the patient's awareness of dying from these almost certain agonal events is quite reasonable, and if the patient dies in a few minutes or hours earlier than without such sedation, that is excusable in most legal systems in the Western world. This is known as the 'doctrine of double effect', in which it is legitimate for a physician to administer a medicine which could possibly cause extreme harm (i.e. death), if the primary purpose of it was to alleviate terrible suffering. However, it is a betrayal of this humane doctrine if physicians hide behind the uncertainty of the response to potent drugs in sick patients, *in order deliberately to shorten life*—even if the patient requests it.

Aside from the emergency situations described above, there is a trend towards increasing use of 'sedation' by drugs such as benzodiazepines and barbiturates—sometimes with opioids—to reduce a person's terminal distress by rendering him or her unconscious. If the response to distress is 'palliative' and 'proportionate', i.e. matching the degree of sedation to symptom level, then this can be part of good symptom management. When it becomes fixed and continuous, maintaining deep unconsciousness without offering hydration until the patient inevitably dies, this can be comparable to active euthanasia, but at a slower rate (51).

Ultimately, the response to extreme suffering is primarily not a medical issue, but one in which societies have to make general statements, and specific judgements in particular cases. It is not desirable for healthcare workers with access to potent drugs to bring it on themselves to step beyond the law of their country. There cannot be a 'final' solution to this debate, as long as different societies and cultures hold life to be more or less 'sacred' to different degrees. For the purposes of supportive care for patients with respiratory diseases and their families, it should again be emphasized that the goal should be to establish a network of professionals from various disciplines, each contributing to relieving suffering as far as is humanely possible and then staying quietly with the patient and family. That will always be preferable to the spectre of the lone doctor or nurse, standing by the bed of a sick patient and making unilateral decisions which involve the premature taking of a life.

References

1. Moinpour CM, Feigl P, Metch B, *et al.* Quality of life endpoints in cancer clinical trials: review and recommendations. *J Natl Cancer Inst* 1989; **81**(7):485–95.
2. Ahmedzai S. Palliative care in oncology: making quality the endpoint. *Ann Oncol* 1990; **1**:396–8.
3. MacDonald N. A proposed matrix for organisational changes to improve quality of life in oncology. *Eur J Cancer* 1995; **31A**(Suppl 6):S18–21.
4. Al Husaini H, Wheatley-Price P, Clemons M, Shepherd FA. Prevention and management of bone metastases in lung cancer: a review. *J Thorac Oncol* 2009; **4**(2):251–9.
5. Milisen K, Steeman E, Foreman MD. Early detection and prevention of delirium in older patients with cancer. *Eur J Cancer Care* 2004; **13**:494–500.

6. Kim H, Neubert JK, San Miguel A, *et al.* Genetic influence on variability in human acute experimental pain sensitivity associated with gender, ethnicity and psychological temperament. *Pain* 2004; **109**:488–96.

7. Lötsch J, Geisslinger G. Current evidence for a genetic modulation of the response to analgesics. *Pain* 2006; **121**:1–5.

8. Clark D, Seymour J. History and development. In Clark D, Seymour J (eds) *Reflections on palliative care*, pp. 65–78. Buckingham: Open University Press, 1999.

9. Giddens A. *Modernity and self-identity: self and society in the late modern age.* Cambridge: Polity Press, 1991.

10. Rajagopal MR, Kumar S. Global exchange. A model for delivery of palliative care in India –The Calicut experiment. *J Palliat Care* 1999; **15**(1):44–9.

11. The Poznan Declaration (1998). *Eur J Palliat Care* 1999; **6**(2):61–3.

12. WHO. *Cancer pain relief and palliative care: report of a WHO expert committee* (Technical Report Series No. 804). Geneva: WHO, 1990.

13. Sepúlveda C, Marlin A, Yoshida T, Ullrich A. Palliative Care: The World Health Organization's Global Perspective. *J Pain Symptom Manage* 2002; **24**:91–6.

14. Heaven CM, Maguire P. Disclosure of concerns by hospice patients and their identification by nurses. *Palliat Med* 1997; **11**(4):283–90.

15. Puhan MA, Behnke M, Devereaux PJ, *et al.* Measurement of agreement on health-related quality of life changes in response to respiratory rehabilitation by patients and physicians–a prospective study. *Respir Med* 2004; **98**:1195–202.

16. Ahmedzai S, Brooks D. Transdermal fentanyl versus sustained-release oral morphine in cancer pain: preference, efficacy, and quality of life. *J Pain Symptom Manage* 1997; **13**(5):254–61.

17. Bottomley A, Efficace F, Thomas R, Vanvoorden V, Ahmedzai SH. Health-related quality of life in non-small cell lung cancer: methodologic issues in randomised controlled trials. *J Clin Oncol* 2003; **21**(15):2982–92.

18. Ahmedzai SH, Costa A, Blengini C, *et al.* A New international framework for palliative care. *Eur J Cancer* 2004; **40**:2192–200.

19. Ahmedzai SH, Gomez-Batiste X, Engels Y, *et al.* (eds). *Assessing organisations to improve palliative care in Europe.* Nijmegen: Vantilt Publishers, 2010.

20. MacDonald N. Oncology and palliative care: the case for co-ordination. *Cancer Treat Rev* 1993; **19**(Suppl A):29–41.

21. Partridge MR, Khatri A, Sutton L, Welham S, Ahmedzai SH. Palliative care services for those with chronic lung disease. *Chron Respir Dis* 2009; **6**(1):13–7.

22. Beattie J, Goodlin SJ. *Supportive care in heart failure.* Oxford: Oxford University Press, 2008.

23. Klastersky J. Supportive care in cancer. *Curr Opin Oncol* 1997; **9**:313.

24. Ahmedzai SH, Walsh D. Palliative medicine and modern cancer care. *Semin Oncol* 2000; **27**(1):1–6.

25. Temel JS, Greer JA, Muzikansky A, *et al.* Early palliative care for patients with metastatic non-small-cell lung cancer. *N Engl J Med* 2010; **363**(8):733–42.

26. Bromley L. Pre-emptive analgesia and protective premedication. What is the difference? *Biomedicine Pharmacotherapy* 2006; **60**:336–40.

27. Kissane DW, Bloch S, Burns W, McKenzies D, Posternino M. Psychological morbidity in the families of patients with cancer. *Psycho-Oncology* 1994; **3**:47–56.

28. Rock LK, Schwartzstein RM. Mechanisms of dyspnea in chronic lung disease. *Curr Opin Support Palliat Care* 2007; **1**(2):102–8.

29. Duggleby WD, Penz KL, Goodridge DM, *et al.* The transition experience of rural older persons with advanced cancer and their families: a grounded theory study. *BMC Palliat Care* 2010; **9**:1–5.

30. Davis MP. Integrating palliative medicine into an oncology practice. *Amer J Hospice Palliat Med* 2005; **22**(6):447–56.

31. Haraoui B, Pope J. Treatment of early rheumatoid arthritis: concepts in management. *Semin Arthritis Rheum* 2011; **40**:371–88.

32. Bredin M, Corner J, Krishnasamy M, *et al.* Multicentre randomised controlled trial of nursing intervention for breathlessness in patients with lung cancer. *BMJ* 1999; **318**(7188):901–4.

33. Keeley V. Pharmacological treatment for chronic oedema. *Br J Community Nurs* 2008; **13**(4):S4, S6, S8–10.

34. Ream E, Blows E, Scanlon K, Richardson A. An investigation of the quality of breast cancer information provided on the internet by voluntary organisations in Great Britain. *Patient Education and Counseling* 2009; **76**(1):10–15.

35. Johnson, IS, Rogers C, Biswas B, Ahmedzai, S. What do hospices do? A survey of hospices in the United Kingdom and Republic of Ireland. *BMJ* 1990; **300**:791–3.

36. Partridge MR, Khatri A, Sutton L, Welham S, Ahmedzai SH. Palliative care services for those with chronic lung disease. *Chron Respir Dis* 2009; **6**; 13.

37. Small N. HIV/AIDS: Lessons for policy and practice. In Clark D (ed) *The future for palliative care*, pp. 80–97. Buckingham: Open University Press, 1993.

38. Willard C. Cardiopulmonary resuscitation for palliative care patients: a discussion of ethical issues. *Palliat Med* 2000; **14**:308–12.

39. Clemens KE, Klaschik E. Symptomatic therapy of dyspnea with strong opioids and its effects on ventilation in palliative care patients. *J Pain Symptom Manage* 2007; **33**:473–81.

40. Clemens KE, Klaschik E. Morphine in the management of dyspnoea in ALS. A pilot study. *Eur J Neurology* 2008; **15**:445–50.

41. Jenkins V, Fallowfield L, Saul J. Information needs of patients with cancer: results from a large study in UK cancer centres. *Br J Cancer* 2001; **84**(1):48–51.

42. Butow PN, Maclean M, Dunn SM, Tattersall MH, Boyer MJ. The dynamics of change: cancer patients' preferences for information, involvement and support. *Ann Oncol* 1997; **8**(9):857–63.

43. Hellbom M, Bergelt C, Bergenmar M, *et al.* Cancer rehabilitation: a Nordic and European perspective. *Acta Oncologica* 2011; **50**:179–86.

44. Delbrück H. Concepts and structures of cancer rehabilitation in Germany: present and a possible future. *Rehabilitacija* 2009; **VIII**:102–5.

45. Deimling GT, Bowman KF, Sterns S, Wagner LJ, Kahana B. Cancer-related health worries and psychological distress among older adult, long-term cancer survivors. *Psycho-Oncology* 2006; **15**:306–20.

46. Maguire MF, Ravenscroft A, Beggs D, Duffy JP. A questionnaire study investigating the prevalence of the neuropathic component of chronic pain after thoracic surgery. *Eur J Cardiothorac Surg* 2006; **29**:800–5.

47. Wildgaard K, Ravn J, Kehlet H. Chronic post-thoracotomy pain: a critical review of pathogenic mechanisms and strategies for prevention. *Eur J Cardiothoracic Surg* 2009; **36**:170–80.

48. Hanks GW, Cherny NI, Christakis NA, Fallon M, Kaasa S, Portenoy RK (eds). *Oxford Textbook of Palliative Medicine.* Oxford: Oxford University Press, 2009.

49. Twycross R, Wilcock A, Toller CS (eds). *Symptom management in advanced cancer.* Oxford: Radcliffe Medical, 2009.

50. Walsh TD, Caraceni AT, Fainsinger R, *et al.* (eds). *Palliative Medicine.* Philadelphia, PA: Saunders, 2009.

51. Hasselaar JG, Verhagen SC, Vissers KC. When cancer symptoms cannot be controlled: the role of palliative sedation. *Curr Opin Support Palliat Care* 2009; **3**(1):14–23.

52. Clark D, Dickinson G, Lancaster CJ, *et al.* UK geriatricians' attitudes to active voluntary euthanasia and physician-assisted death. *Age Ageing* 2001; **30**:395–8.

53. Seale C. Legalisation of euthanasia or physician-assisted suicide: survey of doctors' attitudes. *Palliat Med* 2009; **23**(3):205–12.

Chapter 2

Anatomy and physiology

Martin F. Muers

This chapter is intended to be an aide-memoire for the reader who wishes to be reminded of the normal state of the respiratory system before considering a particular symptom or condition. It is not intended to be comprehensive, and readers who wish to have more complete accounts should consult the Further Reading list. Descriptions refer principally to the adult lung. The basic features apply to children, but the dimensions and normal values are different. More detailed accounts of the mechanisms of some common respiratory symptoms, e.g. cough, are given elsewhere in this book.

Ribcage, respiratory muscles, and respiratory 'pump'

The basic arrangements for the 12 vertebrae and ribs, the manubrium, and sternum, are shown in the radiograph (Figure 2.1). The ribs articulate by means of facet (flat) joints on each of two adjoining vertebral bodies and with another facet joint of a vertebral spine. The anterior ends of ribs 1–10 are attached by costal cartilages to the manubrium and sternum. During inspiration, rotation of the rib necks causes the shafts to move outwards and forwards increasing thoracic diameter. The combination of this and more importantly, the diaphragm excursion, produces an increase in thoracic volume.

Diaphragm

This consists of a central fibrous disc-like tendon and peripheral skeletal muscle innervated by the phrenic nerves (C3–5). It is attached to the first three lumbar vertebrae behind and to the xiphisternum and the upper margins of the bottom six ribs laterally and anteriorly. Physiology of diaphragmatic contraction is complex. Essentially, muscle contraction causes the dome to move downwards. The abdomen is a fluid-filled bag and this downward movement of the diaphragm has to be balanced by an outward movement of the anterior abdominal wall because the abdomen and contents are fixed in volume. As a result, the lower ribs move outwards during inspiration, firstly because of the way the diaphragm muscles are attached and secondly, because abdominal pressure pushes them out.

Diaphragm paralysis causes 'paradoxical' *inward* movement of the abdominal wall in inspiration. A hyperinflated chest cannot expand further and sometimes diaphragmatic contraction causes unexpected *inward* movement of the lower ribs—leading to 'Harrison's sulcus' in children and is seen in adults with severe chronic obstructive pulmonary disease (COPD).

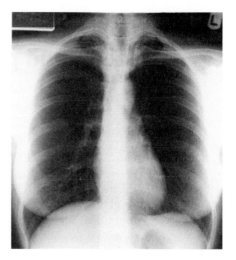

Fig. 2.1 A postero-anterior (PA) chest radiograph of a normal woman. Conventionally, x-rays are taken on full inspiration, and therefore the diaphragms are contracted and are flatter than in expiration. The natural lung markings are the bronchovascular bundles, effectively the pulmonary arteries.

Intercostal muscles

These are two sheets of muscles between adjacent ribs. The externals are predominantly inspiratory and the internals expiratory as they have opposing effects on rib movement. Their contribution to this in quiet breathing is small. Innervation is by segmental T1–12 intercostal nerves running along the inferior border of each rib; irritation of these causes pleurisy.

Accessory muscles

The three scalene muscles run from the cervical vertebrae to the anterior first and second ribs and are primary muscles of inspiration. The abdominal muscles (rectus abdominis, external and internal transverse abdominis) connect the lower ribs and pelvis. Contraction increases abdominal pressure and this forces the lower ribs outwards (inspiration). However, because of their insertions to the lower ribs, these muscles assist in expiration as well, and they are particularly important during activities such as coughing and speaking.

Pleura, pleural space, and pleural fluid

The pleural membrane consists of a layer of mesothelial (pavement) cells on a thin basement membrane and loose connective tissue. The visceral (lung) and parietal (chest wall, diaphragm, and mediastinal) pleura are similar. For the most part, the 'pleural space' in health is a potential one as there is a continuous flow of pleural fluid from capillaries below the parietal pleura into the space between the two layers of pleura whence it passes through the visceral pleura into subpleural lymphatics within the lung. The volume of this fluid is only a few millilitres. The practical effects of pleural disease are that a pleural effusion compresses lung tissue. Pleural inflammation or tumour may be painful because of irritation of the intercostals nerves. Diffuse pleural thickening can both decrease the compliance of the chest wall making it stiffer, and can restrict lung expansion, and these two actions can cause breathlessness.

Airways

Upper airways

The upper airways are comprised of the nasal passages, pharynx, and larynx (Figure 2.2).

The upper airways have no rigid wall, being bounded by muscle and connective tissue. This means that when the pressure within it drops during inspiration as air is drawn into the lungs, it tends to collapse. Reflex muscular tone prevents this. However, if the airway is narrow (as in obesity), or if the muscle tension is reduced (as in sleep), closure can occur. This is the mechanism of obstructive sleep apnoea. The anatomy of the aryepiglottic fold, the false cords, and the vagal cough reflexes involving the true cords, are powerful protective mechanisms preventing the inhalation of oral contents, particularly during eating and drinking. This protection is decreased after, for example, denervation of the larynx as by a thoracic tumour causing recurrent laryngeal nerve palsy, or bilateral strokes causing pseudo-bulbar palsy.

Lower airways

The lower airways consist of the trachea and all bronchi and bronchioles. The trachea is about 10cm long in adults, with its bifurcation at the level of the manubriosternal junction. It consists of a series of anterior horseshoe-shaped cartilaginous rings, connecting to an elastic and muscular membrane posteriorly. Inside these, there is connective tissue, a web of spiral smooth muscle which can narrow the airway, a submucosa which is vascular and contains bronchial glands; and in contact with the air there is a complex pseudo-stratified ciliated epithelium (the mucus membrane) (Figure 2.3a). The trachea is mobile, shortening and becoming crescent-shaped during cough. Bronchi have a similar structure and divide 'dichotomously'—i.e. always into two (although the division may be asymmetrical)—into two main, five lobar and 19 segmental ones. The cartilage support

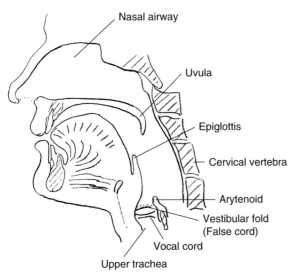

Fig. 2.2 Sagittal section through the nose, pharynx, and larynx. The upper airway extends from the nares to the vestibular folds. Because it is bounded by muscles and connective tissues, it acts as a partially collapsible tube. During inspiration the upper airway narrows slightly and on expiration it widens. Muscular contraction during swallowing moves the epiglottis backwards and the arytenoids upwards and forwards to close off the glottis and prevent aspiration of contents passing to the oesophagus, behind the trachea.

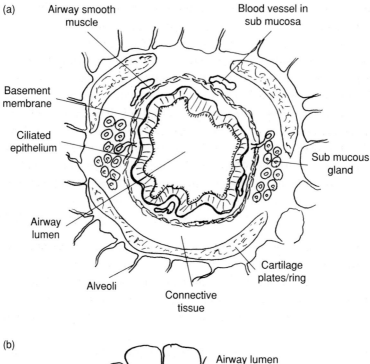

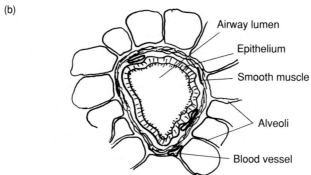

Fig. 2.3 Cross-sectional diagrams of (a) bronchus and (b) a bronchiole. The airway smooth muscle is arranged in a spiral fashion around the submucosa and epithelium and causes narrowing of the airway when it constricts. Bronchial submucous glands are complex tubular structures below the smooth muscle and secrete mucus into the airways. The rigidity of the airway is ensured by cartilage rings which diminish to separate plates as the airways narrow. By contrast, the bronchiole is a simpler structure lacking cartilage, submucous glands, and lymphatics. Smooth muscle is present, but the alveoli are much more closely applied to the bronchiolar wall and exert tension on it, keeping the airway open.

dwindles to an occasional plate with progressive subdivisions as the bronchi reduce in size. Bronchioles begin at about 1mm diameter (Figure 2.3b).

The terminology of the finer anatomy of the lung is confusing (see Box 2.1 for some simple definitions). *Terminal bronchioles* (0.5mm in diameter) are the smallest which act purely to conduct air. These branch to *'respiratory'* bronchioles which have alveolar ducts and alveoli in their walls and participate in gas exchange. There are about 300 million *alveoli*, each approximately 250µm in diameter. They are lined by a very thin epithelium (type I alveolar cells) which are continuous with the epithelium of the bronchioles. A basement membrane separates these from attached capillary endothelial walls. Parts of each alveolus have an *interstitium* where there is a bigger gap between them and the capillaries which is filled by connective tissue and interstitial cells such as fibroblasts, lymphocytes, macrophages, and nerve fibres (Figure 2.4). Type II alveolar cells are found in the corners of alveoli and secrete surfactant. Without this, the lung would not be expandable.

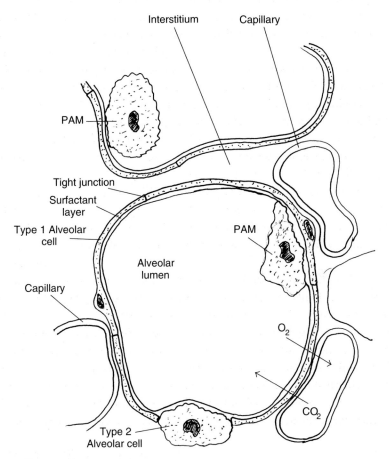

Fig. 2.4 Alveoli consist principally of large flat type I alveolar cells with tight junctions between them. Type II cells are secretory, forming surfactant which is present as a film lining the alveolar surface. Pulmonary alveolar macrophages (PAMs) migrate from the blood to the interstitium, into the alveoli. They are scavenger cells. Below the type I cells is a basement membrane (not shown) and a thin loose interstitium which may contain occasional inflammatory cells such as neutrophils and eosinophils. There are tight junctions between the adjacent cell walls of alveoli and of capillaries. Gas exchange between the alveolar lumen and the capillaries occurs by diffusion.

Alveoli contain a few cells, notably pulmonary alveolar macrophages (PAMs), which are phagocytic and metabolically active. A small quantity of fluid containing proteases regularly extravasates from the capillaries into the alveoli and this moves with the PAMs up the bronchial tree.

The most practically useful subunit of the lung is the *secondary lobule*. This contains a bronchiole and arteriole at its centre and is bounded by loose connective tissue septa. It has pulmonary venules and lymphatics at the edges (Figure 2.5). These lobules are about 1–2.5cm in diameter and are easily seen as 'hexagons' on computed tomography (CT) scanning, particularly when lymphatics are enlarged.

Bronchioles depend upon the tension of their alveolar wall attachments to keep them open during respiration. If the alveoli are damaged, as in emphysema, this tension is lost and the small airways then easily collapse in expiration. This is the major cause of respiratory airflow limitation and hence breathlessness in COPD. By contrast, an increase in the thickness of alveolar walls, as in fibrosing alveolitis, makes the lungs stiffer and elastic recoil is increased but expiratory airflow limitation is low.

Lymph

The lymphatics draining the pleura accompany the pulmonary venules and veins at the edges of the secondary lobules (see Figure 2.5). Proximally, the channels converge on perihilar and then mediastinal nodes, eventually forming the thoracic duct which runs posteriorly in the mediastinum and enters the left subclavian vein. Lymph channels are the principal means whereby the lung is kept dry. They are overwhelmed in heart failure and pulmonary oedema results.

Pulmonary vessels

The gross anatomy of these vessels is demonstrated on angiography (Figure 2.6). Pulmonary arteries course and branch with bronchi so that they accompany each other down to the alveoli and are at the centres of the secondary lobules. Pulmonary veins form at the periphery of acini and interlobular septa and then run separately to drain via the four main pulmonary veins, two from the upper lobes and the right middle lobe and two from the lower lobes, into the left atrium.

Bronchial circulation

Bronchial arteries provide oxygenated blood to lung structures. Arising from the aorta on the left and from the intercostal artery on the right, they accompany the bronchi as they divide within the lungs. There is, as a result, a very rich vascular network within airway walls. The bronchial circulation supplies abnormal tissue too, such as tumours and bronchiectatic segments. In the latter condition the bronchial arteries may enlarge and severe haemoptysis from them may require bronchial artery embolization (block) to control it.

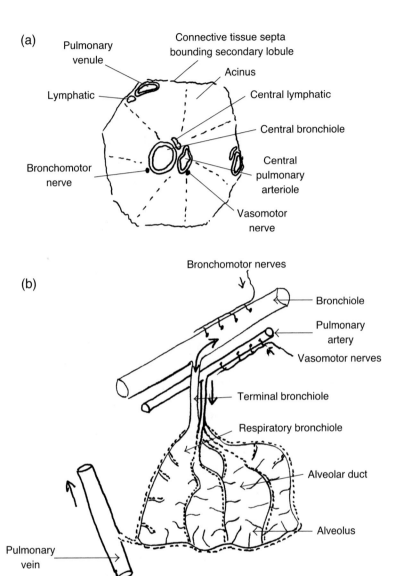

Fig. 2.5 Fine structure of the lungs. (a) Cross-sectional diagram of a secondary lobule. This has a pulmonary arteriole and a bronchiole at its centre together with small lymphatics, nerves and bronchial vessels (not shown). It is about 1–2cm across, bounded by loose connective tissue septa. Pulmonary venules (veins) are at the edge of the secondary lobules with accompanying lymphatics. (b) The anatomy of an acinus. A terminal bronchiole with an accompanying arteriole divides into a number of respiratory bronchioles and then alveolar ducts off which the alveoli open. Innervation is by the vagus and sympathetic nerves.

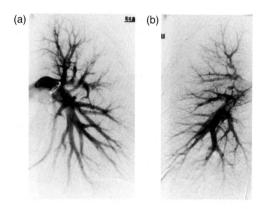

Fig. 2.6 Arteriograms of the pulmonary vessels. (a) A left lung pulmonary arteriogram showing the anatomy of the pulmonary arteries which accompany the bronchi as they subdivide into lung tissue. (b) The venous phase of the arteriogram (right lung)—the venules run from the edges of the secondary lobules and coalesce to form larger vessels which enter the left atrium.

Innervation

The lung is innervated by the parasympathetic vagal nerves and sympathetic nerves from the paravertebral sympathetic chain and the stellate ganglia at the lung apices. There are no somatic nerves and thus, no localization of lung sensation is possible. The parasympathetic nerves cause cholinergic bronchoconstriction of airway smooth muscle and stimulate secretion from submucus glands and constrict subepithelial blood vessels. Sympathetic and purinergic (non-adrenergic, non-cholinergic) nerves supply the airways smooth muscle causing relaxation and the submucosa and vessels where they have opposite effects to the parasympathetic supply.

Afferent, or sensory fibres, come from three types of nerve endings: rapidly adapting type I receptors instigating cough and irritant reflexes; slowly adapting nerve endings type II giving rise to the Hering–Breuer reflex (inhibition of inspiration at high lung volume) and lastly type III receptors (J receptors) which are found in the lung periphery and are sensitive both to mechanical distortion and chemical stimuli. Type I cough receptors are concentrated at branching points within the airways and particularly around the larynx. Cough is also instigated by non-specific stimulation of temperature-sensitive nerve endings, which are also especially found in the larynx.

Integration

Ventilation

During inspiration, as the volume of the chest is increased, a negative pressure relative to the atmosphere develops in the pleural space. It is typically -10 to $-20cmH_2O$ (1–$2kPa$) at the bases and $-5cmH_2O$ ($0.5kPa$) at the apices. The negative pressure encourages movement of air into the lungs as they expand. The force required to expand them, however, must overcome:

- Resistance to airflow in the airways.
- Stiffness or compliance of the lung tissue.
- Stiffness of the chest wall and abdomen.
- Inertia of the whole system.

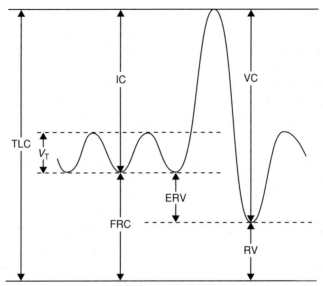

Fig. 2.7 Subdivisions of lung volume. Inspiration upwards, expiration downwards. The volume of air breathed in and out during quiet respiration (tidal volume, V_T is shown on the left. At the end of quiet expiration, the forces of the chest wall tending to move the lungs outwards and the stretching of the lung itself tending to move the lungs inwards, are balanced and this volume is known as the functional residual capacity (FRC). If a maximal inspiration is taken from FRC (inspiratory capacity, IC), and then a forced full expiration is done, the total expired volume is known as the vital capacity (VC). At the end of this forced expiration, the volume of air left in the lungs is called residual volume (RV). The combination of the VC and the RV is the total lung capacity (TLC). The expiratory reserve volume is similar to the inspiratory capacity and simply represents the volume in reserve after a tidal expiration. These lung volumes can change with chronic disease (see Table 2.1).

At rest, the lungs tend to collapse as is evident when there is a complete pneumothorax. This tendency is counter-acted by the chest wall tending to move *outwards*. The thoracic volume where these two forces are equal, is at 'resting' lung volume, i.e. the *functional residual capacity* (FRC) (Figure 2.7, Table 2.1).

Work is needed either to increase the thoracic gas volume above this, for example, to breathe in from FRC to total lung capacity (TLC) or to breathe out further to residual volume (RV). Expiration during tidal breathing is a passive relaxation using stored energy in which the elasticity of the chest wall and lungs (stretched during inspiration) returns them to resting dimensions as air is expelled.

More muscular work has to be done to achieve a tidal volume if the lungs are hyperinflated as in COPD or abnormally stiff or compressed as with diffuse pleural thickening, ankylosing spondylitis, or kyphoscoliosis.

Airway resistance

This is clinically important. Airway narrowing increases the resistance to airflow within the airways and increases the work of breathing. In quiet breathing, surprisingly, the

Table 2.1 Differing effects of obstructive versus restrictive chronic lung disease on pulmonary function. A. Changes in lung function in a 60 year old woman with COPD; predicted values for a person of her age and height, then her observed value and then her values expressed as a percentage of the predicted value. It can be seen that her total lung capacity (TLC) is increased as are her functional residual capacity (FRC) and residual volume (RV) showing gas trapping in the lungs. The FEV$_1$ is low at 36% of predicted, as is the FEV$_1$/FVC ratio. The transfer factor and coefficient are low because of emphysema which reduces the area of alveolar wall available for gas exchange. B. By contrast, this shows the percentage predicted values of a 47-year-old man with severe fibrosing alveolitis—restrictive lung disease. The lung volumes are reduced but the FEV$_1$/FVC ratio is better than predicted. The transfer factor and coefficient are reduced because inflammation and scarring of the alveolar walls which interferes with gas exchange.

	A			B
	Predicted	**Observed**	**% Predicted**	**% Predicted**
Lung volumes (L)				
Vital capacity	2.8	3.3	115	42!
TLC	4.9	6.0	123!	52!
FRC	2.7	5.8	216!	78!
RV	2.1	4.6	220!	87!
Mechanics				
FEV$_1$	2.3	0.83	36!	51!
FVC	2.7	2.8	103	42!
Ratio FEV$_1$/VC	77	29	37	97!
Transfer factor	7.5	38	50!	25!
Transfer coefficient	1.5	0.64	41!	47!

(! denotes an abnormal value (> 2 SD below or above predicted)

major resistance to airflow is in the nose, and in mouth breathing, the larynx. Conversely, resistance within healthy small airways contributes only about 25% to total airway resistance because there are so many of them and their total cross-sectional area is very high. The airway resistance of the bronchi is affected by many things, including airway smooth muscle and oedema or mucus in them. In some diseases, these factors and airway collapse in expiration due to alveolar destruction as in COPD, can hugely increase the resistance to expiration. Likewise, a tumour narrowing a major airway can increase resistance throughout the breathing cycle. The physiology of forced expiration is described in Figure 2.8.

Pulmonary gas exchange

The purpose of ventilation is to achieve gas exchange. Oxygen from the air enters the alveoli by convection (bulk flow) and then diffuses down a molecular concentration gradient from the alveolar gas across the alveolar cell and capillary cell membranes, to attach

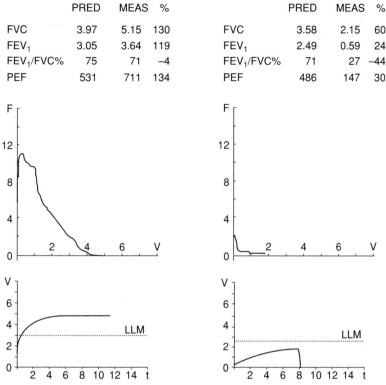

	PRED	MEAS	%
FVC	3.97	5.15	130
FEV$_1$	3.05	3.64	119
FEV$_1$/FVC%	75	71	−4
PEF	531	711	134

	PRED	MEAS	%
FVC	3.58	2.15	60
FEV$_1$	2.49	0.59	24
FEV$_1$/FVC%	71	27	−44
PEF	486	147	30

Fig. 2.8 Physiology of forced expiration. This shows spirometer readings from, on the left, a healthy 45-year-old man and on the right a 70-year-old man with severe COPD. Upper panels are flow-volume plots (F-V) and the lower plots are spirograms plotting volume against time (F-t). The healthy man rapidly reaches a high peak flow of about 11L/s and as expiration continues, flow rate declines in a straight line towards residual volume which is reached at about 5L. The spirogram shows that the FEV$_1$ is approximately 3.6L. The vital capacity is reached in about 5s. By contrast, the patient has a lower peak flow rate of about 3L/s and the flow rate is reduced very abruptly. It continues at a *very* low rate thereafter. Similarly, the spirograms shows the FEV$_1$ is approximately 0.6L and even at 8s expiration is still continuing. The abrupt decline in peak flow rate during a forced expiration in these patients occurs because of the loss of lung elasticity which causes the small airways to close. This is known as pressure-dependent airway narrowing. In asthma, the pattern of expiratory flow is similar to normal, although at much lower flow rates (volume-dependent airway narrowing).

to haemoglobin molecules in the capillary red cells. Conversely, carbon dioxide diffuses from the capillary plasma down a concentration gradient to the alveolar gas and is then expelled by ventilation. Efficient exchange between alveolar gas and pulmonary capillary blood, needs 'matching' between air and blood throughout the lungs—i.e. there needs to be an appropriate supply of each in all alveoli. However, even in health this does not happen with alveoli being relatively over-perfused at the lung bases because of gravity, or over-ventilated at the lung apices. Changes in alveolar perfusion to improve matching, probably occur in health as a result of local regulation of arteriolar tone (and hence flow

Box 2.1 Lung structure: simple definitions

- Lobe: separate bits of each lung, e.g. right upper.
- Segment: subdivision of a lobe (usually 2–5).
- Bronchi: tubes with cartilage.
- Bronchioles: small tubes without cartilage.
- Terminal bronchiole: last one, 0.5mm in diameter.
- Respiratory bronchiole: where alveoli and gas exchange begin.
- Alveoli: gas-exchanging sac (parenchyma).
- Secondary lobule: smallest bit of lung surrounded by connective tissue. About 1–2.5cm in diameter and contains about five terminal bronchioles and the alveoli connected to them. Each terminal bronchiole and alveoli is called an acinus (7mm diameter).
- Primary lobule: one-eighth of an acinus; one respiratory bronchiole + alveoli.

in pulmonary arterioles) as a result of hypoxic vasoconstriction which is mediated by nitric oxide. A crude clinical estimate of this inhomogeneity is the alveolar-arterial oxygen gradient as a measure of the lungs' efficiency at gas exchange. It is normally approximately 2kPa. Lung damage increases this.

If the lungs are inefficient, an increase in alveolar ventilation may help to correct any consequent hypoxaemia—because this increases the oxygen uptake in the alveoli with low ventilation, but there is a concomitant reduction in alveolar PCO_2 and therefore in arterial $PaCO_2$ as more than the physiologically required carbon dioxide is expelled.

A clinical measure of the lungs' capacity for alveolar gas exchange is the transfer coefficient for carbon monoxide (a marker gas) i.e. the TLCO. This measure is sometimes called the diffusing capacity—DLCO (Table 2.1). Typically, this might be reduced in diseases where there is alveolar inflammation, as in fibrosing alveolitis, or when the alveoli are damaged, as in emphysema. It is usually normal in pure airway diseases such as asthma.

Carbon dioxide is carried in the blood principally as dissolved bicarbonate:

$$CO_2 + H_2O \approx H_2CO_3 \approx HCO_3 + H^+$$

Blood has a high capacity for bicarbonate and acts as a buffer against big changes of blood pH. In health, ventilation is regulated to maintain the $PaCO_2$ at 40mmHg (5.3kPa) and the pH of blood at 7.4. Lung damage can result in an inability to ventilate alveoli sufficiently to remove the body's carbon dioxide load. $PaCO_2$ rises as a consequence as does the bicarbonate. This combination is seen typically in the type II hypercapnic respiratory failure of COPD, where, although the pH may be normal, the $PaCO_2$ may, for example, be 60mmHg (8.0kPa) and the bicarbonate 40mmol/L rather than 24mmol/L.

Regulation of breathing

Breathing is regulated by an exquisite but incompletely understood neuronal control system. Peripheral aortic and carotid chemoreceptors, together with medullary chemoreceptors, regulate ventilation in response to changes in $PaCO_2$, in the case of the latter as a result of subsequent changes in cerebrospinal fluid pH. This drive interacts with any hypoxia sensed by the peripheral chemoreceptors. Short-term changes in ventilation, however, usually occur in response to the need to control $PaCO_2$ and hence blood pH. It appears that in addition, the activity of inspiratory neurones in the medulla is modulated by a variety of other inputs, e.g. nerve traffic from pharyngeal and chest wall stretch receptors, which contribute not only to the overall level of ventilation, but also the pattern of breathing. This automatic control of breathing is subconscious and is susceptible to many changes that reduce overall drive, e.g. the use of hypnotics. Central conscious respiratory drive can over-ride the usual medullary automatic control. The resultant breathing pattern is usually less regular and the blood $PaCO_2$ is often reduced because of hyperventilation which is the usual pattern.

Breathing during exercise

Ventilation is increased in steady-state exercise because muscles require additional oxygen to generate the ATP for muscle contraction from carbohydrate fuel and ADP. The resultant increase in carbon dioxide production stimulates the medullary and peripheral chemoreceptors. If anaerobic metabolism occurs, it generates lactate and hydrogen irons reducing blood pH and again, this stimulates chemoreceptors. As the intensity of exercise increases, tidal volume also increases so that the rapidity and depth of breathing approaches 75% of the maximal flow-volume loop. In disease states, however, the limits of expiratory flow may be reached far more quickly.

The work of breathing is hugely increased in exercise; for example, the measured average intrapleural pressure changes may rise to +20cmH$_2$O (2kPa) compared with 5cmH$_2$O (0.5kPa) at rest.

The sensation of dyspnoea is complex (see Chapter 5, this volume) but may be present even at rest in very disabled people. The factors limiting exercise are not fully understood. However, there is usually a component of peripheral muscle discomfort sensed as fatigue and the respiratory muscles may contribute to this. Measures of exercise capacity in the laboratory range from bicycle or treadmill tests, which enable accurate plots of tidal volume, frequency, oxygen consumption, and carbon dioxide production, to less formal tests of capacity such as a 6-minute walking distance or the shuttle walk test. The latter are, however, perfectly suitable for much clinical work in patients with respiratory disease (for more details see Chapter 6, this volume).

Obesity

More and more respiratory patients are obese with a body mass index greater than 30. As obesity increases, the lungs are progressively compressed. Vital capacity and total lung capacity remain well preserved but FRC and expiratory reserve volume are reduced and small airways are narrowed. The work of breathing is increased and poor ventilation perfusing matching may lead to persistent hypoxaemia even at rest.

Lung defence mechanisms

The lungs are open to the air with its contained particles and we inhale 10,000L every day. They need protection against inhaled dust, fumes and micro-organisms as well as oral fluids and solids. The defences are physical, cellular, and humoral.

The nose acts as a crude particulate filter, and the same occurs in the mouth and in the larynx where narrowing of the airway generates turbulence and increases impaction. Within the lung, vortices occur at bifurcations of the large airways but beyond this gas flow becomes so low as the cross-sectional area of the airways increases, that fine particles of less than 2.5μm diameter can only leave the inspired air by sedimentation.

Absorbed particles are removed from the lung by means of the mucociliary escalator. Airway-lining fluid (ALF) is secreted predominantly by the submucous glands which occur about every square millimetre of membrane. About 10mL is produced per 24 hours in health with an upwards flow rate of about 5mm/min. This fluid is swallowed or expectorated when it reaches the larynx.

Additional fluid is secreted by the goblet cells of the airway (Figure 2.9). Respiratory mucus is a highly complex liquid containing macromolecules and proteins which give it physical properties suitable for its function as a protective layer over the underlying cells.

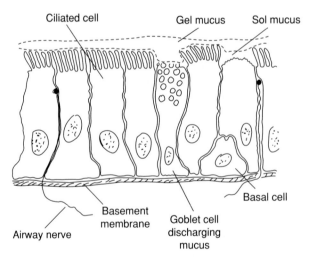

Fig. 2.9 Ultrastructure of the bronchial epithelium. Most of the cells are ciliated; the cilia beat towards the mouth in a coordinated fashion in a sol of bronchial fluid with the more tenacious gel phase at their tips. Bronchial mucus is secreted by goblet cells and also by submucous bronchial glands (not shown). The mucus membrane regenerates from basal cells. Airway nerves penetrate the tight junctions between adjacent epithelial cells. Below the basement membrane is the submucosa where there are blood vessels, fibroblasts, neutrophils, and eosinophils (not shown).

The cilia of the epithelial cells beat in a coordinated fashion in a sol of fluid and the mucus forms a thicker layer above them (gel). The water and ion content of ALF is regulated by cellular protein pumps on the apical and basal surfaces of airway epithelial cells. There is movement of sodium and chloride ions and water determined by an ATPase pump at the base of the epithelial cells. Active secretion of chloride ions can, however, increase the water content of ALF. Genetic defects of this chloride pump (CFTR or cystic fibrosis transmembrane regulator) are the primary lesion in cystic fibrosis where the airway mucus is characteristically extremely thick and tenacious. Genetic defects in ciliary structure (primary ciliary dyskinesias), e.g. as in Kartagener's syndrome, are associated with mucus retention, secondary infection, and resulting bronchiectasis.

Particles deposited in alveoli are cleared differently. The majority are phagocytosed by PAMs (see Figure 2.4), which subsequently pass to the bronchi. However, in addition the lining cells of the alveoli can 'unzip' allowing cells and particles to pass across the membrane and PAMs can migrate in this way in the opposite direction through the epithelium and into lymphatics. Other particles are caught in surfactant and moved up the mucociliary escalator and others may be engulfed by epithelial type I cells which subsequently die and are in their turn phagocytosed. Clearance of particle loads may take many days, and some particles cannot be cleared. Asbestos fibres may be detected in the lungs 50 or more years after inhalation and coal dust may accumulate around bronchioles (causing emphysema) and in submucosal lymphoid tissue. Some soluble inhaled substances can pass directly across the alveolar membrane into the circulation—which is the basis of using inhalation as a route for systemically active medication (e.g. insulin).

In addition to these physical mechanisms, the lungs are protected by airway proteins present either as a result of diffusion through the mucus membrane from the blood (e.g. α_1-antiprotease or albumin) or as a result of secretion by airway cells, e.g. the components of complement. Examples of protective proteins are lysozyme and immunoglobulin. These are particularly important for neutralizing bacterial pathogens and congenital lack of surface-acting immunoglobulin A (IgA), for example, causes bronchiectasis. Cytokines are involved in the exceedingly complex activation of IgE-dependent reactions in response to some inhaled molecules. This may be physiologically appropriate as for parasite control, or inappropriate as in allergy to house dust mite particles and other allergens.

Airway cells (PAMs, lymphocytes, neutrophils, and eosinophils) have two roles in lung defence. They may initiate an immune response (afferent limb) or function as 'effector' cells contributing to an inflammatory response once an immune response has been elicited. In addition, PAMs and neutrophils act as airway scavengers ingesting particles, microbes, and proteins. Defects in cell function (e.g. T-cell defects of HIV) allow lung infection with 'opportunist' organisms which are usually prevented from lung colonization by immune and cellular surveillance.

Lung inflammation

Inflammation is a 'normal' host defence response to persistent antigens in lung tissue. It is stimulated either directly by foreign proteins or by cytokines deriving from antigen–macrophage interaction. Neutrophils adhere to pulmonary capillary endothelium and migrate into lung tissue. They release a large array of cytokines and proteins which recruit more cells and alter vessel permeability leading to protein and fluid accumulation in the inflamed area. The mechanisms underlying inflammatory response are very complex and are incompletely understood. We also do not understand why the results of inflammation vary. In some cases, it terminates and resolves with lung repair, leaving normal tissue—as after a streptococcal pneumonia. In other cases, however, lung destruction occurs as, for example, after a *Klebsiella* pneumonia or tuberculosis, and this leads to permanent scarring. In other instances, inflammation continues chronically as in fibrosing alveolitis. Much lung disease is a result of persistent chronic inflammation—COPD, chronic severe asthma, Acute respiratory distress syndrome (ARDS), cystic fibrosis and the alveolitis of systemic vasculitis as examples. Thus, a chronically ill patient may have lung tissue which is scarred, secondarily infected, or persistently inflamed as a result of an initial event. Unfortunately, at present few of these processes can be directly modulated.

Key points

- An adult breathes 10,000L of air in 24 hours.
- The primary inspiratory muscles are the diaphragm and internal intercostals.
- Expiration is mainly a passive act during tidal breathing.
- The bronchial tree branches dichotomously to about 30,000 terminal bronchioles 0.5mm in diameter.
- There are approximately 300 million alveoli lined by type I pavement cells with type II secretory surfactant cells at intervals.
- The interstitium of the lung consists of basement membrane, connective tissues with protein matrix, and inflammatory cells.
- Important changes in the airways of obstructive lung disease are hyper-reactive muscle, inflammation of the bronchial walls, and loss of alveolar wall tension so that the small bronchioles collapse in expiration leading to 'trapping' of gas in the lung.
- Gas exchange in emphysema and diffuse parenchymal lung disease is poor because of abnormal ventilation-perfusion matching in the alveoli.
- Obesity causes compression of the lungs, poor ventilation-perfusion matching, hypoxaemia and an increased work of breathing.

Further reading

1. Gibson GJ, Geddes DDDM, Costabel U, Sterk PJ, Corrin B. *Respiratory Medicine*, 3rd edn. London: WB Saunders, 2003. [Part A, 'Structure and function', contains 12 chapters on the anatomy and physiology of the lungs and chest.]
2. Gosselink R, Stan H (eds) Lung function testing. *ERS Monograph* 2005; **31**:1–206. [A Comprehensive modern account of all aspects of the measurement of lung function.]
3. Hansell DM, Lynch DA, McAdams HP, Bankier AA (eds). *Imaging of diseases of the chest*, 5th edn. Philadelphia, PA: Mosby/Elsevier, 2009. [Chapter 2, 'The normal chest', is a well illustrated account of chest anatomy and normal radiology.]

Chapter 3

Quality of life: models and measurement

Michael E. Hyland and Samantha C. Sodergren

The term quality of life (QoL) refers to the patient's subjective experience of life, but beyond that there are a wide variety of interpretations which vary in terms of perspective (see Table 3.1). According to some definitions (1–3), QoL is defined in terms of content or theory by researchers. Other definitions, however, suggest that QoL is something that is defined entirely by the patient (4–6). This difference is by no means trivial, because it has an impact on those aspects of life which, by definition, fall within the remit of QoL. Thus, although the general meaning of QoL is not under dispute, the precise form of meaning and measurement is.

As a general rule, patients value the quality of life much more than its quantity, and place little value on physiological measures of morbidity. In the case of supportive and palliative care, the patient's subjective experience therefore should be one of the most important considerations in determining care. Wherever possible, treatment should be decided by a negotiated agreement between the patient and health professionals. In including the patient's perspective it is important to recognize that this perspective can change as a function of time or health status. Patients who feel that a particular health state is 'not worth living' when they are well may have a very different view of the matter

Table 3.1 Proposed definitions of quality of life

Definition	Authors
Having as much money as possible left over after taking care of basic necessities, and having the necessary time and opportunities for spending it in a pleasant way	Singer (1)
The more or less 'good' or 'satisfactory' character of people's life	Szalai (2)
Patients' performance in four areas: physical and occupational function, psychologic state, social interaction, and somatic sensation	Schipper et al. (3)
The quality of life measure the difference or the gap at a particular period of time between the hopes and expectations of an individual and the individual's present experiences	Calman (4)
An overall evaluation of the subjective experience of life	DeHaes and van Knippenberg (5)
The quality, or value of an individual's life is no more and no less than what she considers it to be	Hayry (6)

when they are ill. Thus negotiations between the doctor and patient must take into account the fact that patients are in a vulnerable state and that this vulnerability extends to decision-making about QoL.

It is important to emphasize that good clinicians have always treated patients as people first and foremost, and hence been sensitive to QoL. The original definition of health given by the World Health Organization in 1947 was: '. . . a state of complete physical, mental and social well-being and not merely the absence of disease and infirmity' (8). Good clinicians have always balanced the physiological needs of the patient against the psychological consequences of different kinds of treatment. However, during the last 20 years there has been a formalization of the process of caring for patients as people. Like treatment guidelines, the definitions, the measures, and all the paraphernalia that go with the QoL approach, all have the aim of providing a more consistent service for the patient.

Measuring quality of life

Information about the patient's QoL can be obtained in many different ways. Talking to the patient and history-taking all provide relevant information. However, questionnaires provide a more structured form of assessment and these can be either self-completed or interviewer administered, depending on the scale and the patient's ability. In addition, if patients are capable of completing a questionnaire, they can be asked to do this before the clinical interview and guide the kind of questions asked by the clinician, thereby achieving a more patient-focused interview.

There is a wide range of QoL questionnaires, which broadly fall into three categories: disease-specific, which are designed for a specific disease; generic scales, designed for any disease; and idiographic scales which, in effect, provide a different scale for each patient.

Disease-specific scales

Disease-specific scales are designed to include items that distinguish patients with the disease from healthy controls. Unlike generic scales, disease-specific scales do not include items that are irrelevant to the disease (e.g. an asthmatic is not given questions about eating problems) and so they often have a high degree of user acceptability. However, either explicitly or otherwise, such scales are also designed for a particular purpose and so the content of the scale also reflects that purpose. Most of these scales (e.g. the Chronic Respiratory Disease Questionnaire (9), the St George's Respiratory Questionnaire (10), and the Asthma Quality of Life Questionnaire (11)) have been designed for clinical trials where a tool is needed to assess outcome in drug treatment. Such scales include a range of items (see subscales in Table 3.2). However, they do not include items that are irrelevant to a clinical trial, e.g. they do not include items about the inconvenience or cost of inhaler, as this is irrelevant to a clinical trial.

One scale (the Asthma Bother Profile (12)) is designed for clinical use and so does include items about convenience and cost of inhalers, as well as items concerning

Table 3.2 Disease-specific scales

Measured and	Author	Mode of administration	Number of items and subscales, target population	Subscales
Asthma Bother Profile	Hyland et al. (12)	Self-complete	22 items 2 sub-scales Adult Asthma	(a) Bother (b) Management
Asthma Quality of Life Questionnaire	Juniper et al. (11)	Self-complete or interviewer administered	32 items 4 sub-scales Adult Asthma	(a) Activity limitations (b) Symptoms (c) Emotional functions (d) Exposure to environmental stimuli
Breathing Problems Questionnaire-Long version	Hyland et al. (16)	Self-complete	32 items 13 or 2 sub-scales COPD	(a) Walking (b) Bending or reaching (c) Washing or bathing (d) Household chores (e) Social interactions (f) Effects of weather or temperature (g) Effects of smells and fumes (h) Effects of colds (i) Sleeping (j) Medicine (k) Dysphonic states (l) Eating (m) Excretion urgency
Breathing Problems Questionnaire-Short version Childhood Asthma Questionnaires	Hyland et al. (13) French and Christie (14)	Self-complete	10 items No subscales	(a) Problems (b) Evaluations None
From A (4–7 years)		Completed by the child with assistance	14 items (also 10 questions for parents) 2 sub-scales	(a) Distress (b) Quality of living

Table 3.2 Disease-specific scales (*Cont.*)

Measured and	Author	Mode of administration	Number of items and subscales, target population	Subscales
From B (8–11 years)		Completed independently by the child	Child asthma 38 items (also 6 questions to be completed by parents 3 sub-scales	(a) Distress (b) Severity (c) Active quality of living
From C (12–16 years)		Completed independently by the child	Child asthma 46 items 5 sub-scales Child asthma	(a) Distress (b) Severity (c) Reactivity (d) Active quality of living (e) Teenage quality of living
Chronic Respiratory Disease Questionnaire	Guyatt *et al.* (9)	Interviewer administered	20 items 4 sub-scales Chronic obstructive pulmonary disease	(a) Dyspnoea (b) Fatigue (c) Emotional function (d) Mastery
European Organization for Research and Treatment of Cancer QLQ-C30	EORTC *et al.* (19)	Self-complete or interviewer administered	30 items 6 sub-scales 3 symptoms scales Cancer	(a) Physical (b) Role (c) Cognitive (d) Emotional (e) Social (f) Global QOL (g) Fatigue (h) Nausea and vomiting
Living with Asthma Questionnaire	Hyland *et al.* (20)	Self-complete	68 items 11 or 4 sub-scales Adult asthma	(a) Social and leisure (b) Sport (c) Holidays (d) Sleep (e) Works and other activates (f) Colds (g) Mobility (h) Effects on others (i) Medication use (j) Sex (k) Dysphonic states and attitudes

Table 3.2 Disease-specific scales (*Cont.*)

Measured and	Author	Mode of administration	Number of items and subscales, target population	Subscales
				(l) Activities
				(m) Avoidance
				(n) Preoccupation
				(o) Distress
Pediatric Quality of Life Questionnaire	Juniper *et al.* (17)	Interviewer administered	23 items 3 sub-scales Child asthma	(a) Activity limitation (b) Symptoms (c) Emotional function
Pediatric Asthma Caregiver's Quality of Life Questionnaire	Juniper *et al.* (18)	Self-complete	13 items 2 sub-scales Adult caregiver	(a) Activity limitation (b) Emotional function
St George's Respiratory Questionnaire	Jones *et al.* (10)	Self-complete	76 items 3 sub-scales Adult asthma or COPD	(a) Symptoms (b) Activity (c) Impact

perceived care. Items include: 'How much does the cost of your asthma medicines bother you?' and 'My doctor/nurse has carefully explained how I should manage my asthma'. However, a scale designed for clinical use may be less sensitive as a clinical trial tool. Another scale (a shortened version of the Breathing Problems Questionnaire (13)) was designed for evaluating the outcome of pulmonary rehabilitation, and so may be less sensitive to outcome changes produced by other means. Thus, the different disease-specific scales are by no means equivalent in terms of item content, because they have been designed for different purposes. In addition, one scale (the St George's Respiratory Questionnaire (10)) was designed for asthma and chronic obstructive pulmonary disease (COPD), whereas the other scales have been designed for either asthma or COPD, and again, this is reflected in item content.

Finally, scales for children require very different items compared to those for adults, and in one case, different scales are used for children of different ages (Childhood Asthma Questionnaire (14)). Young children are asked to respond to questions using 'smiley faces', with questions such as: 'Which picture describes how you feel about running around at playtimes?' and 'Which picture describes how you feel when you cough?'.

Generic scales

Generic scales are designed for any disease and may therefore contain items that are irrelevant to a particular patient group. This fact, coupled with their weaker sensitivity to change, may lead some to conclude that generic scales have little clinical use. This, however, is not the case as some generic scales include items which, for one reason or another, are missing from disease-specific scales. Thus, one questionnaire appropriate for advanced illness (the McGill Quality of Life Questionnaire (21)) measures the existential or spiritual domain of life quality that is neglected in the disease-specific scales. Items include: 'My personal existence is utterly meaningless and without purpose'; 'In achieving life goals I have made no progress whatsoever'; and 'I feel good about myself as a person'. Another palliative care questionnaire applicable to any illness (the Missoula-VITAS quality of life index (22)) includes items describing positive experiences in a number of dimensions including transcendence which are not measured in disease-specific questionnaires, simply because the disease-specific questionnaires are not designed to assess QoL in palliative care. For example, items in this questionnaire include: 'I have a greater sense of connection to all things now than I did before my illness'; 'I have a better sense of meaning in my life now than I have had in the past'; and 'I am more satisfied with myself as a person now than I was before my illness'. Finally, the Silver Lining Questionnaire (23) also includes items that measure the extent to which illness has been a positive experience (rather than being less of a negative experience) and thus provides an entirely different perspective on QoL, but one which may be very relevant to the patient. Items include: 'I appreciate life more because of my illness'; 'My illness made me a better person'; and 'My illness helped me find myself'. Thus, although not all generic scales provide a more sensitive measure of QoL than disease-specific scales in respiratory disease, some undoubtedly do so.

Idiographic scales

The Schedule for the Evaluation of Individual Quality of Life (SEIQoL) (27) is the best-known example of an idiographic approach. Patients are asked to nominate five aspects of their life which best characterizes their quality of life to them. Then patients are asked to rate each of those five aspects in terms of how good or bad they are. The result of this procedure is that there is a unique scale of QoL for each patient, because the meaning of QoL differs between patients. That is, the measurement of QoL is individualized rather than normative.

Critics of the individualized approach suggest that a scale which differs between patients is not particularly useful in making the between-patient comparisons needed for clinical trials, though certainly this approach has value as a clinical tool. Critics of the more conventional normative approach, however, argue that although the same questionnaire is given to different patients, in practice different patients interpret that same questionnaire differently so in practical terms the patients are actually receiving different questionnaires (28). These different views are currently unresolved. Perhaps there is room for both approaches.

Implications of QoL for treatment selection and patient management: the individualized perspective

Whether it is measured by a normative scale or an individualized scale, QoL is something which is highly individual. What is important for one patient may not be important for another. This means that in order to optimize QoL for an individual patient, the clinician needs to individualize treatment rather than to select treatment on a routine basis.

Aggressive treatment is more burdensome for some patients than for others. Indeed, intentional non-compliance can be the consequence of patients judging that the burden of treatment outweighs its benefit. For some patients, improvement in physiology has little benefit in terms of QoL. Individualization of treatment and management based on careful assessment of patients' needs (29) is the best strategy for improving quality of life in patients who are terminally ill.

Key points

♦ Management of a patient's QoL requires an individualized approach to treatment. This approach can be assisted by questionnaires, of which there are many kinds.

♦ There is no substitute for careful, humane understanding of the patient.

♦ The clinician needs to find a way of managing the patient where multiple objectives are affected differently by different courses of action.

♦ Good QoL is just one objective, albeit an important one, in the clinical management of patients.

References

1. Singer, cited in *The quality of life concept*. Washington, DC: United States Environmental Protection Agency Office of Research and Monitoring Environmental Studies Division, 1974.
2. Szalai A. The meaning of comparative research on the quality of life. In Szalai A, Andrews FM (eds) *The quality of life, comparative studies*, pp. 7–21. London: Sage Publications, 1980.
3. Schipper H, Clinch J, Powell V. Definitions and conceptual issues. In Spilker B (ed) *Quality of life assessments in clinical trials*, pp. 11–24. New York: Raven Press, 1990.
4. Calman KC. Quality of life in cancer patients – an hypothesis. *J Med Ethics* 1984; **10**:124–7.
5. DeHaes JCJM, van Knippenberg FCE. The quality of life of cancer patients: a review of the literature. *Soc Sci Med* 1985; **20**:809–17.
6. Hayry M. Measuring the quality of life: Why, how and what ? *Theoret Med* 1991; **12**:97–116.
7. Clinch JJ, Schipper H. Quality of life assessment in palliative care. In: Doyle D, Hanks GWC, MacDonald N (eds) *Oxford textbook of palliative medicine*, pp. 61–9. Oxford: Oxford University Press, 1993.
8. World Health Organization. The constitution of the World Health Organization. *WHO Chron* 1947; **1**:29.
9. Guyatt GH, Berman LB, Townsend M, Pugsley SO, Chambers LW. A measure of quality of life for clinical trials in chronic lung disease. *Thorax* 1987; **42**:773–8.

10. Jones PW, Quirk FH, Baveystock CM. The St George's Respiratory Questionnaire. *Respir Med* 1991; **85**(suppl B):25–31.

11. Juniper EF, Guyatt GH, Epstein RS, *et al.* Evaluation of impairment of health related quality of life in asthma: Development of a questionnaire for use in clinical trials. *Thorax* 1992; **47**:76–83.

12. Hyland ME, Ley A, Fisher DW, Woodward V. Measurement of psychological distress in asthma and asthma management programmes. *Br J Clin Psychol* 1995; **34**:601–11.

13. Hyland ME, Singh SJ, Sodergren SC, Morgan MPL. Development of a shortened version of the breathing problems questionnaire suitable for use in a pulmonary rehabilitation clinic: a purpose-specific, disease-specific questionnaire. *Qual Life Res* 1998; **7**:227–33.

14. French DJ, Christie MJ. Developing outcome measures for children: the example of 'Quality of Life' assessment for paediatric asthma. In Hutchinson A, McColl E, Christie MJ, Riccalton CL (eds) *Health outcomes in primary and outpatient care.* Chur, Switzerland: Harwood Academic, 1995.

15. Hyland ME, Finnis S, Irvine SH. A scale for assessing quality of life in adult asthma sufferers. *J Psychosom Res* 1991; **35**:99–110.

16. Hyland ME, Bott J, Singh S, Kenyon CAP. Domains, constructs and the development of the breathing problems questionnaire. *Qual Life Res* 1994; **3**:245–56.

17. Juniper EF, Guyatt GH, Feeny DH, *et al.* Measuring quality of life in children with asthma. *Qual Life Res* 1996; **5**:35–46.

18. Juniper EF, Guyatt GH, Feeny DH, *et al.* Measuring quality of life in the parents of children with asthma. *Qual Life Res* 1996; **5**:27–34.

19. EORTC. The European Organisation for Research and Treatment of Cancer QLQ-C30: a quality of life instrument for use in international clinical trials in oncology. *J Natl Cancer Inst* 1993; **85**:365–76.

20. Hyland ME. The Living with Asthma Questionnaire. *Respir Med* 1991; **85**(suppl B):13–16.

21. Cohen SR, Mount BM, Strobel MG, Bui F. The McGill Quality of Life Questionnaire: a measure of quality of life appropriate for people with advanced disease. A preliminary study of validity and acceptability. *Palliative Med* 1995; **9**:207–19.

22. Byock IR, Merriman MP. Measuring the quality of life for patients with terminal illness: the Missoula-VITAS® quality of life index. *Palliative Med* 1998; **12**:231–44.

23. Sodergren SC, Hyland ME. What are the positive consequences of illness? *Psychol Health* (in press).

24. Ware JE, Sherbourne CD. The MOS 36 item Short-Form Health Survey. *Med Care* 1992; **30**:473–83.

25. Bergner M, Bobbit RA, Carter WB, Gilson BS. The Sickness Impact Profile: Development and final revision of a health status measure. *Med Care* 1981; **19**:787–805.

26. Hunt S, McEwen J, McKenna S. *Measuring health status.* London: Croom Helm, 1986.

27. O'Boyle CA, McGee H, Joyce CRB. Quality of life: assessing the individual. In Fitzpatrick R (ed) *Advances in medical sociology,* pp. 159–80. Greenwich, CT: JAI Press, 1994.

28. Hyland ME. Defining and measuring quality of life in medicine. *JAMA* 1998; **279**:430–1.

29. Fitzsimons D, Mullan D, Wilson JS, *et al.* The challenge of patients' unmet palliative care needs in the final stages of chronic illness. *Palliat Med* 2007; **21**:313–22.

Chapter 4

Principles of economic evaluation

Sarah Willis

Containing the cost of healthcare has always been high on the agenda, in developed and developing countries alike. The financial pressures of recent times and the increasing strain on healthcare budgets only serve to highlight the importance of spending resources wisely.

Most clinicians know how it feels to have some of their options constrained by concerns about cost. Attempts at assessing the cost of a particular treatment frequently raise suspicion and the expectation that results of formal analyses will be used to constrain the clinical options further still.

For health economists it is of utmost importance to stress to clinicians and patients that economics is not just about cost. Economics, as a scientific discipline, is based on the insight that resources are scarce. The resources that are committed to achieve a certain end cannot be put to other uses. There is an inevitable trade-off; when seeking one particular objective, others have to be sacrificed in the process. Economists view this sacrifice as the real cost of using resources for a particular purpose, known more formally as the notion of *opportunity cost*.

Economic evaluation is an explicit way of valuing an intervention in terms of its opportunity cost. It is a transparent framework that helps us determine the relationship between outcomes, in terms of patients' health, and cost, in terms of resources used. The analysis attaches equal importance to the expected health benefits and the cost of obtaining them and therefore makes explicit the health benefits achieved from a given amount of resources. The ultimate aim of economic evaluation is thus to ensure that the available resources are used in such a way that overall health is maximized for the entire population.

This chapter sets out the essential steps in carrying out an economic evaluation in practice. The principles are not particular to any field of medicine, nor are they confined to healthcare. Supportive care interventions have tended to receive less attention in terms of economic evaluations than those involving pharmaceuticals and steps requiring particular care in their assessment are highlighted below.

Economic evaluation is a methodological approach to assess the *relative* worth of different activities. In other sectors this assessment would be performed by the normal market mechanisms. The important word to note is that the assessment is a *relative* one. Economic evaluation is comparative and incremental by nature. Thus, it will always compare two or more alternative ways of achieving a particular objective, taking both the costs and the benefits of each alternative into account. The results should always be incremental (though you may sometimes come across results that are not). In other words the results of an economic evaluation will always tell us how much more 'health' one intervention yields over another and at what cost. This is why caution is always expressed when interpreting results of published economic evaluations, particularly when the interventions in the published analysis are slightly different to those of interest.

Every economic evaluation starts with the basic steps of having to systematically identify, measure, and value all the relevant costs and health effects of the interventions. Whilst the costs of a course of action might sometimes be difficult to capture, they are easy to conceptualize. Health on the other hand is much more difficult to define and measure. There are four different types of economic evaluation in healthcare, which essentially are based on different methods of measuring health: cost-benefit analysis, cost-effectiveness analysis, cost-utility analysis and cost-minimization analysis.

In cost-benefit analysis, treatment outcomes are directly valued in monetary terms. In this way, costs and benefits become commensurable, and the net benefit of a treatment may be determined as total benefits minus total costs. Only treatments with positive net benefit should be implemented.

In cost-effectiveness analysis, the health outcomes of an intervention are measured by means of a single natural physical unit, such as life years gained or even the reduction in the number of episodes of serious dyspnoea. Cost-effectiveness analysis is also commonly used as a generic label to also refer to a cost-utility analysis.

In cost-utility analysis, outcomes are valued by estimating the impact of the treatment on the patients' quality of life, thereby trying to overcome the problems in cost-effectiveness analysis engendered by the fact that outcome assessment is restricted to one single dimension.

Cost-minimization analysis is only considered a partial economic evaluation. In this form of analysis, alternative interventions are considered identical in terms of the health outcomes for patients, so that only costs need to be assessed. As such cost-minimization analysis is rarely seen since there are very few interventions that can be shown to be equivalent in all outcomes. For example, two chemotherapy regimens may have been shown to provide a similar mean duration of progression-free survival but could have very different toxicity profiles.

Cost-utility analysis: step-by-step

This section outlines the basic steps of a cost-utility analysis. This type of analysis is preferred by the National Institute of Health and Clinical Excellence (NICE) and is likely to be the most suitable method for evaluating supportive care interventions as it takes into account the quality as well as quantity of a patient's life. The other types of economics evaluations follow essentially the same steps with modifications concerning the valuation of health outcomes.

Step 1: define the clinical question and identify all relevant comparisons

The task of defining the question is often relatively neglected, but it is the most fundamental part of any evaluation. Framing the clinical question involves defining precisely what the intervention involves and highlighting the relevant clinical alternatives to be used as comparisons in the evaluation. Any course of action aimed at improving health outcomes for patients can be assessed using economic evaluation, so intervention is used here in its widest sense.

Economic evaluation is a comparative exercise, so including all clinically relevant comparators in the analysis is vital to ensure the results are not biased. This is often ignored in practical evaluations, which are often limited to comparing two treatments of immediate interest, such as a standard and an experimental treatment.

Defining the intervention is particularly important in the case of supportive care when there may be several different configurations of care that may all be loosely covered by the same description. 'Best supportive care' is often used to refer to standard practice, which is misleading when studies such as Temel et al. (1) have shown a marked survival difference between early palliative care integrated with standard oncological care or standard oncological care alone. Indeed almost all NICE cancer technology appraisals refer to best supportive care, when in most cases this is never fully described, thus leading to potentially biased results.

Standard practice is to group complex interventions into different categories based on clinically relevant or well-established lines. In a recent study on smoking cessation interventions for patients with chronic obstructive pulmonary disease in the Netherlands, counselling interventions were grouped into minimal or intensive categories, using a 90-minute threshold (2). The pharmacotherapy interventions were considered for subdividing by type, intensity, and duration but lack of detailed reporting in the clinical studies made this difficult. The availability of data from clinical studies usually drives how the question is framed and ultimately what conclusions can be drawn from the results.

Step 2: determine the viewpoint and the time-horizon of the analysis

The viewpoint or perspective of the analysis determines which costs and health outcomes are relevant to the analysis. The classic example to underline the importance of the viewpoint is the question of inpatient treatment versus home care. Several studies (3) show that, from a societal perspective which includes all costs, home care does not result in a significant reduction in cost compared to inpatient care, but there is a significant shift in costs from the hospital to patients, their relatives and social services.

Conventionally, it is recommended that the analysis should be carried out from a societal viewpoint, to ensure that all costs are taken into account, no matter who bears them. What matters most is whether the chosen perspective is appropriate for its intended audience. Most evaluations are carried out from a narrower viewpoint, typically that of the decision-makers such as the National Health Service in the UK.

The time horizon should be chosen to ensure that all differences between the intervention and the comparator are captured. It is important to identify costs and health benefits that not only result from the intervention, but also from longer-term consequences that may not initially be thought of as relating to the intervention of interest. Diagnostic procedures, for example, will not only determine the diagnosis of a patient, but will also impact on the choice of treatment, which in turn will result in different overall outcomes for patients. Similarly for chronic conditions the appropriate time horizon will usually be for the whole lifetime of the patients.

Step 3: measuring and valuing health outcomes

When carrying out a cost-utility analysis, using the primary clinical endpoint to capture health outcomes is not sufficient. Secondary endpoints such as the incidence, severity, and duration of adverse events should also be identified, as these are likely to impact on quality of life or may be associated with varying levels of resource use.

Finding comparative evidence of any clinical endpoint on all the interventions identified as clinically relevant may be difficult, as the interventions of interest are rarely compared in the same trials. Consideration should be given to methods to draw all relevant evidence together whilst maintaining the randomization of trials, such as network meta-analysis (4–6).

The advantage of conducting a cost-utility analysis is that health is measured using a common metric which facilitates a comparison of health interventions across different disease areas. For analyses conducted in developed countries, the quality-adjusted life year (QALY) is the most common metric. A QALY is a measure of a person's length of life weighted by a valuation, on a scale of 0–1 (0 = nil, 1 = no deficit) of their health-related quality of life (HRQL) over that period.

HRQL can be measured in several ways, and different systems produce different utility values. Values resulting from the use of different systems cannot always be compared. In the UK, NICE has stated a preference for the measurement of changes in HRQL to be reported directly from patients and valued using a choice-based method in a representative sample of the UK population to capture public preferences, and states a preference for the use of EQ-5D (7).

HRQL data is notoriously difficult to collect from patients with poor prognosis. As such, questions have been raised about the robustness of the utility values used to calculate QALYs in many NICE assessments, including all recent NICE guidance on lung cancer (8–11).

QALYs will usually be calculated within an economic evaluation as they are rarely reported as the outcome of a clinical trial. Usually HRQL weights from published literature will be used to calculate QALYs. The availability of this data will often direct the design of the economic evaluation, as in its absence a complication model design will lack credibility.

Step 4: measuring and valuing resource use

There are two steps to characterize the difference in cost between the alternative interventions. Firstly the resource use associated with each intervention needs to be identified followed by application of appropriate unit costs for all the resources used. These will again depend on the perspective chosen for the analysis. Both resources and unit costs need to be reported separately to facilitate a judgement to be made by the reader about whether the results of the economic evaluation are applicable to their situation.

If an economic evaluation is being carried out as a substudy within a clinical trial, it is important not to assume the only difference in cost will be for the intervention and immediate healthcare resource use. It may be possible to collect utilization data prospectively alongside the clinical data for the patients in the trial and so in principle, all the necessary data may be collected at the individual patient level. However, the resource use data from a randomized control trial may not always be the same as the intended clinical situation. Other possible sources of relevant data should always be considered, and in most analyses data must in any case be collected outside a trial context, particularly because the time horizon of interest for an economic evaluation is usually longer than that for a clinical trial.

Identifying appropriate unit prices for the resources used is often difficult for hospitals in a system with global hospital budgets funded by general tax revenue. The accounting principles conventionally used do not provide the kind of cost figures ideally needed for an economic evaluation, and there are very few incentives for the decision-makers to determine the real opportunity cost of the various services and procedures. In most cases, the analyst will have to make do with the figures collected on a national level (often collected for different purposes), while being aware of the limitation of these data and making any assumptions explicit in the write-up of the analysis.

It is well known that the charges for clinical services reimbursed by a public or private health insurer do not always relate directly to the cost for the provider of the service. In the UK, there is a decision to be made about using the Payment by Results (PbR) tariff or the National Reference costs. The most appropriate source of unit costs will depend on who the economic evaluation is for; if the decision is to be made on behalf of the NHS (e.g. by NICE), National Reference costs are more appropriate than the PbR tariff.

It is worth noting that cost data are usually positively-skewed because some patients have very high costs, so the mean is higher than the median. The mean values are always used as point estimates in economic evaluation, because the expected total costs of a given treatment option are the most relevant for decision-making.

Step 5: calculating, comparing, and presenting cost and effects

The most important results of an economic evaluation are the incremental costs and the incremental health outcomes. To produce these results, the analyst must first decide which intervention is the baseline against which the other(s) is/are compared. Usually the interventions are compared against the alternative considered to represent standard clinical practice. Where this judgement is difficult, the cheapest option is usually chosen as the baseline. The methods and results of an incremental analysis are best explained when plotted graphically on the same standard axis, known as the cost-effectiveness plane (Figure 4.1). Sometimes a dominant solution may exist, which would lie in either the

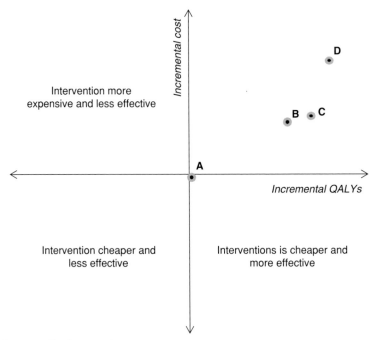

Fig. 4.1 The cost-effectiveness plane.

north-west quadrant of the cost-effectiveness plane when the intervention is more effective yet cheaper than its comparator or in the south-east quadrant where the comparator is cheaper and more effective than the intervention. In either of these cases, the choice of which treatment to choose is simple.

Most reimbursement decisions are focused around results which show no dominant solution, plotted in the north-east quadrant where the intervention is more effective but more expensive than its comparator (less often in the south-west quadrant where the intervention is cheaper but less effective than the comparator). In this case we can present the decision-maker with some data on the trade-off between better health outcomes and higher cost. The results would normally be presented as an incremental cost-effectiveness ratio (ICER), the difference in costs divided by the difference in QALYs. On the cost-effectiveness plane, the ICER is the slope of the line linking the two points.

When more than two interventions are being compared, interventions which are dominated are ruled out of the incremental analysis so each intervention can be compared to the 'next best' in terms of cost-effectiveness. In Figure 4.1, intervention B is ruled out of the analysis due to *extended dominance*. Theoretically it would be possible for resources to be spent on a combination of intervention A and intervention C, which would result in more QALYs than if we invested in intervention B alone. Alternatively, you can see on Figure 4.1 that a line could be drawn linking intervention A and C, to which intervention B would lie to the left. The choice of which intervention to implement lies between interventions A, C, and D. The decision will partly depend on the two ICERs, to determine whether the additional cost of C is worth the extra QALYs than would be produced using intervention A, or whether the additional health benefit from intervention D is worth the extra money than would be required to implement intervention C.

Step 6: interpreting cost-effectiveness

The ICER cannot be interpreted without being related to some external standard. Just presenting a cost per QALY gained does not allow one to determine whether this gain is actually worth obtaining. Ideally, it would be possible to determine a societal trade-off, i.e. the increase in costs that society is willing to accept for a particular gain in outcome. NICE have a threshold of £20,000 per QALY, although allowing for weight to be given to other considerations in the case that the ICER is slightly above this value (7). This and other reference values were not based on empirical data, although some data from Primary Care Trusts (PCTs) in the UK suggest they are operating a lower threshold (12).

It has been suggested that QALYs discriminate against supportive care interventions, particularly those given in a palliative setting. As described above, QALYs use time metrics and assume a degree of linearity (e.g. on the value of life), which do not conform to the palliative care context and literature where values and priorities appear to change with impending death (13). In addition, QALYs have been criticized on the basis that they may not be sensitive enough to capture effects of complex interventions (13, 14). Work is ongoing into eliciting values from the public on additional weighting, if any, they may put on end of life. NICE has adopted a position where their decision making committees can make exceptions in certain circumstances when there may be cause to suspect that benefits have not been adequately captured in the standard methodology used for NICE technology appraisals. These circumstances relate to small populations where treatment is indicated for patients with a short life expectancy (normally less than 24 months) and where there is sufficient evidence to indicate that the treatment offers an extension to life, normally of at least an additional 3 months compared to current NHS treatment (15).

Step 7: analysing the impact of uncertainty

No matter how data for an economic evaluation are collected, they will be surrounded by significant uncertainty. Often no data exist to inform a particular parameter, so assumptions are necessary to fill in the gaps. No analysis can be considered complete without an analysis of how sensitive the results are to plausible changes in the values of the variables in the analysis. The impact these changes have on the results can inform decision-makers, as they will be able to suggest whether a particular variable is a key driver of the total costs or total QALYs. If the results are very sensitive, the analysis will probably have little impact on decision-making and an effort at finding improved data with less uncertainty would be indicated. If the results are robust to changes, the analysis will appear more convincing and probably have a greater impact.

Probabilistic sensitivity analysis (PSA) is required to properly characterize parameter uncertainty—uncertainty that arises from sampling variation. This form of sensitivity analysis requires distributions to be fitted around parameters instead of point estimates and several thousand simulations to be run to propagate the uncertainty through the model. This allows the analyst to provide an estimate of the probability an intervention is cost-effective, recognizing that uncertainty in the data may lead to the wrong decision.

Economic studies of supportive care have tended to focus on cost-of-illness and other cost analyses. The problem with these types of studies is that although they are concerned with identifying and determining costs, they completely ignore the health outcomes of the healthcare interventions considered. From an economic point of view, the value of these interventions can only be properly assessed by relating outcomes with the costs involved in obtaining them. Only by performing a full economic evaluation following the steps briefly introduced in this chapter, which attach as much importance to the assessment of the outcomes of healthcare interventions as to the determinations of their costs, can economic analysis provide the kind of information which is valuable for making decisions about healthcare interventions.

References

1. Temel JS, Greer JA, Muzikansky A., Gallagher ER, *et al.* Early palliative care for patients with metastatic non–small-cell lung cancer. *N Engl J Med* 2010; **363**:733–42.

2. Hoogendoorn M, Feenstra TL, Hoogenveen RT, *et al.* Long-term effectiveness and cost-effectivness of smoking cessation interventions in patients with COPD. *Thorax* 2010; **65**:711–18.

3. Shepperd S, Doll H, Broad J, *et al.* Early discharge hospital at home. *Cochrane Database of Systematic Reviews* 2009; **21**(1):CD000356.

4. Caldwell DM, Ades AE, Higgins JPT. Simultaneous comparison of multiple treatments: combining direct and indirect evidence. *BMJ* 2005; **331**: 897–900.

5. Lu G, Ades AE. Combination of direct and indirect evidence in mixed treatment comparisons. *Stat Med* 2004; **23**:3105–24.

6. Song F, Altman DG, Glenny MA, Deeks JJ. Validity of indirect comparison for estimating efficacy of competing interventions: empirical evidence from published meta-analyses. *BMJ* 2003; **326**:472–6.

7. National Institute for Health and Clinical Excellence. *Guide to the methods of technology appraisal.* London: NICE, 2008. Available at: http://www.nice.org.uk/aboutnice/howwework/devnicetech/technologyappraisalprocessguides/guidetothemethodsoftechnologyappraisal.jsp?domedia=1&mid=B52851A3–19B9-E0B5-D48284D172BD8459.

8. National Institute for Health and Clinical Excellence. *Erlotinib for the treatment of non-small cell lung cancer. NICE TA 162.* London: NICE, 2008. Available at: http://guidance.nice.org.uk/TA162.

9. National Institute for Health and Clinical Excellence. *Pemetrexed for the first-line treatment of non-small-cell lung cancer. NICE TA 181.* London: NICE, 2009. Available at: http://guidance.nice.org.uk/TA181.

10. National Institute for Health and Clinical Excellence. *Topotecan for the treatment of relapsed small-cell lung cancer. NICE TA184.* London: NICE, 2009. Available at: http://guidance.nice.org.uk/TA184.

11. National Institute for Health and Clinical Excellence. *The diagnosis and treatment of lung cancer. NICE Lung cancer guideline.* London: NICE, 2005. Available at: http://guidance.nice.org.uk/CG24.

12. Martin S, Rice N, Smith PC. Further evidence on the link between health care spending and health outcomes. *CHE Research Paper 32.* York: Centre for Health Economics, University of York, 2007.

13. Gomes B, Harding R, Foley KM, Higginson IJ. Optimal approaches to the health economics of palliative care: report of an international think tank. *J Pain Symptom Manage* 2009; **38**(1):4–10.

14. Hughes J. Palliative care and the QALY problem. *Health Care Anal* 2005; **13**(4):289–301.

15. National Institute for Health and Clinical Excellence. *Supplementary advice to the Appraisal Committees: Appraising life-extending, end of life treatments.* London: NICE, 2009. Available at: http://www.nice.org.uk/media/E4A/79/SupplementaryAdviceTACEoL.pdf.

Part 2

Mechanisms and assessment of dyspnoea

The genesis of breathlessness: what do we understand?

Jeremy B. Richards and Richard M. Schwartzstein

Understanding the mechanisms of breathlessness: Why should we care?

Ms Smith is a 72-year-old former smoker with end-stage chronic obstructive pulmonary disease (COPD) who comes to see her physician for a routine visit. She says she feels much worse as of late. Her last spirometry testing revealed her one-second forced expiratory volume (FEV_1) to be 600mL, a decline in her lung function brought on by her smoking three packs of cigarettes per day for 50 years. She now must wear oxygen even at rest. Even when she feels her best, she is only able to walk up one flight of stairs before she must stop and catch her breath. Over the past few weeks she can only go up a few steps at a time.

In this chapter we review the physiological and pathophysiological mechanisms that contribute to the sensation of breathlessness; our goal is to improve one's understanding of the processes and signals that cause this symptom so that the practising physician will be able to apply these principles when evaluating and treating a patient who complains of shortness of breath. We define dyspnoea or breathlessness as 'breathing discomfort'. As discussed later in the chapter, the language used to describe dyspnoea is important in understanding underlying pathophysiological processes; therefore, we define dyspnoea in terms that are as generic as possible to avoid presumptions about the quality of the sensation.

We will follow Ms Smith throughout the chapter and we will frame relevant physiological processes in the context of her clinical course. For example, Ms Smith's COPD is characterized by impaired gas exchange, airway obstruction, and hyperinflation of the lungs—all three of these processes can contribute to dyspnoea. With activity, her damaged lungs may be unable to meet the oxygen demands of metabolically active tissue or to eliminate carbon dioxide produced by aerobic activity. The normal physiological response to hypoxaemia and hypercarbia is to increase both the rate of breathing and the volume of each breath. In patients with obstructive pulmonary disease, this causes worsening hyperinflation of the lungs (due to airway obstruction) and an increased demand on the respiratory muscles. Both worsening hyperinflation and increased demand on respiratory muscles can result in dyspnoea.

While hypoxaemia and/or hypercarbia are potentially life-threatening, they alone do not explain all breathing discomfort. Many patients are limited by breathlessness yet have normal oxygen levels and arterial PCO_2 ($PaCO_2$). Similarly, work of breathing cannot fully explain all dyspnoea. Studies have shown that the intensity of breathing discomfort may vary for a given individual maintaining constant ventilation while other variables are modified (1, 2). Thus, comprehensive consideration of multiple physiological processes is necessary when investigating the cause(s) of dyspnoea. In Ms Smith's case, her known COPD is certainly contributing to her symptoms. Understanding of the pathophysiology of dyspnoea can help clinicians determine if further investigation for alternative, contributing diagnoses should be pursued and what treatments may provide symptom relief.

The natural course of many cardiopulmonary diseases that cause dyspnoea is a slow steady progression, with superimposed acute episodes of worsening symptoms and physiological changes that are variably reversible. Given the incurable nature of most of these processes, healthcare providers are left with a finite number of therapies to direct at alleviating symptoms, such as supplemental oxygen to correct gas exchange abnormalities or bronchodilators to lessen airway obstruction. Treatments can also be targeted towards secondary processes such as muscle deconditioning or acute infection. Skeletal muscle deconditioning due to increasingly sedentary lifestyles of dyspnoeic patients is a progressive and severely debilitating component of almost every cardiopulmonary disease and can be improved with exercise rehabilitation programmes (3, 4). Whether addressing the slow steady progression of a chronic condition or when treating an acute insult, understanding and identifying the physiological derangements that contribute to dyspnoea can allow for the development and application of treatment strategies to address symptoms even when the underlying disease cannot be corrected. Ultimately, our goal is to alleviate suffering and improve the quality of life for patients with chronic cardiopulmonary disorders.

The multiple origins of breathlessness

Differentiating between the different physiological mechanisms responsible for dyspnoea is necessary to design effective treatment strategies. In Ms Smith's case, we suspect that airway obstruction, hyperinflation, and/or deconditioning are contributing to her presentation. Understanding how dyspnoea arises from these processes can allow for a focused intervention and, ideally, meaningful symptom relief.

In contrast to the sensation of pain, which is typically mediated by stimulation of a single receptor, dyspnoea arises from the complex integration of information from a multitude of receptors located throughout the respiratory system. Mechanoreceptors (in the airways, lungs, and chest wall) and central and peripheral chemoreceptors provide sensory signals that may contribute to the sensation of dyspnoea. Information from these receptors, along with sensory signals associated with motor output from the cortex and brainstem, result in the sensation of breathing discomfort that we term dyspnoea. Figure 5.1 provides an overview of the multiple interactions involved in the development of dyspnoea.

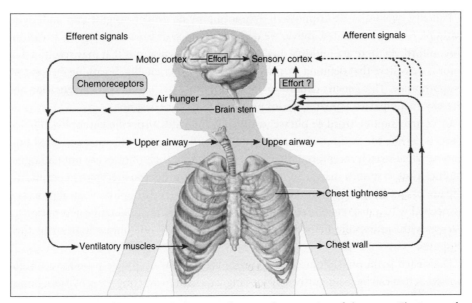

Fig. 5.1 Efferent and afferent signals that contribute to the sensation of dyspnoea. The sense of respiratory effort is believed to arise from a signal transmitted from the motor cortex to the sensory cortex coincidently with the outgoing motor command to the ventilatory muscles (corollary discharge). The arrow from the brainstem to the sensory cortex indicates that the motor output of the brainstem may also contribute to the sense of effort. The sense of air hunger is believed to arise, in part, from increased respiratory activity within the brainstem, and the sensation of chest tightness probably results from stimulation of pulmonary receptors. Although afferent information from airway, lung and chest wall passes through the brainstem before reaching the sensory cortex, the dashed lines indicate uncertainty about whether some afferents bypass the brainstem and project directly to the sensory cortex. Used from (12) with permission of SAGE.

A patient's qualitative description of dyspnoea can indicate that a specific physiological process is causing their symptoms. For example, if Ms Smith characterizes her dyspnoea as 'chest tightness', it may indicate that stretch receptors in the lung parenchyma are activated and contributing to her symptoms. If she complains of a sensation of 'air hunger', central or peripheral chemoreceptors (sensing hypercarbia and/or hypoxaemia) may be causing her symptoms. These qualitative descriptors may provide clinicians with insight into the underlying physiological process causing a patient's dyspnoea.

Language of breathlessness

Patients are asked to characterize chest pain by its 'quality'. Is the chest pain burning, aching, pressure-like, or sharp? These qualitative descriptions of chest pain are associated with causative pathophysiological mechanisms: burning chest pain may indicate gastro-oesophageal reflux, pressure-like pain may suggest myocardial ischaemia, and sharp pain may indicate pleural or pericardial inflammation.

Patients' qualitative descriptions of dyspnoea provide similar insights into underlying pathophysiology. As noted above, we define dyspnoea or breathlessness as 'breathing discomfort'. As there are multiple qualitatively distinct sensations that may result in dyspnoea, we believe that defining dyspnoea broadly as experiencing 'breathing discomfort' is appropriate. This generic definition does not imply a particular, specific sensation and thereby encompasses a broad range of processes that cause dyspnoea.

Of course, no one word or phrase universally indicates a specific pathophysiological process. While Ms Smith may complain of 'chest tightness', indicating activated lung parenchymal stretch receptors and airways obstruction, such phrases are not pathognomonic. That dyspnoea may arise from integration of numerous receptors complicates the use of qualitative descriptions. As such, even if a given pathophysiological process is associated with a discrete sensation (and even with a discrete qualitative description), a patient with cardiopulmonary disease may use more than one phrase to describe their dyspnoea.

Does each pathophysiological mechanism that causes dyspnoea produce a unique sensation that can be distinguished by the language used to describe the sensation? Simon et al. subjected normal subjects to eight breathing tasks that were believed to stimulate different receptors in the cardiopulmonary system and induced dyspnoea (5). The breathing tasks ranged from breath-holding, to breathing with a restricted minute ventilation during induced hypercapnia, to breathing with a resistive load, to exercise. Without exception, all subjects volunteered that the varying respiratory tasks could easily be distinguished by the sensations they produced, an observation that was manifest in the finding that each breathing task was associated with a unique set of phrases. In addition, in some cases subjects used the same phrases to describe two or more breathing tasks, perhaps indicating the presence of common mechanisms of disease. Finally, and equally important, each breathing task (and associated sensation of breathlessness) had *more than one* descriptor associated with it. This study provides clear evidence that there are multiple sensations that contribute to the symptom we call 'breathlessness', rather than a single sensation with variable intensity.

Subsequent survey-based studies of patients with a variety of cardiopulmonary diseases and dyspnoea demonstrated that distinct groups of phrases qualitatively describing a patient's dyspnoea were associated with specific disease states. Of note, one of these studies also included healthy women who experienced breathing discomfort during pregnancy (6, 7).

These qualitative descriptions of dyspnoea in patients with cardiopulmonary disease were demonstrated to be relatively consistent over time; when patients completed a symptom survey on two separate occasions one week apart, there was a significant correlation between the phrases chosen to describe dyspnoea on the two occasions (8). These data indicate that different disease states, with different underlying pathophysiological processes, are associated with qualitatively distinct sensations. Furthermore, these studies suggest that attention to the words and phrases patients use to describe dyspnoea may provide meaningful clues for diagnosing the cause of their dyspnoea.

Table 5.1 Descriptors of breathlessness in certain conditions (data adapted from (4))

Descriptors	Asthma	COPD	CHF	ILD	Neuromuscular/ chest wall	Pregnancy	Pulmonary vascular disease
Rapid breathing			x				x
Incomplete exhalation	x						
Shallow breathing				x			
Increased work or effort	x	x		x	x		
Feeling of suffocation			x				
Air hunger		x	x			x	
Chest tightness	x						

COPD, chronic obstructive pulmonary disease; CHF, chronic heart failure; ILD, interstitial lung disease.

Physiology of breathlessness

Ms Smith describes experiencing 'heavy breathing' and 'having to work harder' when she climbs more than a few stairs. She feels that it is difficult to get air in and finds herself using her abdominal muscles to forcibly exhale. These sensations are disconcerting and profoundly uncomfortable. Thankfully, these symptoms subside with several minutes of rest.

Understanding how the complex interactions of receptors and neural pathways cause dyspnoea depends on familiarity with three concepts that form a model of how we perceive the intensity and qualities of breathlessness. The first concept we will address is termed a 'corollary discharge', a model in which a sensory 'copy' of efferent motor output signals is sent from the motor cortex and brainstem respiratory centres to the sensory cortex, imparting a conscious awareness of respiratory effort. The second concept, called 'efferent-reafferent dissociation', describes how the sensory cortex compares efferent signals from the motor cortex (the above-mentioned 'corollary discharge') with afferent signals from peripheral mechanoreceptors that monitor the flow of air into the lungs and the depth of breathing. The quality and intensity of dyspnoea appear to correlate, in part, with the match or mismatch of these signals, hence the terminology 'efferent-reafferent dissociation'. The greater the dissociation between the efferent and afferent signals, the greater the intensity of the breathing discomfort; it is as if the brain recognizes that the respiratory system is not responding appropriately to the signals being sent to the ventilatory muscles and sounds a 'warning alarm', which we perceive as dyspnoea. Finally, the third concept incorporates the notion that certain peripheral mechanoreceptors and chemoreceptors are responsible for discrete, unique sensations such as 'chest tightness' and 'air hunger'.

Increased work of breathing: the corollary discharge

Due to her obstructed airways disease and associated dynamic hyperinflation (see 'Dynamic hyperinflation' section) with exercise, Ms Smith's dyspnoea worsens with exertion.

Her respiratory musculature is at a mechanical disadvantage due to hyperinflation, and the normally automatic process of moving the diaphragm and chest wall becomes progressively more difficult.

The concept of 'corollary discharge' explains the perception of this increased motor effort. As the motor cortex sends efferent commands to the ventilatory muscles, a neurological 'copy' of these commands is simultaneously sent to the sensory cortex (9). This efferent signal from the motor cortex to the sensory cortex is called a corollary discharge and is thought to be the mechanism by which conscious awareness of the effort of breathing occurs. Although increased work of breathing is not the sole physiological explanation for dyspnoea, it is a common contributor to breathing discomfort. Muscle weakness, respiratory muscle mechanical disadvantage (i.e. the shortening of muscles prior to contracting), and increased mechanical loads (airway obstruction and/or stiff lungs) are all processes that can increase the work of breathing and thereby increase the sensation of the work of breathing via corollary discharge.

Descriptors associated with increased ventilatory muscle work

Normal subjects made to breath against a high resistance (pressure work) and/or made to breath at a high minute ventilation (volume work) describe the sensations generated by these tasks with the phrases 'my breathing requires effort' or 'my breathing requires more work' (5). Similarly, patients with cardiopulmonary diseases describe their dyspnoea at peak exertion with the phrases 'my breathing requires effort' and 'I feel out of breath' (8). These findings demonstrate that in both normal subjects and those with cardiopulmonary diseases, the *sense of effort* may be one of the most prevalent types of dyspnoea.

The sense of effort of breathing arises from corollary discharge from the motor cortex. The motor cortex controls voluntary use of respiratory muscles; the brainstem (specifically respiratory centres in the medulla) controls autonomic, reflex control of ventilation. Studies in which subjects breathed with high minute ventilation at varying levels of inhaled carbon dioxide have demonstrated that the corollary discharge from the motor cortex (voluntary control of breathing) is associated with an increased sense of effort and increased dyspnoea (1). With normal $PaCO_2$, subjects experienced an intense sense of effort to sustain high minute ventilation. When inhaled carbon dioxide levels and $PaCO_2$ increased, the intensity of the sense of effort was reduced despite the fact that subjects maintained the same minute ventilation. The increased $PaCO_2$ activates central chemoreceptors, increases brainstem respiratory centre activity, and decreases the 'voluntary' work being done to achieve an elevated minute ventilation. The decrease in motor cortex (voluntary) mediated work of breathing appeared to decrease the sensation of dyspnoea.

Patients with obstructive airways disease, congestive heart failure, interstitial lung disease, and neuromuscular disease all cite increased effort as a factor in their description of breathlessness (8). The mechanism common to all of these disorders is an increased mechanical load on the ventilatory pump (for example, increased airway resistance or decreased respiratory system compliance), which necessitates a greater neural discharge from the brain to the ventilatory muscles to achieve adequate ventilation for a given metabolic demand. One study assessed the neural respiratory drive, as measured by transoesophageal diaphragmatic electromyelogram in 30 obese (body mass index >30kg/m²) and 30 non-obese subjects. At baseline, the obese subjects had greater dyspnoea as compared to the non-obese subjects. The obese and non-obese subjects had similar breathing patterns while sitting and supine, while the obese subjects had higher neural respiratory drive. These findings suggest that the higher neural respiratory drive (in effect, higher corollary discharge) was key to the increased dyspnoea (10); because of the weight of the chest wall, the lungs and chest wall were not moving as expected given the efferent motor messages—efferent-reafferent dissociation was worsened.

The sensation of effort can also be affected by the strength of respiratory muscles. Normal subjects who participated in a 6–18 week inspiratory muscle training programme had a 51% increase in their maximal inspiratory pressure (11). When asked to rate the intensity of effort associated with breathing with elastic and resistive respiratory loads, the intensity after training was less than it had been prior to training. Physiologically, a stronger muscle generates greater tension for a given neurological stimulus than a weaker muscle. Thus, a stronger muscle requires fewer discrete signals from the motor cortex, which results in diminished corollary discharge to the sensory cortex and a lessened sensation of dyspnoea.

Deconditioning, with corresponding loss of muscle strength, results in a return to pre-training levels of the intensity of the sensation of effort. One small study randomly assigned 30 patients with COPD to a 12-week rehabilitation programme or to a control group with no organized rehabilitation. Immediately after completing the 12-week rehabilitation course, the intervention group had a statistically significant improvement in functional capacity (as measured by 6-minute walk distance and performance scores) as well as an improvement in quality of life. Twelve weeks after completing rehabilitation, however, there were no differences between the intervention and control groups, demonstrating the transient nature of clinical gains obtained from rehabilitation without continued exercise and training (12).

Efferent-reafferent dissociation

During a voluntary breathing task, the sensory cortex simultaneously receives information from the motor cortex (via corollary discharge) and afferent information from the peripheral receptors of the respiratory system (reafferent signals). Reafferent signals are neural impulses produced by afferent receptors in response to efferent commands. For example, when you take a voluntary deep breath, efferent signals from the motor cortex descend to the ventilatory muscles prompting muscle contraction with resultant negative intrathoracic pressure and inspiratory flow. The lungs and the chest wall expand. A variety of flow, pressure, and stretch receptors are stimulated by the increasing thoracic volume, and reafferent information from these receptors is transmitted to the brain (9). If the mechanical response to efferent stimuli is impaired, then reafferent signals become dissociated from the efferent output. This concept has been described as efferent-reafferent dissociation (13). When Ms Smith tries to take a deep breath in, her motor cortex produces an enormous efferent signal to her muscles of respiration. However, because her respiratory muscles are weak (due to deconditioning), because they are at a mechanical disadvantage (due to hyperinflation), and because she has an increased mechanical load (due to airways obstruction), the actual chest wall and lung expansion produced by this enormous motor cortex efferent output is reduced. The disparity between the efferent output and actual mechanical results causes dyspnoea.

Several studies have demonstrated that disparity between motor cortex efferent output and actual ventilatory responses result in dyspnoea. Two studies subjected healthy individuals to acute hypercapnia while maintaining different levels of minute ventilation (14, 15). When minute ventilation was maintained below the level normally associated with that degree of hypercapnia, all subjects experienced increasing breathlessness. The motor cortex was sending a strong efferent signal to increase ventilation, but because the subjects were limited with regard to the tidal volume they could actually generate, an efferent-reafferent dissociation resulted with a concomitant sensation of dyspnoea.

The role of respiratory system afferents

Frequently, Ms Smith develops an increase in audible wheezing and a sensation of 'chest tightness'. These symptoms are relieved with use of her inhaled rescue bronchodilator. If she uses the inhaler incorrectly and the majority of the medicine ends up in her mouth or throat rather than being appropriately inhaled to her lower airways, her symptoms are not alleviated.

Peripheral receptors not only contribute to symptoms of dyspnoea via efferent-reafferent dissociation, they may generate distinct independent signals that are interpreted as dyspnoea when processed by the brain. 'Chest tightness' associated with bronchoconstriction is the most studied example of this hypothesis. The sensation of 'chest tightness' is commonly associated with asthma (6), and is thought to arise from the stimulation of receptors in the lung parenchyma (16). Chest tightness associated with bronchoconstriction has also been differentiated from the increased work of breathing and sense of effort seen in this condition (17). The origin of chest tightness may lie with mechanical receptors (rapidly adapting stretch receptors) in the lungs and/or with chemical receptors (C-fibres). Pulmonary receptors may also play a role in dyspnoea associated with pulmonary vascular disease, congestive heart failure, atelectasis (as may occur in association with large pleural effusions), and acute respiratory infections.

Afferent receptors

A well-recognized problem in the study of dyspnoea is that there is no way to localize and stimulate a single receptor and document the resulting sensory response to the stimulus. However, as researchers have been able to distinguish how different tasks and different physiological changes in the respiratory system produce different sensations, the function of individual pulmonary receptors has been better defined.

The following section will review the various receptors that contribute to the sensation of breathlessness. In discussing each type of receptor, we will describe not only the evidence supporting the function of specific receptors, but whether a receptor modulates the intensity of breathlessness via efferent-reafferent dissociation or by producing a distinct independent signal.

Chemoreceptors

When Ms Smith exercises, she notes a sensation of 'not being able to get a deep breath'. When this sensation is severe, she describes a strong 'need for air', or 'air hunger'. When studied during a cardiopulmonary exercise test, it is evident that she is developing dynamic hyperinflation, her inspiratory capacity is diminishing, and her ability to take a deep breath is constrained by the fact that she is breathing near total lung capacity.

Peripheral chemoreceptors, located in the carotid and aortic bodies, produce the afferent response to changes in $PaCO_2$, PaO_2, and arterial hydrogen ion (i.e. pH) (18, 19). The carotid body is sensitive to increases in $PaCO_2$, decreases in PaO_2, or decreases in pH. In humans, the aortic chemoreceptors appear to have a minimal role in the control of ventilation.

Central chemoreceptors located in the medulla respond to changes in $PaCO_2$ and arterial pH. In addition, skeletal muscle is also thought to have metaboreceptors, which are not typically described as chemoreceptors, but appear to be capable of detecting changes in metabolites produced by anaerobic metabolism at the tissue level (20).

Increasing levels of inhaled carbon dioxide in patients with quadriplegia (21) and normal subjects under conditions of total neuromuscular blockade (22) whose minute ventilation is held constant results in increased $PaCO_2$ and end-tidal PCO_2. Under these conditions, subjects describe severe 'air hunger'. These studies demonstrate that acute hypercapnia (independent of ventilatory muscle function) causes stimulation of chemoreceptors, producing a distinct sensation of breathlessness characterized by phrases such as 'air hunger', 'urge to breathe', and 'need to breathe' (21–23). Although patients with high cervical spinal cord injury do not receive sensory information from the chest wall, they are able to monitor inspiratory flow and pulmonary inflation via sensory nerves transmitting to the brain via the vagus nerve; consequently, efferent-reafferent dissociation may contribute to the sense of breathlessness in such patients. Acute hypercapnia with constrained tidal volume produces severe air hunger as efferent-reafferent dissociation amplifies the stimulus provided by the chemoreceptors.

In Ms Smith's case, the dynamic hyperinflation associated with exercise in the setting of expiratory flow limitation leads to constrained tidal volumes as her end-inspiratory volume approaches total lung capacity. As rate and tidal volume increase during exercise, expiratory time decreases and, in the setting of airways' resistance and airflow limitation, lung volumes increase (24). This process may also lead to severe air hunger (see 'Dynamic hyperinflation' section). To the extent that most cardiopulmonary conditions are associated with impaired respiratory system mechanics and increased drive to breathe, air hunger is a very common qualitative element of clinical dyspnoea.

Chronic elevations in $PaCO_2$ do not cause dyspnoea as severe as that experienced with acute elevations in $PaCO_2$. It is likely that the normalization of arterial and central nervous system pH (due to renal compensatory mechanisms) associated with chronic hyper-carbia ameliorates the severity of breathlessness as compared to acute hypercarbia (25).

Acute hypoxaemia produces less intense dyspnoea (and generally smaller increases in ventilation) than acute hypercarbia. It is not uncommon for patients with chronic lung disease to have mild to moderate hypoxaemia without breathlessness. Chronos et al., however, demonstrated that during heavy exercise at a constant workload, subjects were more breathless when they inspired hypoxic gas mixtures compared with air. Subjects were also less breathless when inspiring 100% oxygen as compared to air (2). Although subjects increased their minute ventilation after becoming hypoxemic, the sensation of dyspnoea occurred before the increase in ventilation. Patients with COPD have also been shown to experience increased dyspnoea due to hypoxaemia (26). Again, it appears that the inten-sity of dyspnoea due to hypoxaemia is less severe than dyspnoea due to hypercarbia.

Healthy subjects with normal cardiopulmonary function do not become hypercarbic, hypoxaemic or acidaemic during typical exercise, but they do experience exercise-induced dyspnoea. Metaboreceptors in skeletal muscles may explain this phenomenon. Metaboreceptors are thought to respond to local changes in the tissue environment due to by-products of metabolism, and generate afferent neurological signals that result in a sensation of dyspnoea. Cardiopulmonary exercise that leads to increased metabolic by-products may contribute to the sensation of dyspnoea, both in normal subjects and patients with cardiopulmonary diseases (20). It is unclear if signals generated by metabo-receptors modify other signals that produce dyspnoea (corollary discharge and/or efferent-reafferent dissociation) or whether metaboreceptors generate an independent signal with a unique sense of dyspnoea.

Cardiovascular fitness is characterized by the ability of the heart to deliver oxygen to the muscles and of the ability of the muscles to extract and utilize oxygen for aerobic metab-olism. Patients with chronic cardiopulmonary disease typically become increasingly sed-entary and their cardiovascular fitness deteriorates (they become 'deconditioned'). Deconditioning and chronic cardiopulmonary disease, therefore, synergistically decrease patients' functional capacity. Deconditioning is associated with the qualitative descrip-tors 'heavy breathing' and 'huffing and puffing' (8). Supervised exercise programmes can improve patients' cardiovascular fitness, improve their functional status, and reduce the severity of dyspnoea with exertion.

Mechanoreceptors

Ms Smith's dyspnoea, particularly with exertion, progresses. She describes deteriorating symptom relief from her medications. In addition to beginning a pulmonary rehabilitation programme, her physician arranges for the initiation of nocturnal non-invasive positive pressure ventilation (NIPPV.) After several weeks of rehabilitation and nocturnal NIPPV, she notes a modest improvement in her functional capac-ity and baseline breathlessness.

There are multiple receptors located in the upper airway, lung parenchyma (including stretch receptors and C-fibres), pulmonary vasculature, and chest wall that contribute to dyspnoea.

Upper airway receptors

Upper airway receptors on the face and in the oro- and nasopharyngeal passages monitor the changes of airflow in the upper airway, primarily by detecting air temperature changes. Opening a window or blowing cool air on one's face with a fan activates the sensory receptors of the trigeminal nerve and serves to lessen the intensity of dyspnoea. This was experimentally demonstrated when cool air blown against the cheek reduced the severity of dyspnoea associated with experimentally induced hypercarbia and a resistive ventilatory load in normal subjects (27). Oral mucosal receptors influence dyspnoea as well; after experimentally induced acute hypercarbia, normal subjects and patients with COPD had increased severity of dyspnoea when oral mucosal receptor activity was blunted by breathing through a mouthpiece, applying oral topical lidocaine, and breathing warm, humidified air (28, 29).

Upper airway receptor stimulation may improve dyspnoea by blunting the central respiratory drive. Blowing cool air through the nasal passages attenuates the expected increase in minute ventilation to experimentally induced hypercarbia (30). Stimulation of upper airway receptors has been shown to clinically reduce breathlessness and increase exercise tolerance in patients with COPD (29, 31). This attenuation in dyspnoea by upper airway receptor stimulation is likely due to changes in efferent-reafferent dissociation; greater stimulation of upper airway receptors may be perceived by the sensory cortex as evidence of an enhanced mechanical response of the respiratory system to the efferent messages emanating from the motor cortex, thereby reducing the efferent-reafferent dissociation and the resultant sensation of dyspnoea.

Lower airway receptors

The major receptors in the lung parenchyma are stretch receptors and C-fibres (unmyelinated nerve endings). These receptors detect a wide variety of pathophysiological processes in the lung and transmit information to the central nervous system via the vagus nerve.

Stretch receptors are thought to modulate breathlessness by altering efferent-reafferent dissociation. In a study of ventilator dependent patients with high cervical spinal cord injuries, acute hypercarbia was induced with resultant 'air hunger'. The tidal volume provided by the ventilator was varied (without altering the level of end-tidal PCO_2) and all subjects reported a decrease in the severity of dyspnoea with higher tidal volumes (32). As these patients had high cervical spinal injuries, their chest wall receptors were not providing afferent signals to the brainstem or sensory cortex. Their improved dyspnoea, therefore, was likely due to larger tidal volumes resulting in greater stimulation of intrapulmonary stretch receptors signalling via the vagus nerve.

Causing airways collapse by applying negative pressure at the mouth leads to increased severity of dyspnoea in patients with COPD (33). This increase in dyspnoea may be due to stretch receptors responding to negative transmural pressure and associated airway collapse. NIPPV, the reciprocal of applying negative pressure at the mouth, is used with therapeutic and symptomatic benefit in patients with a variety of respiratory diseases. In addition to improved ventilation and diminished work of breathing, activation of airway stretch receptors may explain the improvement in dyspnoea associated with positive airway pressure. In one study, 37 patients with advanced COPD were randomly assigned to pulmonary rehabilitation and NIPPV while 35 patients were assigned to rehabilitation alone. After 3 months, the patients receiving NIPPV in addition to rehabilitation had improvement in $PaCO_2$, daily step count, and a trend towards improvement in dyspnoea symptoms (34). A prospective observational study of 40 patients with advanced (GOLD stage IV) COPD demonstrated improved health-related quality of life, 6-minute walk distance, FEV_1, and $PaCO_2$ in patients who received NIPPV and pulmonary rehabilitation compared to 40 matched controls who received only pulmonary rehabilitation (35). Finally, a systematic review of six randomized controlled trials and nine non-randomized controlled trials found a significant improvement in dyspnoea and quality of life associated with NIPPV in patients with COPD (36).

Ms Smith experiences benefit from the combination of pulmonary rehabilitation and NIPPV. Pulmonary rehabilitation addresses respiratory muscle deconditioning while NIPPV serves to attenuate episodic airways collapse and the dyspnoea associated with activation of pulmonary stretch receptors. In addition, in patients with COPD in whom there is evidence of intrinsic positive end expiratory pressure (intrinsic PEEP or auto-PEEP), the use of NIPPV reduces the work of breathing and the sense of effort.

After experimentally inducing acute hypercarbia in laryngectomized patients with tracheal stomas, aerosolized bupivacaine was used to block airway receptors. The severity of dyspnoea increased after the administration of bupivacaine, suggesting that inhibition of afferent signalling from lower airway receptors creates a dissociation between efferent and reafferent neural impulses and, thereby, worsens dyspnoea (37).

Inhaled furosemide has been shown to decrease breathlessness in healthy volunteers experiencing experimentally-induced dyspnoea, likely by sensitizing pulmonary stretch receptors, increasing vagus signalling, and decreasing efferent-reafferent dissociation (38). In one study, severe dyspnoea was induced in 12 healthy subjects both by breath-holding and by increased inspiratory resistive load *in association with* induced hypercapnia (by increasing mechanical deadspace) (39). Inhaled furosemide was administered in a double-blinded, placebo-controlled, randomized fashion with cross-over between groups. Both breath-holding time and the time to developing symptoms of breathlessness after 5 minutes of breathing with an increased inspiratory resistive load *and* increased $PaCO_2$ were significantly improved with the administration of inhaled furosemide as compared to placebo.

A second study of ten healthy volunteers assessed a different method of inducing dyspnoea. Subjects underwent constrained ventilation (during which minute ventilation could not exceed ~8L/m) while breathing a gas mixture containing carbon dioxide to produce hypercapnia with an end-tidal CO_2 of 50mmHg (40). Inducing dyspnoea in this fashion resulted in minimal increase in the reported work or effort of breathing. Nine out of ten subjects, however, reported a reduction in dyspnoea with inhaled furosemide while experiencing constrained ventilation and hypercapnia, although the degree of reduction in symptoms was widely variable. Overall, the sensation of breathlessness was reduced by 13% with inhaled furosemide as compared to placebo; however, the reduction was not statistically significant with a P value of 0.052. In addition, inhaled furosemide resulted in a significant increase in diuresis as compared to placebo.

Finally, a third study evaluated the effects of inhaled furosemide on 20 patients with COPD during exercise (41). Inhaled furosemide was administered in a double-blinded, placebo-controlled, randomized fashion (with cross-over between groups) to patients with severe COPD (average FEV_1 15% predicted); 30 minutes after receiving either placebo or inhaled furosemide, the patients performed symptom-limited exercise at 75% of their maximum work rate. Inhaled furosemide was associated with a significant decrease in dyspnoea at peak exercise, as well as improved respiratory mechanics (dynamic inspiratory capacity, tidal volume, and mean tidal expiratory flow rates.) Eight of the 20 patients' exercise time increased by more than 1 minute after inhaled furosemide.

C-fibres (or irritant receptors) are located in the airway epithelium and are thought to respond to both mechanical and chemical stimuli such as bronchoconstriction and inhaled irritants. In normal subjects, the severity of dyspnoea due to experimentally induced bronchoconstriction (secondary to inhaled histamine) is reduced by inhaling aerosolized lidocaine (42). Normal subjects with dyspnoea due to external resistive loading did not experience reduction in the severity of dyspnoea with aerosolized lidocaine. This suggests that airway receptors stimulated by bronchoconstriction modify breathlessness.

Stimulation of pulmonary receptors by bronchoconstriction also appears to produce a qualitatively distinct sensation. The sensation of chest tightness is associated with experimentally induced and naturally occurring bronchoconstriction and is distinct from the sense of effort. Methacholine-induced bronchoconstriction in asthmatics has been described by subjects almost exclusively with the phrases 'chest tightness' or 'constriction', even at levels of lung function that are in the normal or mildly obstructed range (43). In contrast, subjects described external resistive loading and more severe degrees of bronchoconstriction with the additional phrases 'work' or 'effort', which reflect the increased corollary discharge associated with the mechanical load on the respiratory system from external resistive loading and hyperinflation. The specific receptors responsible for the sensation of chest tightness, however, remain to be determined.

Juxtapulmonary or J receptors are a type of C-fibre. The role of J receptors and pulmonary vascular receptors in dyspnoea is unclear; these receptors are thought to be important to respiratory sensations, but their contributions to symptoms of breathlessness are uncharacterized. J receptors are thought to be stimulated by interstitial fluid and probably contribute to the dyspnoea and rapid, shallow breathing pattern associated with pulmonary oedema (25).

The mechanism by which vascular receptors cause dyspnoea is unclear. The clinical observation that dyspnoea due to pulmonary embolism is rapidly relieved by intra-arterial thrombolysis in the absence of hypoxaemia suggests that stimulation of pulmonary vascular receptors may play a role in dyspnoea (J Markis, R Schwartzstein, pers comm); however, we are not aware of any investigational studies of the role of pulmonary vascular receptors. Although hypoxaemia is frequently seen in patients with pulmonary embolism (PE), correction of hypoxaemia with supplemental oxygen usually has minimal impact on dyspnoea. Bronchoconstriction and airflow obstruction may rarely accompany PE but cannot explain the common occurrence of dyspnoea in this disease. Stimulation of vascular receptors may cause dyspnoea in a primary fashion, analogous to chest tightness produced by pulmonary C-fibres during acute bronchoconstriction. A case report of a patient with acute unilateral pulmonary veno-occlusion whose dyspnoea was relieved by ipsilateral vagotomy provides some evidence that dyspnoea may be mediated by pulmonary vascular receptors stimulated by high pulmonary vascular pressures, or by C-fibres stimulated by pulmonary oedema, or by both processes (44).

Chest wall receptors

Receptors located in the joints, tendons, and muscles of the chest wall communicate with the central nervous system and contribute to the sensation of dyspnoea. Physiotherapeutic vibrators placed over parasternal intercostals muscles have been used to investigate the role of chest wall receptors in respiratory sensation. Normal subjects with experimentally-induced dyspnoea due to acute hypercarbia or external resistive loads noted decreased intensity of dyspnoea with stimulation of chest wall receptors (45). The use of chest wall vibrators on patients with COPD has been shown to reduce dyspnoea in these patients (46) but not 'air hunger' associated with breath-holding and hypercarbia (47). Chest wall receptors, like pulmonary stretch receptors, decrease dyspnoea when stimulated. The clinical role of chest wall vibration in patients with chronic dyspnoea remains to be determined.

Dynamic hyperinflation

Patients with expiratory flow limitation breathe at increasingly high lung volumes during exertion; this is a consequence of inadequate expiratory time to accommodate the rising tidal volume and respiratory rate associated with exercise. At higher lung volumes airway diameter is larger and, consequently, airways resistance is reduced, which permits greater expiratory flow. As a consequence of increasing lung volumes, the elastic recoil of the lung increases, and there is a threshold inspiratory load associated with auto-PEEP. The use of NIPPV, as described previously, may alleviate the work of breathing in these circumstances.

   The more severe the airflow obstruction, the more likely that hyperinflation will occur with exertion. This increase in lung volumes during exercise is termed 'dynamic hyperinflation'. In some cases, patients with flow limitation will breathe at lung volumes that approximate total lung capacity. Patients experiencing dynamic hyperinflation use descriptors such as 'I cannot get enough air in' or describe their inspiratory effort as 'unsatisfied' (16, 48). It may be that many patients experiencing significant dynamic hyperinflation literally cannot breathe any more deeply because inspiratory capacity is limited by their maximal lung volume (24). Although dyspnoea in patients with obstructive airways disease can also be attributed to gas exchange abnormalities or increased sense of effort due to weakened muscles, dynamic hyperinflation due to air trapping may be the primary cause of breathlessness in many of these patients, especially during exercise (48).

Evaluation of the affective dimension of dyspnoea

Recent work has demonstrated the importance of psychological factors in the development and severity of dyspnoea. Many sensations may elicit or be associated with a strong emotional component, e.g. fear or anxiety. Sensations that are deemed 'unpleasant' connote a negative affective response. It appears that it may be possible, under laboratory conditions, for subjects to distinguish the intensity of a respiratory sensation from its unpleasantness. In one study of ten healthy volunteers breathing with progressively increasing resistive loads, the authors demonstrated a statistically significant increase in perceived 'unpleasantness' (the affective component) as compared to 'intensity' (the sensory component) as measured by real-time visual analogue scales (49). These findings were expanded upon in a subsequent study in which 12 healthy subjects performed three breathing tasks: 1) maximal voluntary hyperpnoea with an inspiratory load that markedly increased the work of resting breathing while sustaining a normal end-tidal PCO_2, 2) forced decreased minute ventilation with an average elevation in end-tidal PCO_2 of 6.1mmHg greater than baseline, and 3) further decreased minute ventilation with end-tidal PCO_2 7.7mmHg above baseline. Tasks 2 and 3 (with elevated PCO_2 and reduced minute ventilation) generated significantly higher levels of unpleasantness as compared to task 1. This study demonstrated that increased work of breathing (task 1) was less unpleasant than 'air hunger' induced by increased end-tidal PCO_2 (tasks 2 and 3); thus the affective component can be generated and measured separately from the intensity of dyspnoea (50). A model that links the sensory intensity of dyspnoea to two aspects of the emotional response to the sensations has been proposed (51) (Figure 5.2).

A recent study assessed unpleasantness and functional magnetic resonance imaging (fMRI) of 14 healthy subjects breathing with increased resistive loads while viewing a standardized series of pictures designed to precipitate positive and negative emotions. Dyspnoea was induced in all subjects, and unpleasantness was significantly increased

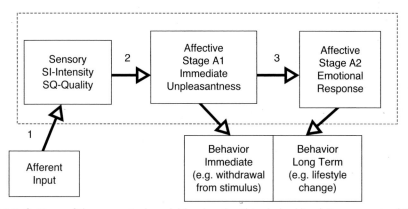

Fig. 5.2 Definitions of the perceptual model (enclosed within dashed line.) Components of the sensory dimension: SI, sensory intensity; SQ, sensory quality; SL, sensory location; ST, time course of sensation. Components of the affective dimension: A1, immediate unpleasantness (first stage of the affective dimension), A2, emotion/evaluation (second stage of the affective dimension.)

when subjects viewed negative emotional pictures. fMRI imaging demonstrated increased neuronal activation of the right anterior insula and right amygdala with increased unpleasantness, suggesting that these areas of the brain may be important in producing the affective sensations associated with dyspnoea (52). As the anterior insula and amygdala are involved in processing emotional states, it is not unreasonable to postulate a potential role for emotional state as a modulator of the perception of dyspnoea.

More work needs to be done to further clarify the role of affective symptoms in the development of breathlessness, particularly as available pharmacological therapies for affective symptoms have limited efficacy. Specifically, benzodiazepines have consistently been shown to have no significant beneficial effect on breathlessness. A recent Cochrane review of seven studies of benzodiazepines in patients with advanced diseases (COPD, chronic heart failure (CHF), advanced cancer, pulmonary fibrosis and motor neuron disease) demonstrated no significant benefit and increased drowsiness (53). The supportive environment offered by pulmonary rehabilitation programmes may alleviate the fear and anxiety associated with exercise, and may partly explain the reduced dyspnoea and improved exercise performance noted in those programmes. Further evaluation of therapies that specifically target affective symptoms and their effect on dyspnoea are of particular interest.

Physiology of breathlessness in advanced disease

Other chapters in this book will address specific types of diseases, such as heart failure, neuromuscular disease, and malignancy. The information presented in this chapter should assist clinicians in approaching individual diseases with an understanding of the underlying physiological and pathophysiological processes that contribute to dyspnoea. The physiological origins of dyspnoea are complex, as individual pathophysiological processes can produce a discrete sense of dyspnoea or can modify dyspnoea produced by a complex, multifaceted network of signals and processes. Ultimately, the perception of breathlessness involves the complex integration of information from throughout the body. Our understanding of how each source of information affects a patient's awareness of breathing discomfort allows a targeted approach to treatment and, in the future, may lead to improved therapeutic options to better alleviate dyspnoea.

References

1. Demediuk BH, Manning H, Lilly J, *et al.* Dissociation between dyspnea and respiratory effort. *Am Rev Respir Dis* 1992; **146**:1222–5.
2. Chronos N, Adams L, Guz A. Effect of hyperoxia and hypoxia on exercise-induced breathlessness in normal subjects. *Clin Sci* 1988; **74**:531–7.
3. Man WD, Polkey MI, Donaldson N, Gray BJ, Moxham J. Community pulmonary rehabilitation after hospitalisation for acute exercerbations of chronic obstructive pulmonary disease: randomised controlled study. *BMJ* 2004; **329**:1209–14.
4. Costi S, Crisafulli E, Antoni FD, Beneventi C, Fabbri LM, Clini EM. Effects of unsupported upper extremity exercise training in patients with COPD: a randomized clinical trial. *Chest* 2009; **136**: 387–95.

5. Simon PM, Schwartzstein RM, Weiss JW, *et al.* Distinguishable sensations of breathlessness induced in normal volunteers. *Am Rev Respir Dis* 1989; **140**:1021–7.

6. Simon PM, Schwartzstein RM, Weiss JW, Fencl V, Teghtsoonian M, Weinberger SE. Distinguishable types of dyspnea in patients with shortness of breath. *Am Rev Respir Dis* 1990; **142**:1009–14.

7. Elliott MW, Adams L, Cockcroft A, MacRae KD, Murphy K, Guz A (1991). The language of breathlessness: use of verbal descriptors by patients with cardiopulmonary disease. *Am Rev Respir Dis* 1991; **144**:826–32.

8. Mahler DA, Harver A, Lentine T, Scott JA, Beck K, Schwartzstein RM. Descriptors of breathlessness in cardiorespiratory diseases. *Am J Respir Crit Care Med* 1996; **154**:1357–63.

9. McCloskey DI, Gandevia S, Potter EK, Colebatch JG. Muscle sense and effort; Motor commands and judgments about muscular contractions. In Desmedt JE (ed) *Motor control mechanisms in health and disease.* New York: Raven Press, 1983.

10. Steier J, Jolley CJ, Seymour J, Roughton M, Polkey MI, Moxham J. Neural respiratory drive in obesity. *Thorax* 2009; **64**: 719–25.

11. Redline S, Gottfried SB, Altose MD. Effects of changes in inspiratory muscle strength on the sensation of respiratory force. *J Appl Physiol* 1991; **70**(1):240–5.

12. Theander K, Jakobsson P, Jorgensen N, Unosson M. Effects of pulmonary rehabilitation on fatirgue, functional status and health perceptions in patients with chronic obstructive pulmonary disease: a randomized controlled trial. *Clin Rehabil* 2009; **23**:125–36.

13. Schwartzstein RM, Manning HL, Weiss JW, Weinberger SE. Dyspnea: A sensory Experience. *Lung* 1990; **169**:185–99.

14. Schwartzstein RM, Simon PM, Weiss JW, Fencl V, Weinberger SE. Breathlessness induced by dissociation between Ventilation and Chemical Drive. *Am Rev Respir Dis* 1989; **139**:1231–7.

15. Chonan T, Mulholland MB, Cherniack NS, Altose MD (1987). Effects of voluntary constraining of thoracic displacement during hypercapnia. *J Appl Physiol* 1987; **63**:1822–8.

16. Manning HL, Schwartzstein RM. Pathophysiology of dyspnea. *N Engl J Med* 1995; **333**:1547–53.

17. Binks AP, Moosavi SH, Banzett RB, Schwartzstein RM. 'Tightness' sensation of asthma does not arise from the work of breathing. *Am J Respir Crit Care Med* 2002; **165**:78–82.

18. Fidone SJ, Gonzalez C. Initiation and control of chemoreceptor activity in the carotid body. In Fishman AP, Cherniack NS, Widdicombe JG, Geiger SR (eds) *The Handbook of Physiology: The Respiratory System.* Section 3, Volume II, Part 2, pp. 247–312. Bethesda, MD: American Physiological Society, 1986.

19. Fitzgerald RS, Lahiri S. Reflex responses to chemoreceptor stimulation. In Fishman AP, Cherniack NS, Widdicombe JG, Geiger SR (eds) *The Handbook of Physiology: The Respiratory System.* Section 3, Volume II, Part 2, pp. 313–63. Bethesda, MD: American Physiological Society, 1986.

20. Scott AC, Davies LC, Coats AJ, Piepoli M. Relationship of skeletal muscle metaboreceptors in the upper and lower limbs with the respiratory control in patients with heart failure. *Clin Sci* 2002; **102**:23–30.

21. Banzett RB, Lansing RW, Reid MB, Adams L, Brown R. 'Air hunger' arising from increased PCO_2 in mechanically ventilated quadriplegics. *Respir Physiol* 1989; **76**:53–68.

22. Banzett RB, Lansing RW, Brown R, *et al.* 'Air hunger' from increased PCO_2 persists after complete neuromuscular block in humans. *Respir Physiol* 1990; **81**:1–18.

23. Shea SA, Andres LP, Guz A, Banzett RB. Respiratory sensations in subjects who lack a ventilatory response to CO2. *Respir Physiol* 1993; **93**(2):203–19.

24. O'Donnell DE. Hyperinflation, dyspnea, and exercise intolerance in chronic obstructive pulmonary disease. *Proc Am Thorac Soc* 2006; **3**:180–4.

25. Manning HL, Schwartzstein RM. Mechanisms of dyspnea. In Mahler DA (ed) *Dyspnea*, pp. 63–95. New York: Marcel Dekker, 1998.

26. Lane R, Cockroft, Adams L, Guz A. Arterial oxygen saturation and breathlessness in patients with chronic obstructive airways disease. *Cli Sci* 1987; **72**:693–8.

27. Schwartzstein RM, Lahive K, Pope A, Weinberger SE, Weiss JW. Cold facial stimulation reduces breathlessness induced in normal subjects. *Am Rev Respir Dis* 1987; **136**:58–61.

28. Simon PM, Basner RC, Weinberger SE, Fencl V, Weiss JW, Schwartzstein RM. Oral mucosal stimulation modulates intensity of breathlessness induced in normal subjects. *Am Rev Respir Dis* 1991; **144**:419–22.

29. Burgess KR, Whitelaw WA. Reducing ventilatory response to carbon dioxide by breathing cold air. *Am Rev Respir Dis* 1984; **129**:687–90.

30. Liss HP, Grant BJB. The effect of nasal flow on breathlessness in patients with chronic obstructive pulmonary disease. *Am Rev Respir Dis* 1988; **137**:1285–88.

31. Spence DPS, Graham DR, Ahmed J, Rees K, Pearson MG, Calverley PMA. Does cold air affect exercise capacity and dyspnea in stable chronic obstructive pulmonary disease? *Chest* 1993; **103**:693–6.

32. Manning HL, Shea SA, Schwartzstein RM, Lansing RW, Brown R, Banzett RB. Reduced tidal volume increases 'air hunger' at fixed PCO_2 in ventilated quadriplegics. *Respir Physiol* 1992; **90**:19–30.

33. O'Donnell DE, Sanii R, Anthonisen NR, Younes M. Effect of dynamic airway compression on breathing pattern and respiratory sensation in severe chronic obstructive pulmonary disease. 1987; *Am Rev Respir Dis* **135**:912–8.

34. Dulverman ML, Wempe JB, Bladder G, *et al*. Nocturnal non-invasive ventilation in addition to rehabilitation in hypercapnic patients with COPD. *Thorax* 2008; **63**:1052–7.

35. Kohnlein T, Schonheit-Kenn U, Winterkamp S, Welte T, Kenn K. Noninvasive ventilation in pulmonary rehabilitation of COPD patients. *Respir Med* 2009; **103**:1329–36.

36. Kolodziej MA, Jensen L, Rowe B, Sin D. Systematic review of noninvasive positive pressure ventilation in severe stable COPD. *Eur Respir J* 2007; **30**:293–306.

37. Hamilton RD, Winning AJ, Perry A, Guz A. Aerosol anesthesia increases hypercapnic ventilation and breathlessness in laryngectomized humans. *J Appl Physiol* 1987; **63**:2286–92.

38. Sudo T, Hayashi F, Nishino T. Responses of tracheobronchial receptors to inhaled furosemide in anesthetized rats. *Am J Respir Crit Care Med* 2000; **162**:971–5.

39. Nishino T, Ide T, Sudo T, Sato J. Inhaled furosemide greatly alleviates the sensation of experimentally induced dyspnea. *Am J Respir Crit Care Med* 2000; **161**:1963–7.

40. Moosavi SH, Binks AP, Lansing RW, Topulos BP, Banzett RB, Schwartzstein RM. Effect of inhaled furosemide on air hunger induced in healthy humans. *Respir Physiol Neurobiol* 2006; **156**:1–8.

41. Jensen D, Amjadi K, Harris-McAllister V, Webb KA, O'Donnell DE. Mechanisms of dyspnoea relief and improved exercise endurance after furosemide inhalation in COPD. *Thorax* 2008; **63**:606–13.

42. Taguchi O, Kikuchi Y, Hida W, Iwase N, Satoh M, Chonan T, Takishima T (1991). Effects of bronchoconstriction and external resistive loading on the sensation of dyspnea. *J Appl Physiol* **71**:2183–90.

43. Moy ML, Weiss JW, Sparrow D, Israel E, Schwartzstein RM. Quality of dyspnea in bronchoconstriction differs from external loads. *Am J Respir Crit Care Med* 2000; **162**:451–5.

44. Davies SF, McQuaid KR, Iber C, *et al*. Extreme dyspnea from unilateral venous obstruction. *Am Rev Respir Diseases* 1987; **136**:184–8.

45. Manning HL, Basner R, Ringler J, *et al*. Effect of chest wall vibration on breathlessness in normal subjects. *J Appl Physiol* 1991; **71**:175–81.

46. Sibuya M, Yamada M, Kanamaru A, *et al*. Effect of chest wall vibration on dyspnea in patients with chronic respiratory disease. *Am J Respir Crit Care Med* 1994; **149**:1235–40.

47. Bloch-Salisbury E, Binks AP, Banzett RB, Schwartzstein RM. Mechanical chest-wall vibration does not relieve air hunger. *Respir Physiol Neurobiol* 2003; **134**:177–90.

48. O'Donnell DE, Webb KA. Exertional breathlessness in patients with chronic obstructive airflow limitation. *Am Rev Respir Dis* 1993; **148**:1351–7.

49. von Leupoldt A, Dahme B. Differentiation between the sensory and affective dimension of dyspnea during resistive load breathing in normal subjects. *Chest* 2005; **128**:3345–49.

50. Banzett RB, Pedersen SH, Schwartzstein RM, Lansing RW. The affective dimension of laboratory dyspnea: air hunger is more unpleasant than work/effort. *Am J Resp Crit Care Med* 2008; **177**:1384–90.

51. Lansing RW, Gracely RH, Banzett RB. The multiple dimensions of dyspnea: review and hypotheses. *Respir Physiol Neurobiol* 2009; **167**(1):53–60.

52. von Leupoldt A, Sommer T, Kegat S, *et al*. The unpleasantness of perceived dyspnea is processed in the anterior insula and amygdala. *Am J Resp Crit Care Med* 2008; **177**:1026–32.

53. Simon ST, Higginson IJ, Booth S, Harding R, Bausewein C. Benzodiazepines for the relief of breathlessness in advanced malignant and non-malignant diseases in adults. *Cochrane Database Syst Rev* 2010; **1**:CD007354.

Chapter 6

Multidimensional assessment of dyspnoea

Ingrid Harle and Deborah Dudgeon

Introduction

Dyspnoea is a common and distressing symptom in people with advanced disease of diverse aetiologies. The American Thoracic Society defines dyspnoea as: 'a subjective experience of breathing discomfort that consists of qualitatively distinct sensations that vary in intensity' (1). This definition suggests that dyspnoea, like pain, is a complex, multidimensional construct that is subjective and cannot be inferred from clinical or laboratory investigations. The quality and intensity of the person's perception of dyspnoea arise from an intricate interplay between physiological mechanisms, and psychological, social, and environmental factors (1–3) which may in turn cause secondary physiological and behavioural responses. Studies show that patients decrease their activities to cope with their breathlessness with a negative impact on their functional status, social activities (4), quality of life (5), and will to live (6). Patients use many terms and phrases to describe their sensation of breathlessness: 'suffocating', 'chest tightness', 'air hunger', and 'an uncomfortable sensation of breathing'. A comprehensive assessment of dyspnoea needs to consider all of these factors (1–3).

The multidimensional assessment of dyspnoea involves both a clinical appraisal and measurement of the different factors that impact on the perception of breathlessness and the effects of shortness of breath on the individual. Prior to embarking on an assessment of a person's dyspnoea it is important to determine what questions you are trying to answer (1) and in the setting of advanced disease which clinical assessments and measurements are reasonable to consider given the patient's diagnosis, prognosis, functional abilities, setting, and goals of care. Clinical assessments are usually to determine the underlying pathophysiology, the most effective treatments, and subsequently the response to the interventions. Measurement instruments or tools are used to bring some objectivity and precision to the evaluation of clinical assessments or interventions and to answer research questions.

Clinical assessment

From a clinical perspective it is important to determine the underlying diagnosis and pathophysiology responsible for a person's breathlessness so that appropriate interventions are initiated and the response appropriately evaluated. To determine an accurate diagnosis and the underlying pathophysiology a thorough history, complete physical examination, and different appropriate diagnostic tests are needed.

History

A complete history is paramount in the initial clinical evaluation of a person's shortness of breath. Questions should be directed at delineating the following features:

- The temporal onset—is it acute, subacute, or chronic?
- Qualities of the breathlessness
- Variability of the symptom—does it stay the same or change in intensity or severity?
- What are the aggravating factors—different positions or activities?
- Are there associated symptoms—cough, sputum, fever?
- Previous episodes of dyspnoea?
- Alleviating factors—response to medications or non-pharmacological measures?
- The impact on functional abilities?

The impact on psychosocial well-being, spiritual well-being, and quality of life?

Other important features to elicit include: history of smoking, underlying cardiac, pulmonary disease or other comorbid medical conditions, significant weight loss, possible deconditioning, allergies, medications, and other treatments to date (7, 8).

The temporal onset of the breathlessness—whether it is an acute, subacute, or chronic problem—helps to tailor further questioning and determine the differential diagnosis. In the setting of acute dyspnoea, the differential diagnosis is relatively short and includes pneumonia, pulmonary embolism, acute congestive heart failure, or myocardial infarction (9). However, in persons with subacute or chronic breathlessness the diagnostic possibilities are much greater and the dyspnoea may be related to the underlying disease and thus potentially irreversible (i.e. a patient with chronic obstructive pulmonary disease (COPD) receiving optimal medical management) or alternatively, there may be a potentially curable and unrelated cause of the dyspnoea, such as pneumonia.

Physical examination

A thorough physical examination should be performed focusing on the possible underlying aetiologies identified in the history and looking for clinical signs associated with any of these (i.e. elevated jugular venous pressure, S3 heart sound, pulmonary crackles in congestive heart failure (CHF)) (10).

As stated earlier, dyspnoea is a subjective experience and may not be evident to the observer. People can have a normal respiratory rate and feel breathless and conversely be tachypnoeic without a sensation of discomfort with breathing. As clinicians, we must accept the patient's own assessment of whether he/she feels short of breath. Gift et al. (11) assessed patients with COPD experiencing mild, moderate, and severe levels of dyspnoea and studied the physiological factors associated with the breathlessness. The only significant difference was in the use of accessory muscles seen in patients with high levels of dyspnoea and not in those with low levels of breathlessness. Respiratory rate, depth of respiration, and peak expiratory flow rates were not significantly different between the three levels of dyspnoea. These results suggest that the extent of use of accessory muscles is a physical finding that reflects the intensity of dyspnoea and is therefore helpful when assessing breathlessness (particularly in those persons who are not able to rate their breathlessness).

Investigations

Clinical investigations are useful to help determine whether the underlying pathophysiology is a result of increased ventilatory demands, impaired mechanical responses, or a combination of the two. The choice of appropriate laboratory investigations to assist in determining the underlying aetiology of dyspnoea, should not be made in isolation, but needs to take into account the stage of the person's disease, the prognosis, the desires of the patient/family, and the risk:benefit ratio of performing the specific test or intervention (10).

Oxygen saturation is a non-invasive test commonly used in evaluating causes for dyspnoea in the clinical setting. At high oxygen saturations pulse oximetry is reasonably accurate ($\pm$ 3%), but the accuracy decreases with saturation levels below 80% (12). It is important to remember that an individual may have normal (or near normal) oxygen saturations, but may still experience dyspnoea secondary to inadequate ventilation and subsequent hypercapnia. In such circumstances, arterial blood gases would be beneficial as they provide information regarding oxygenation (pO_2), ventilation (pCO_2), and acid–base balance (pH).

Blood tests that are potentially useful to consider are: complete blood count (CBC) to diagnose possible infection, anaemia or polycythaemia; metabolic parameters to look for hypocalcaemia, hypokalaemia, hypomagnesaemia, and hypophosphataemia which can impair respiratory muscle function, and may require correction, if deemed clinically appropriate (13).

Radiological investigations might include a chest x-ray, ventilation/perfusion scan, computed tomography (CT) scan, CT angiogram, magnetic resonance imaging (MRI), or echocardiogram. Lung function tests such as spirometry and standardized pulmonary function tests (PFTs) are performed at rest and may be helpful in diagnosing the underlying disease process or in evaluating response to therapies. Spirometry is least cumbersome and can differentiate between an obstructive disorder or restrictive disorder of the lungs. Full PFTs can be useful in diagnosing the underlying problem and determining its severity and assessing the response to treatments. The severity of the abnormality in pulmonary function tests does not necessarily reflect the intensity of dyspnoea that a person will experience. The relationship of abnormal pulmonary function and the severity of breathlessness is strongest within a specific disease state (14). Mahler and Wells demonstrated a few such relationships (15):

1) In patients with COPD, measurements of maximal expiratory pressure (PEmax) ($r = 0.35$) and maximal inspiratory pressure (PImax) ($r = 0.51$) showed the strongest correlations to the intensity of dyspnoea as measured by the baseline dyspnoea index (BDI).

2) In asthmatics, forced vital capacity (FVC) (r = 0.78) and forced expiratory volume in 1s (FEV$_1$) (r = 0.77) were highly related to BDI.

3) In restrictive pulmonary diseases, such as interstitial lung disease, PImax (r = 0.51) and FVC (r = 0.44) showed significant correlations with intensity of breathlessness.

Other investigators had different results. Epler and colleagues (16) demonstrated that maximal voluntary ventilation (MVV) (r=0.78) exhibited the greatest correlation with breathlessness in persons with COPD; PImax (r=0.51) and FVC (r=0.44) were the best correlates of dyspnoea in interstitial lung disease. Bruera et al. (17) used multivariate analysis to reveal that PImax (p=0.02) was an independent correlate of dyspnoea in the cancer patient experiencing moderate to severe dyspnoea. In general, Mahler et al. noted that standardized pulmonary function tests correlate poorly with the intensity of dyspnoea (18).

Cardiopulmonary exercise tests are performed in the appropriate setting for three reasons: 1) to identify a cardiac or respiratory cause for exercise limitation; 2) to quantify the degree of functional disability; and 3) to assess response to treatment (12). Progressive exercise testing is often used to establish a baseline for entry into a pulmonary rehabilitation programme, or to identify the aetiology of exertional dyspnoea and to assess response to interventions. The person exercises using a cycle ergometer or the treadmill while various parameters are continuously measured in response to increasing workloads (12). Exercise capacity is more simply measured by the use of walking tests; these tests correlate with measures of dyspnoea and exercise capacity (18). In the 6- or 12-min walking test (6MWT, 12MWT), an individual is required to walk as far as they can on a set course, at their own pace, for 6min or 12min. In the shuttle walking test, the person walks around two points at a speed controlled by an audiotape. The speed is gradually increased and the individual continues to walk until they cannot keep up with the tape or need to stop (12). The shuttle walking test was validated against the treadmill exercise test and provides reproducible results when testing functional capacity in the ambulatory patient with advanced cancer (19).

Psychological factors

A number of studies demonstrate that anxiety is significantly correlated with the intensity of dyspnoea (20–23). Many of the correlations are significant but low, with anxiety only explaining nine percent of the variance in the intensity of breathlessness. Tanaka and colleagues also found significant correlations with the Hospital Anxiety and Depression Scale (HADS) depression scores (20, 24, 25). When they combined the HADS anxiety and depression scores the correlation coefficient was r=0.63 (p <0.01), explaining 36% of variance in the intensity of dyspnoea. Henoch et al. (26) studied palliative patients with lung cancer and demonstrated that both coping capacity and anxiety influenced the intensity of dyspnoea negatively. These studies suggest that a comprehensive assessment of factors potentially impacting the perception of dyspnoea should include measurement of anxiety and depression.

Currently there is little agreement on the best instrument to measure anxiety and depression. The HADS is a 14-item questionnaire with two separate subscales that is commonly used to measure these symptoms (24, 25).

Qualitative dimensions

In the assessment of breathlessness, it is important to acknowledge that dyspnoea is not a single sensation. The 'language' of dyspnoea varies with each person describing his/her discomfort with breathing. Studies demonstrate an association between the different phrases or word clusters used by patients to describe their breathlessness, and the various pathophysiological conditions (27–29). Even though descriptor word choices are different between health and disease states, O'Donnell and colleagues found that there was too much overlap to be able to distinguish between COPD, restrictive lung disease and CHF (30–32). Wilcock and colleagues (29) have also suggested that there was not enough robustness and construct validity to use word descriptors or clusters in formulating a differential diagnosis for dyspnoea.

Measurement of dyspnoea

Quantification and analysis of dyspnoea is complex but important, as objective measures allow evaluation of therapeutic interventions and increase our understanding of the neurophysiological basis of the symptom. Research studies show that the patient's rating of the intensity of his/her breathlessness provides a different dimension than what is obtained by measurement of pulmonary function tests or exercise testing which evaluate dysfunction of the respiratory system (14, 33–35). There are many validated measurement tools available and it is important to choose the one which answers the particular clinical or research questions that you want addressed (36). Instruments that are commonly used to measure dyspnoea either evaluate the intensity of shortness of breath exclusively (unidimensional) or are multidimensional questionnaires that evaluate the impact of dyspnoea on other aspects of the person's life.

Unidimensional scales

Visual analogue scale (VAS)

The visual analogue scale (VAS) is perhaps the easiest scale to use and is the most popular tool utilized for measuring the perceived intensity of breathlessness. This scale is a vertical or horizontal line, usually 100mm in length, with descriptive phrases as anchors, indicating the extremes of the sensation (Figure 6.1). At the bottom of the scale is usually

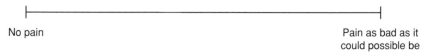

No pain

Pain as bad as it
could possible be

Fig. 6.1 10-cm Visual analogue scale.

'No breathlessness' and at the top is 'Worst possible breathlessness'. The respondents indicate a point on the line that corresponds to their perceived level of dyspnoea, at the time of assessment. The correlation between a vertical and horizontal VAS is high (r=0.97) (37). The VAS is used for the initial assessment, to monitor progress and to evaluate the effectiveness of treatments in an individual patient (37). The VAS is not an appropriate tool for comparing dyspnoea intensity in different patients as there is no standardization. Numerous studies have established the validity of the VAS, with respect to sensitivity and reproducibility (38–40). Test-retest reliability was established in the cancer population (4) and in patients with stable asthma (41). There is high concurrent validity with the modified Borg scale (r ≥0.90) (42, 43). The VAS is reproducible at maximum exercise and the same levels of exercise (43, 44). It is also sensitive to the effects of treatments (7). The vertical VAS had greater sensitivity to change than the horizontal scale in two separate studies (45, 46)

Likert scales

Using a seven-point Likert scale: 1=all the time; 2=most of the time; 3=a good bit of the time; 4=some of the time; 5=a little of the time; 6=hardly any of the time; and 7=none of the time, Guyatt at al. (47) found that this Likert scale was more readily understood than the VAS anchored by the descriptors, 'none of the time' and 'all of the time'. Both techniques, however, measured similar responsiveness to change following enrolment in a pulmonary rehabilitation programme. Dudgeon et al. (48) compared the 0–4 Likert scale (0=none, 1=mild, 2=moderate, 3=severe, and 4=horrible) used by Reuben and Mor (49) in the National Hospice Study, with the VAS in an outpatient cancer population and found good correlation (r=0.82, p=0.0001). See Figure 6.2 for an example scale.

Numeric rating scale (NRS)

The NRS is a ten-point (0–10) scale that correlates well with the VAS and the modified Borg scale (40), however it has not been tested as extensively as other scales (Figure 6.3).

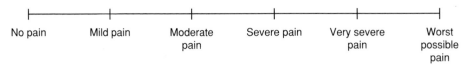

Fig. 6.2 Simple descriptive dyspnoea intensity scale.

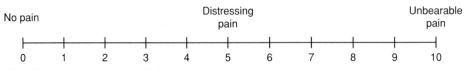

Fig. 6.3 Numeric dyspnoea scale (0–10).

Modified Borg dyspnoea scale (MBS)

The Borg scale was initially developed in 1962 to rate perceived exertion and effort during exercise (50). The Borg Scale correlates with physiological parameters of lung disease during exercise (51). It is usually used in conjunction with an exercise protocol with standardized power output or metabolic loads.

The modified Borg scale is a ten-point category-ratio scale, adapted by Burdon et al. to measure the intensity of dyspnoea (52). The MBS is a non-linear scale with corresponding verbal descriptors of progressively increased sensation intensity (52). The descriptive anchor at the top, 'Nothing at all', corresponds to the number '0',and the anchor at the bottom, 'Maximum', corresponds with the number '10'. This scale has strong and significant correlations with the VAS in COPD patients (r=0.99) (53) with minute ventilation (r=0.98), oxygen consumption during exercise (r=0.95) (54), and moderate correlations with peak expiratory flow rates and oxygen saturation in emergency room patients (55). The modified Borg scale has the following advantages: those with acute dyspnoea report satisfaction with its use, it is conceptually easier for the older patients to use, the descriptors may assist patients in choosing the intensity of the sensation, and direct comparisons between individuals may be more valid (55). A possible disadvantage is that sensitivity may be blunted by the proximity of the words 'slight' and 'severe' on the scale, discouraging patients from using the whole scale. This disadvantage is presumably outweighed by the simplicity of the tool and the reproducibility of results obtained in the short term (42) and with repeated testing over time (56). When O'Donnell and colleagues used the Borg scale to monitor changes in dyspnoea during exercise in the COPD population, measurements obtained were both highly reproducible and responsive to change (57).

Respiratory distress observation scale (RDOS)

There are various reasons why a patient is unable to communicate or self-report the severity of his/her dyspnoea. This can result in unnecessary suffering due to under recognition and under treatment of the symptom. Campbell (58) established the reliability (alpha=0.78), convergent and discriminant validity of the RDOS. The seven behavioural variables assessed in this instrument included: heart rate, respiratory rate, restlessness, accessory muscle use, grunting at end-expiration, nasal flaring, and fearful facial expression. This study suggests that if a person cannot reliably rate his/her dyspnoea, then an observation scale such as the RDOS may be a useful tool for assessment.

Unidimensional instruments anchored to activities

Some scales use a ratio scaling technique that measures the relationship between the intensity of a physical stimulus and its perceived magnitude (59, 60). These scales attempt to estimate the intensity of the sensation and to allow comparison of intensity across individuals (61).

Medical Research Council (MRC) breathlessness scale

The MRC breathlessness scale is a self-report or interview guide based on five grades describing the magnitude of the task required to evoke dyspnoea. The five grades on the scale are:

0: not troubled with breathlessness except with strenuous exercise.

1: troubled by shortness of breath when hurrying or walking up a slight hill.

2: walks slower than people of the same age due to breathlessness or has to stop for breath when walking at own pace on the level.

3: stops for breath after walking—100m or after a few minutes on the level.

4: too breathless to leave the house or breathless when dressing or undressing.

   The instrument has been reported to lack discrimination, but is useful to define and characterize a patient population. It has been used as a simple tool to measure functional dyspnoea (62, 63), as it is noted to be predictive of health-related quality of life (64) and survival (65). Several studies have established content validity (66), inter-rater reliability (15), and concurrent validity (66, 67) for this tool.

Oxygen cost diagram (OCD)

The OCD is a variation on the VAS or the Borg scale, designed for the assessment of dyspnoea in persons with pulmonary disease. The OCD is a self-administered questionnaire with intermediate reproducibility and validity (68). This scale uses a 100mm vertical line, with descriptive phrases representing everyday activities, positioned at various points on either side of the line (Figure 6.4). The descriptions correspond to the oxygen requirements required for each activity. The activities towards the bottom require low energy expenditure (i.e. sitting) and those activities that require the most energy expenditure (i.e. brisk walking) are towards the top of the scale. The patient selects one of the activities on the line during which his/her dyspnoea would be severe enough to prevent them from progressing any further (68). The point indicated on the line is scored in millimetres above zero. McGavin et al. (68) found a significant correlation between the points marked on the oxygen cost diagram and the distance the patients walked (r=0.68, p <0.001). The OCD correlated significantly with the MRC scale and the BDI in patients with cardiopulmonary disease of different aetiologies and variable severity (15). Mahler and Wells suggest that the OCD is the most appropriate assessment tool for statistical comparisons of response to treatment (15). One of the limitations of the scale relates to its heavy reliance on ambulatory activities, and therefore may be of restricted value in subjects who are breathless at rest.

Reading numbers aloud

People with cancer can become breathless at very low levels of exertion, thus limiting their activities. 'Reading numbers aloud' is a test designed as an objective measure of this activity-limiting effect of dyspnoea. The test requests patients to read a grid of numbers as fast and as quickly as possible for 60seconds. The number of numerals read and the number read

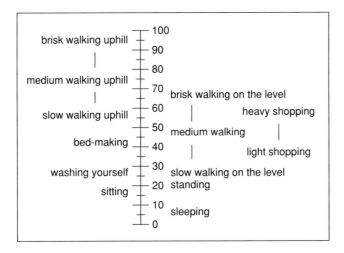

Values for oxygen expenditure

Brisk walking uphill	95	Light shopping	36
Medium walking uphill	75	Washing yourself	27
Brisk walking on the level	69	Slow walking on the level	27
Heavy shopping	58	Standing	21
Slow walking uphill	57	Sitting	17
Medium walking	47	Sleeping	7
Bed-making	42		

Fig. 6.4 Oxygen-cost diagram. Reproduced from (68) with permission from BMJ Publishing Group Ltd.

per breath are recorded. One study revealed good test-retest reliability and construct validity and suggests it may be beneficial to use in a debilitated population (69).

Multidimensional measures of dyspnoea anchored to activities

Baseline dyspnoea index/transitional dyspnoea index (BDI/TDI)

The BDI is a multidimensional assessment instrument administered by an interviewer (18). It uses a five-point scale to quantify functional impairment, magnitude of task, and magnitude of effort to elicit dyspnoea (18). A trained interviewer asks open-ended questions concerning the different dimensions and then, using specific criteria allocates a value between 0 (severe) and 4 (not impaired). By adding the scores together, a total score ranging between 0–12 is obtained, with lower scores indicative of more severe intensity of dyspnoea. The measurements are made at a baseline state and can be repeated after an intervention to generate the TDI (36). The BDI/TDI is a discriminative tool with good reproducibility (18), inter-rater reliability (15, 18), concurrent validity (15, 18, 67, 70), construct validity (15, 67, 70), and sensitivity (71). This instrument has undergone extensive testing and is used in research studies, which allows for patient scores and outcomes to be compared to other studies (10). The TDI was developed to measure changes in dyspnoea rated by the interviewer comparing patient report with the baseline state. The focus is on how an individual's dyspnoea affects their activities. The instrument is responsive to treatment such as exercise training and rehabilitation programmes (72, 73), plus the TDI correlates with changes in quality of life measures (SF 36) (74). The self-administered version of the modified BDI/TDI shows high and significant correlations when compared to the interviewer version of the instrument (75).

Pulmonary functional status and dyspnoea questionnaire (PFSDQ)

The PFSDQ is a self-administered questionnaire rating of breathlessness based on 79 activities, divided into six categories: self-care, mobility, eating, home management, social, and recreational (76). Recently, a modified shorter version was developed, associated with ten activities plus a fatigue component (77). The longer PFSDQ has high test-retest reliability for dyspnoea (r=0.94), high internal consistency (alpha=0.88–0.94) (76) and is responsive over time (77). The shorter PFSDQ has similar reliability, internal consistency and is responsive to change after pulmonary rehabilitation (78). The instrument is sensitive to small changes in dyspnoea with activities, and the level of dyspnoea for specific activities can be followed over time.

University of California, San Diego shortness of breath questionnaire (SOBQ)

The SOBQ is a self-administered six-point scale, easy for patients to understand, with the purpose of measuring dyspnoea with daily activities. Twenty-one activities of daily living are rated, with 0= not all to 5=maximally or unable to do because of breathlessness (79). Three other questions are also posed, regarding limitations due to dyspnoea, fear of harm, and fear of shortness of breath. The SOBQ has good test-retest reliability (r=0.94 over 2 days), good internal consistency (alpha=0.91), moderate correlation with the 6MWT (r =−0.47) (80) and it is responsive to pulmonary rehabilitation (81).

The pulmonary functional status scale (PFSS)

The PFSS is a self-administered questionnaire containing 53 items measuring mental, physical, and social functioning. Ratings of dyspnoea are obtained independent of activities, in relation to several activities, and then placed on a subscale. This scale has a test-retest reliability of 0.67, internal consistency of 0.81 (82), construct validity, moderate correlation with the 12MWT (83) and is responsive to pulmonary rehabilitation (84).

The cancer dyspnoea scale (CDS)

The CDS is a 12-item questionnaire developed to assess the multidimensional nature of dyspnoea in the cancer population (85). Three factors are rated: sense of effort (five items), sense of anxiety (four items), and sense of discomfort (three items). A score of 8/48 is reported to correspond to significant breathlessness. It was evaluated in Japanese and demonstrated some evidence of reliability and validity as a multidimensional instrument, but there is no evidence of responsiveness (86). The scale has been translated into English but still requires evaluation in this version.

The Cancer Dyspnoea Scale

We would like to ask you about your breathlessness or difficulty in breathing. Please answer each question by circling only the numbers that best describes the breathing difficulty that you felt during the past few days. Base your response on your first impression.

	Not at all	A little	Somewhat	Considerably	Very much
1 Can you inhale easily?	1	2	3	4	5
2 Can you exhale easily?	1	2	3	4	5
3 Can you breathe slowly?	1	2	3	4	5
4 Do you feel short of breath?	1	2	3	4	5
5 Do you feel breathing difficulty accompanied by palpitations and sweating?	1	2	3	4	5
6 Do you feel as if you are panting?	1	2	3	4	5
7 Do you feel such breathing difficulty that you don't know what to do about it?	1	2	3	4	5
8 Do you feel your breath is shallow?	1	2	3	4	5
9 Do you feel your breathing may stop?	1	2	3	4	5
10 Do you feel your airway has become narrower?	1	2	3	4	5
11 Do you feel as if you are drowning?	1	2	3	4	5
12 Do you feel as if something is stuck in your airway?	1	2	3	4	5

Calculation method

1. Add the scores for each factor together
   - Factor 1 = (items 4 + 6 + 8 + 10 + 12) − 5   = sense of effort
   - Factor 2 = (items 5 + 7 + 9 + 11) − 4   = sense of anxiety
   - Factor 3 = 15 − (items 1 + 2 + 3)   = sense of discomfort
2. Add the total scores for each factor together   = total dyspnoea

*Subtractions are to make adjustments for 0 as a state of absence of dyspnoea

Fig. 6.5 Cancer dyspnoea scale. Reproduced from (85) with permission from Macmillan Publishers Ltd.

Quality of life instruments

Breathlessness can significantly impact a person's life with potential consequences and so a comprehensive assessment of dyspnoea should include measurement of his/her health-related quality of life (36, 87). There are many quality of life/health status questionnaires that summarize the numerous effects of disease on patients' lives and perceived well being. The reader should refer to Chapter 3 of this volume for discussion of the different types of quality of life instruments. Generic quality of life questionnaires are useful for surveys to document the range of disability in a general population or a specific group. Well-designed quality of life instruments can assist in the design of treatment strategies, analysis of the cost and consequences of disabilities, and to evaluate the effectiveness of treatments (36). The Medical Outcomes Study Short Form (SF-36) and Sickness Impact Profile (SIP) are two generic quality of life instruments that are often used in people with airflow limitation (88).

Sickness Impact Profile (SIP)

The SIP is one of the most commonly used generic quality of life questionnaires. The SIP includes 136 items describing the effect of illness on behavioural function, and assesses many areas including movement, body care, sleeping, eating, recreation, and emotional and social behaviour (36, 89). This tool has been compared with numerous measures of disease and disability; it provides a valid indication of health in the population of patients with airflow limitation (90). It tends to be less sensitive for those individuals with an FEV_1 greater than 50% predicted. Measure of general health studies (88, 90) demonstrated that SIP is able to differentiate between moderate and severe disease, but has very low sensitivity for mild to moderate chronic airflow limitation disease (88). Although the SIP is widely used and well evaluated, it is cumbersome to use (36).

The Medical Outcomes Study Short Form: SF-36

The alternative questionnaire is the SF-36 (36, 91) which is easier to administer than the SIP and is well validated (36, 91, 92). It includes 36 items, with health and functional status assessed across eight subscales: physical function, role disability—physical problems, bodily pain, health perceptions, vitality, social function, role disability—emotional problems, and mental health. Studies have confirmed content, concurrent, construct, criterion, and predictive validity across a variety of illnesses (92).

Disease-specific quality of life instruments

Disease-specific quality of life questionnaires can provide valuable information for the clinician or researcher because they include an assessment of the influence of dyspnoea on the person's life. These disease-specific questionnaires are more sensitive than the generic quality of life tools, and consequently are more useful when evaluating the effectiveness of treatments (36). Currently there is no 'gold standard' available to use as a comparator when measuring the outcomes of care in diseases of the airways (88).

Chronic respiratory disease questionnaire (CRDQ)

The CRDQ was designed for use in clinical trials to measure the quality of life of patients with chronic airflow limitation (93). This instrument focuses on four dimensions of illness: dyspnoea, fatigue, emotional function, and the patient's feeling of control over the disease (mastery) (36, 93). Guyatt et al. developed the CRDQ in 1987 as an interview-based questionnaire requiring 15–25min to complete. It contains a 20-item, self-report tool. The patient is asked to report the dyspnoea related to any five most troublesome activities from personal experience in his/her daily life. The interviewer then reads a list of 26 activities allowing the respondent time to report their level of dyspnoea with these activities. Using a scale of 1 (extreme dyspnoea) to 7 (no dyspnoea), the severity of dyspnoea (over the past 2 weeks) is rated for each activity. The patient is then asked by the interviewer to indicate which of all the activities they have listed is most important to them. This process continues until the five most important activities have been determined. The sum of these scores is then divided by five to obtain the overall score for the CRQ. The questionnaire also asks 15 questions that are identical for each subject (36). Several studies have demonstrated CRQ scores to be sensitive to change. Guyatt also developed a paper and pencil version of the CRQ for use in place of the interview, and it has been validated. Pulmonary rehabilitation programmes use this tool extensively to measure health-related quality of life outcomes which thus allows comparisons between programmes. Stulbarg et al. (94) showed good internal consistency for all four scales in COPD patients, with alpha ranging from 0.71–0.92. This is in contrast to Wijkstra et al. (95) who reported a lower internal consistency (alpha=0.53), probably because activities are individualized; these authors demonstrated acceptable test-retest reliability (r=0.73). The questionnaire has shown response to therapy (96) with the level of change judged to be clinically significant (97).

The St George respiratory questionnaire (SGRQ)

The SGRQ is a self-administered test with 76 items that measure three aspects of a specific disease: symptoms (types, frequency, severity), activity (those that are caused or limited by breathlessness), and the impact of disease on quality of life (looks at a range of factors concerned with social and psychological functioning as a result of airways disease). A score is calculated for each section plus a total score is the summation of these (88). Dyspnoea is not a discretely measured symptom, but it is included with other respiratory symptoms (cough, wheeze, and sputum) in the symptom category. Therefore the dyspnoea response to therapy cannot be measured separately. The test-retest reliability of the questionnaire is good (r=0.92) (98), the instrument is responsive to treatments (99), and thresholds of significant clinical change are reported (100). This instrument is used extensively and has computerized scoring capabilities.

The instruments discussed above, CRQ and SGRQ, were compared by Rutten-van Molken et al. (36, 101) and were deemed similar in terms of reliability, validity, and responsiveness to change. The major difference between these instruments is that the CRQ is interviewer-rated and the SGRQ is self-rated.

Choosing a measurement instrument

When choosing a method to assess dyspnoea, one needs to consider whether the evaluation is for clinical or research purposes, the reliability and validity of the instruments, the setting of the assessment, the acuity of the dyspnoea, the length of time for completion, whether it is 'self' report or 'other' report, and the functional status of the patient.

In the clinical setting, measurement tools serve to establish a baseline against which to measure and evaluate response to therapies or progression of disease. As these assessments are usually done in the context of a busy clinic and are repeated at various intervals, it is important that they are simple to use, do not take very long and have good test-retest reliability (10). It is particularly important that the questionnaire(s) are not too onerous for patients in the palliative phase of their disease.

Research questions may be to determine the prevalence of the symptom and associated factors; to determine the natural history of breathlessness; to establish the underlying pathophysiology; or be related to clinical trials to evaluate different treatments. The selection of measurement tools is determined by the aims of the study but should also consider patient burden.

Studies show that there are significant differences in physicians', nurses' and patients' ratings of the intensity of dyspnoea and other symptoms (102, 103). It is generally accepted that patient's self-assessments are the 'gold standard'.

Conclusions

In summary, dyspnoea is a very complex, subjective experience that is multidimensional in nature and involves many factors that modulate both the quality and intensity of its perception. At the present time there is no single instrument which assesses all components of the sensation of breathlessness. It is important when assessing dyspnoea to choose the appropriate method(s) depending on whether it is for clinical appraisal or research and the questions that you are asking. In the palliative phase of an illness, it is particularly important that the burden of the assessments is not too onerous and they are appropriate to the person's prognosis and stage of disease.

References

1. American Thoracic Society. Dyspnea. Mechanisms, assessment, and management: A consensus statement. *Am J Respir Crit Care Med* 1999; **159**:321–40.

2. Cherniack NS, Altose MD. Mechanisms of dyspnea. *Clin Chest Med* 1987; **8**(2):207–14.

3. Tobin MJ. Dyspnea: Pathophysiologic basis, clinical presentation, and management. *Arch Intern Med* 1990; **150**:1604–13.

4. Brown ML, Carrieri V, Janson-Bjerklie S, Dodd MJ. Lung cancer and dyspnea: The patient's perception. *Oncol Nurs Forum* 1986; **13**(5):19–24.

5. Roberts DK, Thorne SE, Pearson C. The experience of dyspnea in late-stage cancer. Patients' and nurses' perspectives. *Cancer Nursing* 1993; **16**(4):310–20.

6. Chochinov MH, Tataryn D, Clinch JJ, Dudgeon D. Will to live in the terminally ill. *Lancet* 1999; **354**(9181):816–19.

7. Silvestri GA, Mahler DA. Evaluation of dyspnea in the elderly patient. *Clin Chest Med* 1993; **14**(3):393–404.

8. Ferrin MS, Tino G. Acute dyspnea. *AACN Clin Issues* 1997; **8**(3):398–410.

9. Man GCW, Hsu K, Sproule BJ. Effect of alprazolam on exercise and dyspnea in patients with chronic obstructive pulmonary disease. *Chest* 1986; **90**(6):832–6.

10. Carrieri-Kohlman V, Dudgeon D. Multidimensional assessment of dyspnea. In Booth S, Dudgeon D (eds) *Dyspnea in Advanced Disease*, pp. 19–37. Oxford: Oxford University Press, 2005.

11. Gift AG, Plaut SM, Jacox A. Psychologic and physiologic factors related to dyspnea in subjects with chronic obstructive pulmonary disease. *Heart Lung* 1986; **15**(6):595–601.

12. Hancox B, Whyte K. *McGraw-Hill's Pocket Guide to Lung Function Tests*. Roseville NSW: McGraw-Hill, 2001.

13. Lewis MI, Belman MJ. Nutrition and the respiratory muscles. *Clin Chest Med* 1988; **9**(2):337–47.

14. Nguyen HQ, Altinger J, Carrieri-Kohlman V, Gormley JM, Paul SM, Stulbarg MS. Factor analysis of laboratory and clinical measurement of dyspnea in patients with chronic obstructive pulmonary disease. *J Pain Symptom Manage* 2003; **25**(2):118–27.

15. Mahler DA, Wells CK. Evaluation of Clinical Methods for Rating Dyspnea. *Chest* 1988; **93**(3): 580–6.

16. Epler GR, Saber FA, Gaensler EA. Determination of severe impairment (disability) in interstitial lung disease. *Am Rev Respir Dis* 1980; **121**:647–59.

17. Bruera E, Schmitz B, Pither J, Neumann CM, Hanson J. The frequency and correlates of dypsnea in patients with advanced cancer. *J Pain Symptom Manage* 2000; **19**(5):357–62.

18. Mahler DA, Weinberg DH, Wells CK, Feinstein AR. The measurement of dyspnea. Contents, interobserver agreement, and physiologic correlates of two new clinical indexes. *Chest* 1984; **85**(6):751–8.

19. Booth S, Adams L. The shuttle walking test: a reproducible method for evaluating the impact of shortness of breath on functional capacity in patients with advanced cancer. *Thorax* 2001; **56**(2): 146–50.

20. Tanaka K, Akechi T, Okuyama T, Nishiwaki Y, Uchitomi Y. Factors correlated with dyspnea in advanced lung cancer patients: Organic causes and what else? *J Pain Symptom Manage* 2002; **23**(6):490–500.

21. Swinburn CR, Wakefield JM, Newman SP, Jones PW. Evidence of prednisolone induced mood change ('steroid euphoria') in patients with chronic obstructive airways disease. *Br J Clin Pharmacol* 1988; **26**:709–13.

22. Yellowlees PM, Ruffin RE. Psychological defenses and coping styles in patients following a life-threatening attack of asthma. *Chest* 1989; **95**(6):1298–303.

23. Dudgeon D, Lertzman M. Dyspnea in the Advanced Cancer Patient. *J Pain Symptom Manage* 1998; **16**(4):212–19.

24. Hermann C. International experiences with the Hospital Anxiety and Depression Scale – a review of validation data and clinical results. *J Psychosom Res* 1997; **42**(1):17–41.

25. Zigmond A, Snaith RP. The Hospital Anxiety and Depression Scale. *Acta Psychiatr Scand* 1983; **67**(5):361–70.

26. Henoch I, Bergman B, Gustafsson M, Gaston-Johansson F, Danielson E. Dyspnea experience in patients with lung cancer in palliative care. *Eur J Onc Nursing* 2008; **12**:86–96.

27. Simon PM, Schwartzstein RM, Weiss JW, *et al.* Distinguishable sensations of breathlessness induced in normal volunteers. *Am Rev Respir Dis* 1989; **140**:1021–7.

28. Simon PM, Schwartzstein RM, Weiss JW, Fencl V, Teghtsoonian M, Weinberger SE. Distinguishable types of dyspnea in patients with shortness of breath. *Am Rev Respir Dis* 1990; **142**:1009–14.

29. Wilcock A, Crosby V, Hughes AC, Fielding K, Corcoran R, Tattersfield AE. Descriptors of breathlessness in patients with cancer and other cardiorespiratory diseases. *J Pain Symptom Manage* 2002; **23**(3):182–9.

30. O'Donnell DE, Chau LL, Bertley J, Webb KA. Qualitative aspects of exertional breathlessness in CAL: Pathophysiological mechanisms. *Am J Respir Crit Care Med* 1997; **155**:109–15.

31. O'Donnell DE, Chau LKL, Webb KA. Qualitative aspects of exertional dyspnea in interstitial lung disease. *J Appl Physiol* 1998; **84**:2000–9.

32. D'Arsigny C, Raj S, Abdollah H, Webb KA, O'Donnell DE. Ventilatory assistance improves leg discomfort and exercise endurance in stable congestive heart failure (CHF). *Am J Respir Crit Care Med* 1998; **157**:A451.

33. Mahler DA, Harver A. A factor analysis of dyspnea ratings, respiratory muscle strength and lung function in patients with COPD. *Am Rev Respir Dis* 1992; **145**(2 Pt 1):467–70.

34. Eakin EG, Kaplan RM, Ries AL, Sassi-Dambron DE. Patients' self reports of dyspnea: an important and independent outcome in COPD. *Ann Behav Med* 1996; **18**(2):87–90.

35. Hajiro T, Nishimura K, Tsukino M, Ikeda A, Koyama H, Izumi T. Analysis of clinical methods used to evaluate dyspnea in patients with COPD. *Am J Respir Crit Care Med* 1998; **158**(4):1185–9.

36. Harty HR, Adams L. Assessment of dyspnoea in research. In Ahmedzai S, Muers M (eds) *Supportive Care in Respiratory Disease*, pp. 123–34. Oxford University Press, 2005.

37. Gift AG. Validation of a vertical visual analogue scale as a measure of clinical dyspnea. *Rehabil Nurs* 1989; **14**(6):323–5.

38. Mancini I, Body JJ. Assessment of dyspnea in advanced cancer patients. *Support Care Cancer* 1999; **7**(4):229–32.

39. Aitken RCB. Measurement of feelings using visual analogue scales. *Proc R Soc Med* 1969; **62**:989–93.

40. Gift AG, Narsavage GL. Validity of the numeric rating scale as a measure of dyspnea. *Am J Crit Care* 1998; **7**(3): 200–4.

41. Dhand R, Kalra S, Malik SK. Use of visual analogue scales for assessment of the severity of asthma. *Respiration* 1988; **54**:255–62.

42. Wilson RC, Jones PW. A comparison of the Visual Analogue Scale and Modified Borg Scale for the measurement of dyspnea during exercise. *Clin Sci (Colch)* 1989; **76**:277–82.

43. Mador MJ, Kufel TJ. Reproducibility of Visual Analogue Scale measurements of dyspnea in patients with chronic obstructive pulmonary disease. *Am Rev Respir Dis* 1992; **146**:82–7.

44. Muza SR, Silverman MT, Gilmore GC, Hellerstein HK, Kelsen SG. Comparison of scales used to quantitate the sense of effort to breathe in patients with COPD. *Am Rev Respir Dis* 1990; **141**: 909–13.

45. Gift AG. Validation of a vertical visual analogue scale as a measure of clinical dyspnea. *Am Rev Respir Dis* 1986; **133**(4, Part 2): A163.

46. Gift AG. Clinical measurement of dyspnea. *Dimens Crit Care Nurs* 1989; **8**(4):210–16.

47. Guyatt GH, Townsend M, Berman LB, Keller JL. A comparison of Likert and visual analogue scales for measuring change in function. *J Chronic Dis* 1987; **40**(12):1129–33.

48. Dudgeon DJ, Kristjanson L, Sloan JA, Lertzman M, Clement K. Dyspnea in cancer patients: prevalence and associated factors. *J Pain Symptom Manage* 2001; **21**(2):95–102.

49. Reuben DB, Mor V. Dyspnea in terminally ill cancer patients. *Chest* 1986; **89**:234–6.

50. Borg GAV. Psychophysical Basis of Perceived Exertion. *Med Sci Sports Exerc* 1982; **14**(5): 377–81.

51. Wolkove N, Dajczman E, Colacone A, Kreisman H. The relationship between pulmonary function and dyspnea in obstructive lung disease. *Chest* 1989; **96**:1247–51.

52. Burdon J, Juniper E, Killian K, Hargeave F, Campbell E. The perception of breathlessness. *Am Rev Respir Dis* 1982; **126**:825–8.

53. Lush MT, Janson-Bjerklie S, Carrieri-Kohlman V, Lovejoy N. Dyspnea in the ventilator-assisted patient. *Heart Lung* 1988; **17**(5):528–35.

54. Adams L, Chronos N, Guz A. The measurement of breathlessness induced in normal subjects: validity of two scaling techniques. *Clin Sci* 1985; **69**:7–16.

55. Kendrick KR, Baxi SC, Smith RM. Usefulness of the modifed 0–10 Borg Scale in assessing the degree of dyspnea in patients with COPD and asthma. *J Emerg Nurs* 2000; **26**:216–22.

56. Wilson RC, Jones PW. Long term reproducibility of Borg Scale estimates of breathlessness during exercise. *Clin Sci* 1991; **80**:309–12.

57. O'Donnell DE, Lam M, Webb KA. Measurement of Symptoms, Lung Hyperinflation, and Endurance during Exercise in Chronic Obstructive Pulmonary Disease. *Am J Respir Crit Care Med* 1998; **158**:1557–65.

58. Campbell ML. Psychometric testing of a respiratory distress observation scale. *J Palliat Med* 2008; **11**(1):44–50.

59. Wilcock A, Corcoran R, Tattersfield AE. Safety and efficacy of nebulized lignocaine in patients with cancer and breathlessness. *Palliat Med* 1994; **8**:35–8.

60. van der Molen B. Dyspnoea: a study of measurement instruments for the assessment of dyspnoea and their application for patients with advanced cancer. *J Advance Nurs* 1995; **22**:948–56.

61. Killian KJ. Assessment of dyspnoea. *Eur Respir J* 1988; **1**(3):195–7.

62. ATS/ERS. Standards for the diagnosis and treatment of patients with COPD: a summary of the ATS/ERS position paper. *Eur Respir J* 2004; **23**:932–46.

63. Bestall JC, Paul EA, Garrod R, Garnham R, Jones PW, Wedzicha J. Usefulness of the Medical Research Council (MRC) dyspnea scale as a measure of disability in patients with COPD. *Thorax* 1999; **54**(7):581–6.

64. Hajiro T, Nishimura K, Tsukino M, Ikeda A, Oga A, Izumi T. A comparison of the level of dyspnea vs disease severity in indicating the health-related quality of life of patients with COPD. *Chest* 1999; **116**:1632–7.

65. Nishimura K, Izumi T, Tsukino M, Oga A. Dyspnea is a better predictor of 5-year survival than airway obstruction in patients with COPD. *Chest* 2002; **121**:1434–40.

66. Mahler DA, Rosiello RA, Harver A, Lentine T, McGovern JF, Daubenspeck JA. Comparison of clinical dyspnea ratings and psychophysical measurements of respiratory sensation in obstructive airway disease. *Am Rev Respir Dis* 1987; **135**:1229–33.

67. Mahler DA, Harver A, Rosiello RA, Daubenspeck JA. Measurement of respiratory sensation in interstitial lung disease. *Chest* 1989; **96**:767–71.

68. McGavin CR, Artvinli M, Naoe H, McHardy G. Dyspnoea, Disability and distance walked: comparison of estimates of exercise performance in respiratory disease. *Br Med J* 1978; **2**:241–3.

69. Wilcock A, Crosby V, Clarke D, Corcoran R, Tattersfield AE. Reading numbers aloud: a measure of the limiting effect of breathlessness in patients with cancer. *Thorax* 1999; **54**(12):1099–103.

70. Mahler DA, Faryniarz K, Tomlinson D, *et al.* Impact of dyspnea and physiologic function on general health status in patients with chronic obstructive pulmonary disease. *Chest* 1992; **102**(2):395–401.

71. Mahler DA, Matthay RA, Snyder PE, Wells CK, Loke J. Sustained-release theophylline reduces dyspnea in nonreversible obstructive airway disease. *Am Rev Respir Dis* 1985; **131**:22–5.

72. O'Donnell DE, McGuire M, Samis L, Webb KA. The impact of exercise reconditioning on breathlessness in severe chronic airflow limitation. *Am J Respir Crit Care Med* 1995; **152**:2005–13.

73. Reardon J, Awad E, Normandin E, Vale F, Clark B, Zu Wallack RL. The effect of comprehensive outpatient pulmonary rehabilitation on dyspnea. *Chest* 1994; **105**(4):1046–52.

74. Mahler DA, Tomlinson D, Olmstead EM, Tosteson AN, O'Connor GT. Changes in dyspnea, health status, and lung function in chronic airway disease. *Am J Respir Crit Care Med* 1995; **151**(1):61–5.

75. Mahler DA, Ward J, Fierro-Carrion G, Waterman LA, Lentine T, Mejia-Alfaro R. Development of self-administered versions of modified baseline and transition dyspnea indexes in COPD. *J COPD* 2004; **1**(2):165–72.

76. Lareau SC, Carrieri-Kohlman V, Janson-Bjerklie S, Roos PJ. Development and testing of the Pulmonary Functional Status and Dyspnea Questionnaire (PFSDQ). *Heart Lung* 1994; **23**(3): 242–50.

77. Lareau SC, Meek PM, Roos PJ. Development and testing of the modified version of the pulmonary functional status and dyspnea questionnaire (PFSDQ-M). *Heart Lung* 1998; **27**(3): 159–68.

78. Lareau SC, Meek PM, Press D, Anholm JD, Roos PJ. Dyspnea in patients with chronic obstructive pulmonary disease: does dyspnea worsen longitudinally in the presence of declining lung function? *Heart Lung* 1999; **28**(1):65–73.

79. Eakin EG, Sassi-Dambron DE, Ries AL, Kaplan RM. Reliability and validity of dyspnea measures in patients with obstructive lung disease. *Int J Behav Med* 1995; **2**:118–34.

80. Eakin EG, Resnikoff PM, Prewitt LM, Ries AL, Kaplan RM. Validation of a new dyspnea measure: The UCSD Shortness of Breath Questionnaire. University of California, San Diego. *Chest* 1998; **113**(3):619–24.

81. Ries AL, Kaplan RM, Limberg TM, Prewitt LM. Effects of pulmonary rehabilitation on physiologic and psychosocial outcomes in patients with COPD. *Ann Intern Med* 1995; **122**(11): 823–32.

82. Weaver TE, Narsavage GL. Physiological and psychological variables related to functional status in COPD. *Nursing Res* 1992; **43**:286–91.

83. Weaver TE, Richmond RS, Narsavage GL. An explanatory model of functional status in COPD. *Nursing Res* 1997; **46**:26.

84. Normandin E, McCusker C, Connors M, Vale F, Gerardi D, Zu Wallack RL. An evaluation of two approaches to exercise conditioning in pulmonary rehabilitation. *Chest* 2002; **121**(4): 1085–91.

85. Tanaka K, Akechi T, Okuyama T, Nishiwaki Y, Uchitomi Y. Development and validation of the Cancer Dyspnoea Scale: a multidimensional, brief, self-rating scale. *Br J Cancer* 2000; **82**(4): 800–5.

86. Dorman S, Byrne A, Edwards A. Which measurement scales should we use to measure breathlessness in palliative care? A systematic review. *Palliat Med* 2007; **21**:177–91.

87. Mahler DA. How should health-related quality of life be assessed in COPD? *Chest* 2000; **117**: 54–75.

88. Jones PW, Quirk FH, Baveystock CM. The St George's Respiratory Questionnaire. *Respir Med* 1991; **85**(Supplement B):25–31.

89. Bergner M, Bobbitt RA, Carter WB, Gison BS. The Sickness Impact Profile: development and final revision of a health status measure. *Medical Care* 1981; **19**:878–95.

90. Jones PW, Baveystock CM, Littlejohns P. Relationships between general health measured with the Sickness Impact Profile and respiratory symptoms, physiological measures and mood in patients with chronic airflow limitation. *Am Rev Respir Dis* 1989; **140**:1538–43.

91. Ware JE, Sherbourne CD. The MOS 36-item short-form health survey (SF-36). I. Conceptual framework and item selection. *Medical Care* 1992; **30**:473–83.

92. Ware JE, Gandek B. Overview of the SF-36 Health Survey & the International Quality of Life Assessment (IQOLA) Project. *J Clin Epidemiol* 1998; **51**:903–12.

93. Guyatt GH, Berman L, Townsend M, Pugsley S, Chambers L. A measure of quality of life for clinical trials in chronic lung disease. *Thorax* 1987; **42**:773–8.

94. Stulbarg MS, Carrieri-Kohlman V, Demir-Deviren S, *et al.* Exercise training improves outcomes of a dyspnea self-management program. *J Cardiopulm Rehabil* 2002; **22**:109–21.

95. Wijkstra PJ, TenVergert EM, Van Altena R, *et al.* Reliability and validity of the chronic respiratory questionnaire (CRQ). *Thorax* 1994; **49**:405–67.

96. Guyatt GH, Townsend M, Pugsley S. Bronchodilators in chronic airflow limitation: effect on airway function, exercise capacity, and quality of life. *Am Rev Respir Dis* 1987; **135**:1069–74.

97. Jaeschke R, Singer J, Guyatt GH. Measurements of health status: ascertaining the minimal clinically important difference. *Contr Clin Trials* 1989; **10**:407–15.

98. Jones PW, Quirk FH, Baveystock CM, Littlejohns P. A self-complete measure of health status for chronic airflow limitation. The St George's Respiratory Questionnaire. *Am Rev Respir Dis* 1992; **145**:1321–7.

99. Jones PW, Bosh TK. Quality of life changes in COPD patients treated with Salmeterol. *Am J Respir Crit Care Med* 1997; **155**:1283–9.

100. Jones PW. Dyspnea and quality of life in chronic obstructive pulmonary disease. In Mahler D (ed) *Dyspnea*, pp. 199–220. New York: Marcel Dekker, Inc., 1998.

101. Molken MR, Roos B, Van Noord JA. An empirical comparison of the St George's Respiratory Questionnaire (SGRQ) and the Chronic Respiratory Disease Questionnaire (CRQ) in a clinical trial setting. *Thorax* 1999; **54**(11):995–1003.

102. Nekolaichuk CL, Bruera E, Spachinsky K. A comparison of patient and proxy symptom assessments in advanced cancer patients. *J Pain Symptom Manage* 1998; **15**:S10.

103. Higginson IJ, McCarthy M. Validity of the support team assessment schedule: do staffs' ratings reflect those made by patients or their families? *Palliat Med* 1993; **7**(3):219–28.

Part 3

General supportive interventions

Chapter 7

Pharmacological treatment of respiratory symptoms

David C. Currow and Amy P. Abernethy

Dyspnoea: definitions and prevalence

Dyspnoea is a complex, subjective, somatopsychic experience generated by a mismatch of peripheral input with central response; the efferent drive to stimulate muscles or respiration is out of proportion to the afferent signals from chemo or mechanoreceptors (1). Like other symptoms, there are discrete components to the sensation. Work over the last 15 years has progressively established different trajectories for the unpleasantness of breathlessness and its intensity in both healthy volunteers and people with underlying cardiopulmonary pathology (2, 3). Like pain, the interaction of physical, psychological, and existential components of breathlessness are not easily delineated, leading to a concept of 'total breathlessness' (4).

Chronic or episodic breathlessness remains a stark reminder of underlying pathologies. The subjective nature of the sensation means that there is still very poor correlation between objective measures of respiratory compromise, and the measured subjective sensation reported by patients. Gross or rapid changes in homeostasis (increased $PaCO_2$, increased pH, or decreased PaO_2), space-occupying lesions, and substantial fluid accumulation are associated strongly with changes in breathlessness, but in the chronic setting, the way that breathlessness is perceived is still widely variable (5). In a clinical context, breathlessness is an independent prognostic factor; for example, in people with advanced cancer, persistent dyspnoea predicts impending death with a hazard ratio of 2.04 (95% confidence interval (CI), 1.26–3.31; p <0.01) (6).

The prevalence and the intensity of chronic breathlessness experienced across the whole community has been reported independent of health service utilization; population-based data in South Australia suggests that 9% of individuals in the community experience chronic breathlessness that limits exertion (7, 8). In people who have life-limiting illnesses, the prevalence and intensity increases dramatically, especially in the weeks leading to death and despite treatment for the symptom. Among palliative care patients reporting dyspnoea in the 3 months leading to death, the prevalence of 'no breathlessness' decreased from 50% to 35%, and the proportion of patients with 'severe breathlessness' (>7 out of 10 on a numerical rating scale) increased from 10% to 26% (9).

Clinically, severe chronic or episodic breathlessness rarely has a single cause, with multiple organ systems usually involved. Even when there is a single identifiable clinical cause, there are likely to be emotional and social factors that influence the subjective sensation (4). Ultimately, chronic breathlessness is a constant reminder of mortality, and the tenuous nature of existence. The cycle of emotion (anxiety, anger, frustration)/breathlessness/emotion heightens the sense of threat generated by ongoing dyspnoea.

In considering the pharmacological management of chronic dyspnoea, the concept of dyspnoea being 'intractable' or 'refractory' is an important factor to acknowledge (10). When reversible causes have been optimally addressed, the remaining quantum of breathlessness is the 'refractory' or 'intractable' component. Evidence of respiratory effort or distress is a clinical sign and often described as dyspnoea while, by definition, the symptom of breathlessness is entirely subjective. While diagnosing and addressing the aetiologies of breathlessness, it is important to treat the symptom of breathlessness in parallel. When reasonably reversible causes of breathlessness have been excluded, the symptom needs to be treated aggressively given that it intrudes on every aspect of a person's life.

Pharmacological interventions for the symptom of breathlessness are typically divided into those directed at the underlying disease such as steroids, diuretics, and bronchodilators, and more general interventions indicated by the symptom without reference to the underlying disease such as opioids and oxygen. This chapter is about the symptomatic management of breathlessness, not the methods of treating underlying reversible pathologies. Alone, or in combination, the more general interventions have the strongest evidence to support their use in the symptomatic sensation of breathlessness.

Opioids

Regular, low-dose opioids, particularly morphine, have the strongest evidence base underpinning their role in the pharmacological management of dyspnoea, including both basic scientific and clinical research data. Recent major shifts have occurred in how this evidence is viewed by the clinical community, with opioids now receiving endorsement from respiratory physicians in a way that has not been the case before (11).

Systemic opioids
Mechanisms of action
The mechanisms of action through which opioids relieve dyspnoea are still not well defined. There is a central component that helps to reduce breathlessness, but whether part of this is a cortical anxiolytic effect remains unknown. Whether there are additional peripheral actions of opioids is also not clear at this time. Physiologically, opioids can reduce ventilatory response to several stimuli including increased levels of carbon dioxide (12), hypoxaemia (13, 14), exercise (15), and inspiratory flow-resistive loading (16).

The central effect of opioids mediating breathlessness has recently been characterized *in vivo*. A randomized controlled trial comparing naloxone with normal saline explored the exercise capacity of people with moderate to severe chronic obstructive pulmonary disease (COPD) that were *not* on exogenous opioids. Without affecting exercise tolerance, people had more dyspnoea for the same workload when randomized to naloxone. Naloxone is a centrally acting opioid antagonist, and in this trial it is assumed to be antagonizing the effects of endogenous opioids. This landmark study helps to define the role of endogenous opioids, and suggests that exogenous opioids can have a role without necessarily compromising respiratory function (17). These findings corroborate studies from over 30 years ago, where, in healthy volunteers, morphine was demonstrated to reduce oxygen consumption at rest and on exertion (15). Similarly, these findings support data that demonstrate that people with severe COPD have higher circulating levels of beta-endorphins than healthy age-matched controls (18).

Central nervous system areas responding to breathlessness

One mechanism that can create the subjective sensation of breathlessness is air hunger. Functional magnetic resonance imaging (fMRI) has been used *in vivo* to determine the areas of increased neuronal activity in the brain when air hunger is induced in healthy volunteers. Air hunger was generated by reducing tidal volume and several regions were shown to have increased neuronal response: the limbic and paralimbic regions including the insula, cingulate gyrus, and amygdala. These are areas of the central nervous system that share a common response to noxious or threatening stimuli including pain, hunger, and thirst, and are richly invested with opioid receptors (19). Interestingly, the respiratory depressant effect of mu opioid agonists is likely, in part, due to their action on central chemoreceptors in the midline medullary raphe and the nucleus tractus solitarus in the dorsal medulla (20). Painful stimuli appear to reverse the respiratory depressant effects mediated through these pathways by stimulating breathing. Together these fMRI studies of neurocorrelates for dyspnoea and pain suggest similar central neural processing, and support the dual role of opioids in dyspnoea and pain.

Peripherally, opioid receptors are extremely widespread including in the peripheral chemoreceptors in type I glomus cells in the carotid bodies (where hypoxaemic ventilatory suppression is a significant response together with interactions with hypercapnia) the vagus nerve, and mechanosensory receptors throughout the lungs (epithelial, submucosal, and muscularis layers of airways) (21). Any clinical action mediated through peripheral opioid receptors has yet to be elucidated.

Clinical use

Low-dose, regular systemic opioids (orally or parenterally) have been shown to reduce intractable breathlessness in people with a range of underlying aetiologies, but predominantly in people with COPD and cancer. The opioid used almost exclusively in these studies has been morphine. A meta-analysis demonstrated a net clinical benefit of morphine when compared with a placebo (22). The authors found a statistically significant effect of regular oral and parenteral opioids on the sensation of breathlessness (overall pooled effect size, -0.31; 95% CI, -0.50 to -0.13; $p=0.0008$) when compared to placebo. However, the clinical benefit across all participants was relatively modest (approximately 8mm on a 100-mm visual analogue scale (VAS), with baseline breathlessness levels of 50mm) (22).

The magnitude of the findings of the meta-analysis were confirmed by an adequately powered, cross-over, randomized, placebo-controlled, fixed dose trial of 20mg sustained release oral morphine each morning in opioid naïve people with intractable dyspnoea, mostly with COPD as the underlying aetiology (10). For study purposes, intractable or refractory was defined as residual dyspnoea when all underlying causes had been treated optimally. Participants had a mean age of 76 (standard deviation (SD)=5) with 71% already on long-term home oxygen therapy. Eligible patients were clinically stable for at least 1 week preceding randomization, with stable medications and stable oxygen needs. This 8-day study saw people swap between an active arm (morning low dose sustained release morphine) and a placebo. Participants spent 4 days on each arm and key measures were from the last day on each arm to allow for washout after cross-over.

Participants receiving morphine had a significant reduction in breathlessness, with mean improvements in dyspnoea intensity of 6.6mm in the morning (p=0.011; trough plasma levels) and 9.5mm in the evening (p=0.006; peak plasma levels). Relative improvement over baseline dyspnoea was between 15% and 22%. Because it was a cross-over study of relatively short duration, blinded preference by participants was sought. Preference was more likely to be for morphine than for the placebo arm. While on the morphine arm, people also reported significantly better quality of sleep (p=0.039).

The main side effect of opioids was constipation (p=0.021) but importantly, no sedation, obtundation or respiratory depression were reported at this dose, with resting respiratory rates identical on the fourth day. It is critical to treat the constipation expectantly. Unpublished data from this study suggests that breathlessness was not improved until morphine-related constipation was relieved.

Such evidence is shifting the recommendations of key bodies. The Global initiative on Obstructive Lung Disease suggests that opioids should only be used *in extremis*. By contrast, a landmark position statement from the American College of Chest of Physicians for the first time explicitly endorses the use of individually titrated regular opioids in the control of breathlessness for people with advanced cardiorespiratory diseases (11).

In cancer-related dyspnoea, a systematic review concluded that oral or parenteral systemic opioids can be used to manage dyspnoea in cancer patients (23, 24). Although most studies of dyspnoea include participants with a range of underlying aetiologies, the randomized controlled studies testing systemic opioids that exclusively include people with cancer are relatively small (25, 26).

A major continuing concern about the use of opioids for breathlessness has been respiratory depression. When used regularly and in low doses, the literature is absolutely silent on toxicity. The systematic review of opioids for the relief of refractory breathlessness also reports that in 11 of the 18 studies cited, that oxygenation and carbon dioxide levels did not change with the introduction of opioids (22). When data including respiratory rate, oxygen saturation, and carbon dioxide levels are collected, respiratory compromise has not been demonstrated for people receiving low doses of opioids, even when they are opioid naïve when the medications are initiated. Opioids studied with these measures include both morphine and hydromorphone (23–29). Respiratory depression was not reported in a more recent study looking at rapid titration to achieve a 50% reduction in breathlessness over baseline in people who were acutely short of breath in the palliative setting within a 90 minute period (30). To date, the majority of concern about opioid-related respiratory depression has been extrapolated from acute care settings where (relatively) large doses of intravenous opioids are administered to opioid-naïve patients predominantly for pain; to date, there are not compelling data that these risks transfer to the setting of low dose regularly prescribed opioid for dyspnoea (10,31). Rigorous prospective pharmacovigilance studies could help to address such concerns.

The next most widely studied opioid is dihydrocodeine with evidence from four placebo-controlled trials. These are all much older, shorter studies often with much higher doses of medications. There have been no demonstrated advantages in using dihydrocodeine over morphine especially as the only adequately powered study of opioids uses a once daily preparation of oral morphine that was not available in the 1980s (32–35).

Of note, despite a number of small studies, no evidence points to predictable benefit at a population level from nebulized opioids even when the data are brought together in a meta-analysis (22). A definitive study has not been done, nor has the underlying science of airways opioid receptors been resolved in a way that suggests the study is likely to be positive.

Psychotropic medications

Given the complex aetiology of the sensation of breathlessness, it is reasonable to postulate that psychotropic medications may demonstrate some benefits in selected patients. Psychotropic agents have been used to treat refractory dyspnoea based on the assumptions that: 1) dyspnoea contains a large psychological component, and 2) anxiety significantly contributes to the functional impairment associated with breathlessness (36). Psychotropic drugs used in dyspnoea management have included anxiolytics (benzodiazepines, buspirone), phenothiazines (promethazine, prochlorperazine), and selective serotonin reuptake inhibitors (SSRIs). A wide range of study designs and clinical endpoints have been used, making comparisons problematic.

Of these medications, data support the need for further study of sertraline, promethazine and buspirone.

Benzodiazepines

Benzodiazepines are widely used in the treatment of breathlessness especially when the onset is relatively rapid (23, 37). If anxiety is a contributing factor to acute onset of breathlessness, short term use of benzodiazepines seems reasonable. Onset of action and duration of benefit are probably the main factors that help to distinguish the choice of a specific benzodiazepine. Despite widespread use, a recent systematic review concluded that there was insufficient evidence to support the routine use of this class of medications currently for the routine management of breathlessness (37).

The earliest prospective studies suggested that benzodiazepines were likely to have marginal benefit (34, 38). Diazepam has been studied for its anxiolytic effects on breathlessness. A small study by Mitchell-Heggs et al. reported a 'striking reduction in dyspnoea' for four people with severe COPD (39).

Two recent studies by Navigante and his team have explored the role of benzodiazepines for breathlessness in prospective studies (40). In the first of these studies,

101 people in the last days of life with breathlessness who were opioid and benzodiazepine naïve were offered morphine 2.5mg 4-hourly, midazolam 5.0mg 4-hourly, or the combination of both. The study found improved dyspnoea intensity compared with baseline with each medication and the combination of the two. However, there were no between-treatment differences in the three arms. These were relatively large doses for people who had not been exposed to these medications before, and the safety of this approach has been questioned. Importantly, the study was conducted in an inpatient setting where patients were carefully monitored, and patients were very near end of life.

Another study explored relief of acute breathlessness in outpatients with cancer who were undergoing diagnostic work-up to define the cause of worsening breathlessness. Patients with heart failure or worsening COPD were excluded if this was the cause of their progressive dyspnoea (30). This single-blinded, randomized study compared oral midazolam with oral immediate release morphine solution over a 5-day period following a rapid titration phase at the time they presented with shortness of breath for assessment. Titration sought a 50% reduction in baseline breathlessness on a five-point categorical scale. Participants received between 2mg and 7.5mg of oral midazolam over a 1-hour period, or between 3mg and 10.5 mg of immediate release oral morphine solution, with final assessment at 90min after commencing therapy. If already on opioids, participants were offered 25% increments over baseline, but this was not replicated for people on benzodiazepines. All participants responded to the fast titration protocol with a >50% reduction in breathlessness, thereby defining their fourth hourly dose for the remaining 5 days on study.

In the rapid titration phase, participants were much more likely to respond to midazolam with 64% deriving a 50% or greater benefit with the first dose of medication compared with 35% who received morphine (p=0.023). This benefit was maintained across the study period. During follow-up over the next 4 days, there were significantly lower dyspnoea scores for the midazolam group, and significantly fewer breakthrough doses taken.

This paper outlines a very specific type of acute breathlessness and the ability to extrapolate these findings to chronic, intractable breathlessness is limited, especially given the potential for tachyphylaxis in other uses of benzodiazepines. The dose equivalence of the chosen doses of midazolam and morphine solution need to be established in this population in order to ensure the comparison is fair. The number of breakthrough doses taken and the regular doses for each arm are not given, making application of the findings into clinical practice difficult (41).

Man et al. investigated the use of alprazolam, a shorter-acting and theoretically less sedating (but potentially more addictive) medication than diazepam, for reducing breathlessness. This placebo-controlled, double-blind study randomized 24 participants with COPD to alprazolam (0.5mg twice a day) or placebo administered for 1 week, followed by placebo for 1 week, then the opposite arm for the final week. Maximum exercise level attained, distance covered in the 12-minute walk test, and subjective perception of dyspnoea remained unchanged while on alprazolam (42). A study by Eimer et al. of clorazepate was closed due to intolerable side effects (43).

Buspirone

Buspirone, a serotonergic anxiolytic agent, is a respiratory stimulant in animals (44, 45). Two small studies in people with severe COPD (46, 47) evaluated buspirone on exercise tolerance, breathlessness, and anxiety. The study populations differed: Singh et al. (47) required that participants were diagnosed with anxiety (as per the Speilberger State-Trait Anxiety Inventory Scale (STAI)) while Argyropoulou et al. (46) did not assess anxiety. Although Singh et al. found no difference, Argyropoulou et al. documented improvement in all three domains. These data suggest that larger, prospective randomized studies may be justified in people with severe, ongoing breathlessness, but that the studies need to explicitly include assessments of anxiety and stratification by baseline level of anxiety.

Phenothiazines

Promethazine has been suggested as a second-line pharmacological agent in people who have not responded to opioids, or as a first-line therapy in people who have a contraindication to opioids (23). The evidence for this is still extremely limited. Presumably the mechanism of action here is indirect; promethazine blocks dopamine, producing sedation, and thus may alleviate the anxiety that underlies or exacerbates dyspnoea in some patients.

The studies that evaluate this medication are small. Woodcock et al. evaluated diazepam/placebo and then promethazine/placebo in 18 people with COPD in a double blind, placebo-controlled, cross over study. Twenty-five milligrams daily of diazepam caused unacceptable drowsiness while 125mg of promethazine appeared to reduce breathlessness at 2 weeks. Exercise tolerance appeared to be better in the promethazine arm.

Rice et al. investigated 11 participants in a double-blind, randomized, cross-over study of 120mg codeine daily or promethazine 100mg daily each in four divided doses (48). Participants spent 1 month on each arm. No differences were noted between arms in 12-minute walk or subjective breathlessness, and in the absence of a control arm, it is difficult to draw conclusions that can influence practice.

Light et al used a double-blind, cross-over study evaluating exercise tolerance in people with moderate to severe COPD comparing single dose morphine 30mg orally with morphine/promethazine (25mg) and morphine/prochlorperazine (25mg) (49). Exercise tolerance increased in the morphine/promethazine arm, although the total number of participants was only seven.

Antidepressants

There is evidence to suggest that clinically important depression is under-recognized and hence undertreated, especially in people with COPD (50, 51) and that, as such, antidepressants may deliver clinical benefit for the management of dyspnoea. SSRIs have an anxiolytic effect and for many people, progressively worsening breathlessness causes a breathlessness/anxiety/breathlessness cycle that can become overwhelming. A potential target of action for SSRIs has been identified in the brainstem (52). Tricyclics are the other class of medications that have been studied.

For SSRIs, four studies point to potential benefits that need to be confirmed in larger prospective randomized controlled studies: one small, blinded, randomized trial of paroxetine (53) and three case series (even in people who may not be depressed or anxious). These small case series (n=7, 6, and 6) explored paroxetine, sertraline and citalopram (54–56). Optimal dosing or whether the benefit is maintained in the longer term has not been defined for any of the agents studied.

Lacasse et al. enrolled 23 people in a 12-week double-blind, placebo-controlled, parallel arm trial of paroxetine in people with moderate to severe intensity of breathlessness and mild to moderate depression not necessitating treatment immediately (53). Although 105 people were deemed eligible following screening, only 23 people consented of whom only 15 people completed the protocol. In the intervention arm, paroxetine was started at 5mg daily and increased by 5mg weekly to a maximum of 20mg. Lower doses were allowed if side effects precluded the maximum dose. The four subdomains of the Chronic Respiratory Questionnaire were used to assess response. The reported analysis was on a per protocol basis rather than intention-to-treat. In outcomes, subdomains of mastery and emotional function improved significantly in the intervention group, while dyspnoea and fatigue trended in the direction of benefit. This may well be a type I error that can be directly addressed with a larger study sample in the future. (Of note, the proposed sample size for this study was for 126 completed participants.) There is still much to be learned about potential role in SSRIs contributing to the management of breathlessness, and more clinical studies are warranted.

Among tricyclic antidepressants, two studies stand out both suggesting that this class of antidepressants probably does not have the same magnitude of benefit as SSRIs. In a double-blind, parallel arm, randomized trial involving 30 people with moderate to severe COPD as their most significant medical problem and depression diagnosed by a psychiatrist using Diagnostics and Statistical Manual (DSM) III criteria, nortriptyline up to 1mg/kg/day was compared with placebo (57). After 4 weeks of upward titration, 8 weeks of steady state administration followed. Breathlessness was assessed using the Pulmonary Functional Status Instrument (PFSI) and standardized exercise testing. There were no differences in dyspnoea at rest or after a 12-minute walk test. Distressing respiratory sensations including feelings of suffocation and exhaustion were less in the nortriptyline arm than the control arm (5.4 ± 0.6 mm reduction; p=0.04). Activities of daily living that cause low levels of breathlessness were statistically significantly better in the intervention arm; however, there were a large number of factors analysed and few significant findings leaving open the risk that this was a type II error. The unpleasantness of breathlessness (compared with the intensity of breathlessness) may be a target for further studies of antidepressants (2).

Another study examined protriptyline 10mg nocte in a multisite, double-blind, placebo-controlled, parallel arm study in people with COPD and mild or moderate hypoxaemia (58). Participants were recruited to a 16-week study with 4 weeks of upward titration and 12 weeks of steady state medication. The primary outcomes included dyspnoea scores, quality of life, and changes in spirometry. A total of 19 people of the 45 enrolled were withdrawn from the study during titration because of worsening partial pressure of arterial oxygen during titration. The report of the study fails to make clear whether this was a clinically significant deterioration, especially given that tricyclics are not contraindicated in people with COPD. Twelve people were evaluable in each arm. Dyspnoea was measured on a seven-point categorical scale and no differences were seen between the groups to justify a larger study.

Inhaled furosemide

Although known for its diuretic properties, separately furosemide has been suggested as a theoretical intervention for breathlessness given its documented ability to prevent bronchoconstriction (59) and to limit vagally-mediated afferent input (60). Nebulized furosemide also has the potential to lessen the cough response (61). In healthy volunteers, documented differences after the administration of inhaled furosemide include improved breath-holding ability and a higher threshold before breathing is perceived as uncomfortable during loaded breathing (62). A recent systematic review suggested that there are not enough data to draw clinically applicable conclusions about the use of nebulized furosemide in relieving breathlessness (63).

In people with moderate or severe COPD (forced expiratory volume in 1s (FEV_1) <70%) and accompanying symptomatic breathlessness (n=19), a randomized study evaluated the effects of inhaled furosemide compared to placebo on exercise-induced dyspnoea (64). After exercise, average breathlessness scores on a visual analogue scale were lower in the furosemide group (34mm (SD 25) vs. 42 (SD 24); p=0.014). Exercise-related FEV_1 and forced vital capacity (FVC) also improved after furosemide inhalation (p=0.038 and 0.005, respectively) but not after placebo. This latter observation again raises the question of whether part of the perceived benefit is a bronchodilator effect.

Conclusions

The pharmacological management of breathlessness continues to evolve. Opioids have demonstrated benefit without documented respiratory toxicity. Several psychotropic agents and nebulized furosemide have sufficient promise to warrant rigorous prospective studies. Ultimately, reducing the frightening sensation of breathlessness is something that can be achieved predictably with medications currently available.

References

1. Mahler DA. Mechanisms and measurement of dyspnea in chronic obstructive pulmonary disease. *Proc Am Thorac Soc* 2006; **3**(3):234–8.
2. O'Donnell D, Banzett BB, Carrieri-Kohlman V *et al.* Pathophysiology of dyspnea in chronic obstructive pulmonary disease. A roundtable. *Proc Am Thorac Soc* 2007; **4**:145–68.
3. Williams MT, Cafarella P, Olds T, Petkov J, Frith P. The language of breathlessness differentiates between patients with chronic obstructive pulmonary disease and age-matched adults. *Chest* 2008; **134**:489–96.
4. Abernethy AP, Wheeler JL. Total dyspnoea. *Curr Opin Support Palliat Care* 2008; **2**(2):110–13.
5. Anon. Dyspnea. Mechanisms, assessment, and management: a consensus statement. American Thoracic Society. *Am J Respir Crit Care Med* 1999; **159**(1):321–40.

6. Hardy JR, Turner R, Saunders M, A'Hern R. Prediction of survival in a hospital-based continuing care unit. *Eur J Cancer* 1994; **30A**(3):284–8.

7. Hammond E. Some preliminary findings on physical complaints from a prospective study of 1,064,004 men and women. *Am J Pub Health* 1964; **54**:11–23.

8. Currow DC, Plummer J, Crockett A, Abernethy AP. A community population survey of prevalence and severity of dyspnoea in adults. *J Pain Symptom Manage* 2009; **38**(4):533–45.

9. Currow DC, Smith J, Davidson PM, Newton PJ, Agar MR, Abernethy AP. Do the trajectories of dyspnoea differ in prevalence and intensity by diagnosis at the end of life? A consecutive cohort study. *J Pain Symptom Manage* 2010; **39**(4):480–90.

10. Abernethy AP, Currow DC, Frith P, Fazekas BS, McHugh A, Bui C. Randomised, double blind, placebo controlled crossover trial of sustained release morphine for the management of refractory dyspnoea. *BMJ* 2003; **327**(7414):523–8.

11. Mahler DA, Selecky PA, Harrod CG, *et al.* American College of Chest Physicians consensus statement on the management of dyspnea in patients with advanced lung or heart disease. *Chest.* 2010; **137**(3):674–91.

12. Eckenhoff JE, Oech SR. The effects of narcotics and antagonists upon respiration and circulation in man. A review. *Clin Pharmacol Therapeut* 1960; **1**:483–524.

13. Santiago TV, Pugliese AC, Edelman NH. Control of breathing during methadone addiction. *Am J Med* 1977; **62**(3):347–54.

14. Weil JV, McCullough RE, Kline JS, Sodal IE. Diminished ventilatory response to hypoxia and hypercapnia after morphine in normal man. *N Engl J Med* 1975; **292**(21):1103–6.

15. Santiago TV, Johnson J, Riley DJ, Edelman NH. Effects of morphine on ventilatory response to exercise. *J Appl Physiol: Resp, Environ Ex Physiol* 1979; **47**(1):112–18.

16. Kryger MH, Yacoub O, Dosman J, Macklem PT, Anthonisen NR. Effect of meperidine on occlusion pressure responses to hypercapnia and hypoxia with and without external inspiratory resistance. *Am Rev Resp Dis* 1976; **114**(2):333–40.

17. Mahler DA, Murray JA, Waterman LA, Ward J, Kraemer WJ, Zhang X, Baird JC. Endogenous opioids modify dyspnoea during treadmill exercise in patients with COPD. *Eur Respir J* 2009; **33**(4):771–7.

18. Hjalmarsen A, Viitanen M, Jenssen T, Jorde R, Johansen O. Plasma beta-endorphin concentrations are increased in chronic obstructive pulmonary disease patients. *Scand J Clin Lab Invest.* 2000; **60**(6):501–6.

19. Evans KC, Banzett RB, Adams L, McKay L, Frackowiak RSJ, Corfield DR. BOLD fMRI identifies limbic, paralimbic, and cerebellar activation during air hunger. *J Neurophysiol* 2002; **88**(3):1500–11.

20. Bailey PL, Lu JK, Pace NL, *et al.* Effects of intrathecal morphine on the ventilatory response to hypoxia. *N Engl J Med* 2000; **343**:1228–34.

21. Pattinson KTS. Opioids and the control of respiration. *Br J Anaesth* 2008; **100** (6):747–58.

22. Jennings AL, Davies AN, Higgins JPT, Gibbs JSR, Broadley KE. A systematic review of the use of opioids in the management of dyspnoea. *Thorax* 2002; **57**(11):939–44.

23. Viola R, Kiteley C, Lloyd NS, *et al.* The management of dyspnea in cancer patients: a systematic review. *Support Care Cancer* 2008; **16**(4):329–37.

24. Ben-Aharon I, Gafter-Gvili A, Paul M *et al.* Interventions for alleviating cancer-related dyspnea: a systematic review. *J Clin Oncol* 2008; **26**:2396–404.

25. Bruera E, MacEachern T, Ripamonti C, Hanson J. Subcutaneous morphine for dyspnea in cancer patients. *Ann Intern Med* 1993; **119**(9): 906–7.

26. Mazzocato C, Buclin T, Rapin CH. The effects of morphine on dyspnea and ventilatory function in elderly patients with advanced cancer: a randomized double-blind controlled trial. *Ann Oncol* 1999; **10**(12):1511–14.

27. Clemens KE, Klaschik E. Symptomatic therapy of dyspnoea with strong opioids and its effect on ventilation in palliative care patients. *J Pain Symptom Manage* 2007; **33**(4):473–81.

28. Clemens KE, Klaschik E. Effect of hydromorphone on ventilation in palliative care patients with dyspnoea. *Support Care Cancer* 2008; **16**:93–9.

29. Estfan B, Mahmoud F, Shaheen P, *et al*. Respiratory function during parenteral opioid titration for cancer pain. *Pall Med* 2007; **21**:81–6.

30. Navigante AH, Castro MA, Cerchietti LC. Morphine versus midazolam as upfront therapy to control dyspnea perception in cancer patients while its underlying cause is sought or treated. *J Pain Symptom Manage* 2010; **39**(5):820–30.

31. Pauwels RA, Buist AS, Calverley PM, Jenkins CR, Hurd SS, Committee GS. Global strategy for the diagnosis, management, and prevention of chronic obstructive pulmonary disease. NHLBI/WHO Global Initiative for Chronic Obstructive Lung Disease (GOLD) Workshop summary. *Am J Resp Crit Care Med* 2001; **163**(5):1256–76.

32. Buck C, Laier-Groeneveld G, Criee CP. The effect of dihydrocodeine and terbutaline on breathlessness and inspiratory muscle function in normal subjects and patients with COPD (abstract). *Eur Respir J* 1996; **9**:344S.

33. Chua TP, Harrington D, Ponikowski P, Webb-Peploe K, Poole-Wilson PA, Coats AJ. Effects of dihydrocodeine on chemosensitivity and exercise tolerance in patients with chronic heart failure. *J Am Coll Cardiol* 1997; **29**(1):147–52.

34. Woodcock AA, Gross ER, Geddes DM. Drug treatment of breathlessness: contrasting effects of diazepam and promethazine in pink puffers. *Br Med J (Clin Res Ed)* 1981; **283**(6287):343–6.

35. Johnson MA, Woodcock AA, Geddes DM. Dihydrocodeine for breathlessness in 'pink puffers'. *Br Med J (Clin Res Ed)*. 1983; **286**(6366):675–7.

36. Kim HF, Kunik ME, Molinari VA, *et al*. Functional impairment in COPD patients: the impact of anxiety and depression. *Psychosomatics* 2000; **41**:465–71.

37. Simon ST, Higginson IJ, Booth S, Harding R, Bausewein C. Benzodiazepines for the relief of breathlessness in advanced malignant and non-malignant diseases in adults. *Cochrane Database Syst Rev* 2010; 1:CD007354.

38. Sen D, Jones G, Leggat PO. The response of the breathless patient treated with diazepam. *Br J Clin Pract* 1983; **37**(6):232–3.

39. Mitchell-Heggs P, Murphy K, Minty K, *et al*. Diazepam in the treatment of dyspnoea in the 'Pink Puffer' syndrome. *Quar J Med* 1980; **49**(193):9–20.

40. Navigante AH, Cerchietti LC, Castro MA, *et al*. Midazolam as adjunct therapy to morphine in the alleviation of severe dyspnea perception in patients with advanced cancer. *J Pain Symptom Manage* 2006; **31**(1):38–47.

41. Currow DC, Abernethy AP. Potential opioid sparing effects of benzodiazepines in breathlessness. *J Pain Symptom Manage* 2011; **41**(4):e2–3.

42. Man GC, Hsu K, Sproule BJ. Effect of alprazolam on exercise and dyspnea in patients with chronic obstructive pulmonary disease. *Chest* 1986; **90**(6):832–6.

43. Eimer M, Cable T, Gal P, Rothenberger LA, McCue JD. Effects of clorazepate on breathlessness and exercise tolerance in patients with chronic airflow obstruction. *J Fam Prac* 1985; **21**(5):359–62.

44. Garner SJ, Eldridge FL, Wagner PG, Dowell RT. Buspirone, an anxiolytic drug that stimulates respiration. *Am Rev Respir Dis* 1989; **139**(4):946–50.

45. Mendelson WB, Martin JV, Rapoport DM. Effects of buspirone on sleep and respiration. *Am Rev Respir Dis* 1990; **141**(6):1527–30.

46. Argyropoulou P, Patakas D, Koukou A, *et al*. Buspirone effect on breathlessness and exercise performance in patients with chronic obstructive pulmonary disease. *Respiration* 1993; **60**(4): 216–20.

47. Singh NP, Despars JA, Stansbury DW, *et al.* Effects of buspirone on anxiety levels and exercise tolerance in patients with chronic airflow obstruction and mild anxiety. *Chest* 1993; **103**(3):800–4.

48. Rice KL, Kronenberg RS, Hedemark LL, Niewoehner DE. Effects of chronic administration of codeine and promethazine on breathlessness and exercise tolerance in patients with chronic airflow obstruction. *Br J Dis Chest* 1987; **81**(3):287–92.

49. Light RW, Stansbury DW, Webster JS. Effect of 30 mg of morphine alone or with promethazine or prochlorperazine on the exercise capacity of patients with COPD. *Chest* 1996; **109**(4):975–81.

50. Light RW, Merrill EJ, Despars JA, Gordon GH, Mutalipassi LR. Prevalence of depression and anxiety in patients with COPD. Relationship to functional capcity. *Chest* 1985; **87**(1): 35–8.

51. Lacasse Y, Rousseau L, Maltais F. Prevalence of depressive symptoms and depression in patients with severe oxygen-dependent chronic obstructive pulmonary disease. *J Cardiopulm Rehabil* 2001; **21**:80–6.

52. Mueller RA, Lundberg DB, Breese GR, Hedner J, Hedner T, Jonason J. The neuropharmacology of respiratory control. *Pharmacol Rev* 1982; **34**(3):255–85.

53. Lacasse Y, Beaudoin L, Rousseau L, Maltais F. Randomized trial of paroxetine in end-stage COPD. *Monaldi Arch Chest Dis* 2004; **61**(3):140–7.

54. Smoller JW, Pollack MH, Systrom D, Kradin RL. Sertraline effects on dyspnea in patients with obstructive airways disease. *Psychosomatics* 1998; **39**(1):24–9.

55. Papp LA, Weiss JR, Greenberg HE, *et al.* Sertraline for chronic obstructive pulmonary disease and comorbid anxiety and mood disorders. *Am J Psychiatry* 1995; **152**(10):1531.

56. Perna G, Cogo R, Bellodi L. Selective serotonin re-uptake inhibitors beyond psychiatry: are they useful in the treatment of severe, chronic, obstructive pulmonary disease? *Depress Anxiety* 2004; **20**(4):203–4.

57. Borson S, McDonald GJ, Gayle T, Deffeback M, Lakshminarayan S, VanTuinen C. Improvement in mood, physical symptoms, and function with nortriptyline fo r depression in patients with chronic pulmonary disease. *Psychosomatics* 1992; **33**(2):190–210.

58. Ström K, Boman G, Pehrsson K, *et al.* Effect of protryptiline, 10mg daily, on chronic hypoxaemia in chronic obstructive pulmonary disease. *Eur Respir J* 1995; **8**:425–9.

59. Robuschi M, Gambaro G, Spagnotto S, Vaghi A, Bianco S. Inhaled frusemide is highly effective in preventing ultrasonically nebulised water bronchoconstriction. *Pul Pharmacol* 1989; **1**(4):187–91.

60. Chung KF, Barnes PJ. Loop diuretics and asthma. *Pul Pharmacol* 1992; **5**(1):1–7.

61. Ventresca PG, Nichol GM, Barnes PJ, Chung KF. Inhaled furosemide inhibits cough induced by low chloride content solutions but not by capsaicin. *Am Rev Resp Dis* 1990; **142**(1):143–6.

62. Nishino T, Ide T, Sudo T, *et al.* Inhaled furosemide greatly alleviates the sensation of experimentally induced dyspnea. *Am J Resp Crit Care Med* 2000; **161**(6):1963–7.

63. Newton PJ, Davidson PM, Macdonald P, Ollerton R, Krum H. Nebulized furosemide for the management of dyspnea: does the evidence support its use? *J Pain Symptom Manage* 2008; **36**(4):424–41.

64. Ong KC, Kor AC, Chong WF, Earnest A, Wang YT. Effects of inhaled furosemide on exertional dyspnea in chronic obstructive pulmonary disease. *Am J Resp Crit Care Med* 2004; **169**(9):1028–33.

Chapter 8

Oxygen and airflow

Christine McDonald and James Ward

Dyspnoea is one of the most distressing symptoms experienced by those with respiratory disease, impacting significantly upon the quality of their lives. Characterized as a subjective experience of breathing discomfort consisting of qualitatively distinct sensations that vary in intensity, dyspnoea appears to derive from interactions among multiple physiological, psychological, social, and environmental factors, and may induce secondary physiological and behavioural responses (1). In the last year of their lives as many as 94% of patients with chronic lung disease and 78% of patients with cancer will experience dyspnoea (2). As well as causing suffering to the person with the disease, the presence of dyspnoea in a loved one or patient can be extremely distressing to carer and clinician alike, causing frustration at their inability to adequately treat this most troubling of symptoms.

Oxygen is often used for relief of dyspnoea not responding to treatment of the underlying disease, even if the patient is not hypoxaemic. Despite the fact that various international consensus guidelines support this practice (1, 3, 4), evidence for the use of oxygen in this situation is sparse. Stronger evidence does exist for the use of oxygen therapy in those whose chronic dyspnoea is associated with hypoxaemia. However, the relationship between hypoxaemia and dyspnoea is not fully understood, with it being well recognized that chronic hypoxaemia is not always associated with dyspnoea and, similarly, that the dyspnoea experienced by such individuals may not relate to hypoxaemia.

In this chapter we will discuss the uses of oxygen therapy in the supportive care setting. This includes management of patients with conditions such as terminal cancer as well as those with long-term life-limiting respiratory conditions, including chronic obstructive pulmonary disease (COPD). We will address briefly the proven benefits of long-term oxygen therapy in hypoxaemic patients and then discuss the more vexed question of the role of oxygen therapy in relieving dyspnoea in a more general sense. As discussed in previous chapters, oxygen therapy, if appropriate, should always be given as part of comprehensive supportive care, with maximal pharmacotherapy directed at the underlying disease, pulmonary rehabilitation, occupational therapy, psychosocial supports, nutritional support, as well as consideration of specific palliative pharmacotherapy such as the use of opiates.

Definitions

Refractory dyspnoea: breathlessness that does not respond to treatment of the underlying cause of the breathlessness (for example, COPD, cancer, heart failure, interstitial lung disease).

Palliative oxygen: oxygen that is given for relief of refractory dyspnoea, where relief of breathlessness is the primary aim of the oxygen therapy.

Domiciliary oxygen therapy: supplemental oxygen provided for ongoing home use. In this setting oxygen is delivered at normal pressure with increased concentrations, most commonly via nasal prongs but also via oxygen masks.

Long-term oxygen therapy (LTOT): supplemental oxygen used for more than 15 hours (ideally up to 24 hours) per day.

Ambulatory oxygen: oxygen delivered by equipment that can be carried by most patients.

Measuring oxygen levels

In order to use oxygen correctly, it is important to have an understanding of some basic physiology concerning oxygen and its measurement.

Air comprises 21% oxygen, 79% nitrogen, and 0.04% carbon dioxide. The fraction of inspired air that is oxygen (FiO_2) is thus 0.21. Measuring a patient's oxygen levels can be done either invasively (arterial blood gases) or non-invasively (pulse oximetry). In the later stages of the supportive care setting, invasive measures may not be appropriate and decisions about oxygen therapy are often based on pulse oximetry measurements alone.

Pulse oximetry measures oxygen bound to haemoglobin using a detector placed on the finger or ear lobe. Two light-emitting diodes measure the differential absorption of oxy-haemoglobin and haemoglobin in the arterial blood of the capillary bed. This measures the proportion of oxygenated haemoglobin molecules compared with the total amount of haemoglobin molecules, giving the SpO_2 value as a percentage. It measures the functional saturation of the haemoglobin, however it cannot differentiate between oxygenated haemoglobin (oxyhaemoglobin) and carboxyhaemoglobin (carbon monoxide bound to oxygen binding sites on the haemoglobin). It is therefore not accurate in carbon monoxide poisoning which increases the proportion of carboxyhaemoglobin thus giving a falsely elevated reading. False low readings can occur with hypotension, darkly painted nails, some haemoglobinopathies, hyperbilirubinaemia, and movement artefact.

Arterial blood gas (ABG) analysis is more accurate but involves an arterial puncture, usually obtained from the radial artery. From this, the partial pressure of oxygen dissolved in arterial blood (PaO_2) is obtained, as is additional information such as arterial oxygen saturation (SaO_2), the partial pressure of carbon dioxide dissolved in arterial blood ($PaCO_2$) and pH. Levels of blood glucose, bicarbonate, and haemoglobin varieties (carboxyhaemoglobin and methaemoglobin) may also be measured, depending on the blood gas analyser used.

Normal oxygen levels for PaO_2 in a young adult is about 95mmHg (range 85–100mmHg), with the corresponding SpO_2 >95%. The normal SpO_2 value decreases gradually with age but still ranges between 93–98% in those aged over 65 years. In a healthy individual, oxygen levels do not generally fall during exercise, although some degree of desaturation may occur in fit, healthy subjects at extremes of exertion (48). A small degree of desaturation also occurs during sleep in normal subjects, with PaO_2 falling by 5mmHg or less, and SpO_2 falling by 2% or less.

Low oxygen levels

Respiratory failure is defined as a PaO_2 <60mmHg or a SpO_2 <90%, and can be either acute or chronic. *Type 1 respiratory failure* is hypoxaemia with a normal or low $PaCO_2$. Oxygen therapy (providing increasing concentrations of oxygen) is often adequate to treat this. *Type 2 respiratory failure* is hypoxaemia with an elevated $PaCO_2$, which reflects hypoventilation. Oxygen therapy alone is normally insufficient and ventilation (either invasive or non-invasive) should be considered.

In severe stable lung disease, PaO_2 values may be as low as 45–60mmHg and SpO_2 80–90%. In these patients any acute deterioration can see values fall as low as a PaO_2 of 30mmHg and a SpO_2 65–80%.

The effects of hypoxaemia are well documented (see Box 8.1). Acute hypoxaemia in those with compromised lung function may result in dyspnoea along with confusion and elevation in pulmonary and systemic blood pressure. Patients are usually unconscious when PaO_2 reaches 30mmHg or SpO_2 drops to 60% (49).

Chronic hypoxaemia results in pulmonary hypertension, right heart failure (termed cor pulmonale when it is secondary to lung disease) and secondary polycythaemia, but if the problem develops insidiously over time patients may adjust to the hypoxaemia and complain of few symptoms, particularly if they do not exert themselves.

Box 8.1 Summary of effects of hypoxaemia

Acute

- Dyspnoea
- Tachycardia
- Confusion
- Nausea/vomiting
- Confusion
- Poor judgment
- Loss of consciousness
- Pulmonary vasoconstriction

Chronic

- Pulmonary hypertension
- Right heart failure
- Polycythaemia

Oxygen and dyspnoea

Our ability to understand interventions, such as oxygen, which aim to relieve dyspnoea, depends largely on our ability to define dyspnoea and to understand the mechanism underlying this symptom.

The definition of dyspnoea along with its underlying pathophysiology and the language of dyspnoea have been discussed in previous chapters. As discussed in Chapter 6, dyspnoea is a combination of a sensory experience and also the patient's perception of that sensation. It is therefore influenced by many factors including the patient's underlying disease, their ethnic and cultural background, their past experiences and their psychological state.

The development of a 'language of dyspnoea' is an attempt to develop verbal descriptors of dyspnoea in order to help characterize this symptom and perhaps to assist in elucidating its underlying pathophysiology. Numerous studies (5–11) are starting to define distinct qualities of dyspnoea which can be differentiated by patients with different underlying disease conditions and indeed by healthy individuals. For example, patients with COPD may use terms such as 'work', 'effort', 'heavy' or 'shallow breathing' to describe their dyspnoea, while patients with asthma may describe their dyspnoea as 'chest tightness', 'work', or 'effort'. It is hoped that developing verbal descriptors will aid in identifying underlying pathophysiology and disease processes behind the dyspnoea reported and thus help with targeting specific treatments.

Little is known about the neural pathways that lead to dyspnoea. It is known to be a complex sensory modality that includes several qualitatively distinct sensations that probably arise from different pathophysiological mechanisms (1). There are inputs from numerous receptors (chemoreceptors, vagoreceptors, mechanoreceptors, pulmonary stretch receptors, and muscle receptors) interacting with numerous central pathways but the exact nature of these signals and their interactions is yet to be clearly defined. Conditions that cause dyspnoea most likely do so by more than one mechanism, the unique combination of which determines the quality and intensity of the dyspnoea in the individual patient (See chapter 5).

The contribution of hypoxaemia to dyspnoea is uncertain. Not all people with hypoxaemia experience dyspnoea and many people with dyspnoea may have normal oxygen levels, leading to the assertion that there is 'very little correlation between blood oxygen saturation of a subject and presence or absence of breathlessness' (12). When dyspnoea occurs in the setting of hypoxaemia it is thought that the hypoxaemia may cause dyspnoea through its effects on peripheral chemoreceptors triggering the body to increase ventilation (14). It is not known whether this is the only mechanism causing the dyspnoea, or whether the hypoxaemia is but one of the pathophysiological processes at play leading to the dyspnoea. Certainly, in most situations where hypoxaemia occurs, there will be an underlying pathology which may itself contribute in a variety of ways to dyspnoea.

The mechanisms by which oxygen therapy reduces the sensation of dyspnoea also remain unclear. It is known that supplemental oxygen may decrease minute ventilation and therefore the work of breathing (13–15), which may explain the relief of dyspnoea that occurs in some patients with only mild hypoxaemia when oxygen is administered. Other potential mechanisms include: an altered perception of dyspnoea, independent of the drop in ventilation; improved respiratory and peripheral muscle function and possible cardiovascular effects (37).

There are many unanswered questions remaining regarding dyspnoea and the role of oxygen in its management. It perhaps oversimplifies medical care to assume that all patients with dyspnoea are experiencing the same sensation and that if oxygen benefits one patient with dyspnoea this can be generalized to all patients. It may be that as our knowledge of dyspnoea expands, oxygen use will be found to be beneficial only in dyspnoea of certain pathophysiological subtypes.

Role of oxygen therapy

Oxygen therapy has been used as a therapeutic tool since 1917 when Haldane first used it in treating World War I gas inhalation injuries. Since then its use has expanded such that it has become the treatment of choice for hypoxaemia from all causes. In the acutely ill medical patient its use is well validated with the primary aim being to achieve near normal oxygen levels (PaO_2 >60mmHg (8 kPa), SpO_2 >90%). This is appropriate as the consequences of acute hypoxia are well documented (see Box 8.1).

Documentation of the efficacy of oxygen therapy in the chronically ill patient or the patient requiring supportive care for end-stage respiratory disease is more limited. Currently its use in these patients is twofold: firstly, in correcting chronic hypoxaemia with LTOT; and secondly, in providing relief of dyspnoea. In this section we will discuss the evidence behind the use of oxygen in both of these settings. In the first setting, there is evidence showing the benefit of oxygen therapy in improving survival. In the second setting, the goal for use of oxygen therapy is typically as a palliative intervention for dyspnoea refractory to maximal medical therapy, and, as described below, there is limited evidence to support its use.

Benefits of long-term oxygen therapy

LTOT is a recognized treatment in hypoxaemic patients, irrespective of whether or not they are dyspnoeic. International guidelines reflect this and LTOT is reimbursed in most healthcare systems. These guidelines are based mainly on two landmark multicentre studies reported in the early 1980s which examined the use of LTOT in COPD patients with chronic hypoxaemia.

These trials, the Nocturnal Oxygen Therapy Trial (NOTT) (16) and the Medical Research Council (MRC) (17) study, showed that LTOT when given for greater than 15 hours per day improved survival in patients with COPD and chronic hypoxaemia (PaO_2 ≤55–60mmHg (7.33 - 8 kPa)), with or without hypercapnia. Based on these studies, most national and international guidelines on home oxygen therapy have subsequently recommended that such patients should receive oxygen for at least 15 hours per day. A subsequent trial reported by Gorecka and colleagues (18) found that LTOT had no effect on survival in patients with COPD and only moderate hypoxaemia (56–65mmHg (7.5 - 8.5 kPa)), thus explaining the cut-off points for many of the guidelines.

There is little convincing evidence from studies to date that LTOT has significant benefits other than on survival. Indeed, the mechanism for the improvement in survival with oxygen therapy remains unclear, despite the observation of small improvements in some haemodynamic parameters in the NOTT (11). Endpoints in the MRC study were physiological characteristics and mortality. In the NOTT, neuropsychological tests were assessed in both continuous and nocturnal oxygen groups at baseline and at 6 months. Only 42% of patients showed improvements in the battery of tests at 6 months and there were no differences between the continuous and nocturnal groups (50). There was no true control group (intranasal air) in this or in the MRC study.

Although various other studies have suggested benefits from oxygen therapy such as reduced pulmonary artery pressures (19, 20), increased exercise capacity (21), and improvements in cognitive function (22) it is notable that many of these studies have not used a randomized controlled format, as such a methodology would be considered unethical given the demonstrated mortality benefit with oxygen. Many have a pre–post design or even use historical data as a form of 'control' and, thus, any improvements observed may relate to the Hawthorne effect of being in a clinical trial or to the more intensive medical and nursing attention received from being in a study. It is also likely that the clinical benefits seen depend on treatment compliance, the duration of treatment, and adequate correction of hypoxaemia.

Based on the observed mortality benefits in patients with COPD, LTOT is widely used in conditions other than COPD associated with chronic hypoxaemia. However, evidence for a survival benefit from this practice is lacking. There have been no published randomized controlled trials on the use of LTOT in other chronic lung diseases that lead to chronic hypoxaemia, such as interstitial lung disease and bronchiectasis. LTOT is also used in hypoxaemic patients with heart failure and in lung conditions requiring palliative therapy, but again this is without any evidence for a mortality benefit and is extrapolated from benefits seen in patients with hypoxaemia and COPD.

Oxygen therapy to treat dyspnoea

Oxygen is often prescribed for management of refractory dyspnoea in the home setting even when the criteria for LTOT are not met. As discussed, the guidelines for use of long-term oxygen are based on survival benefits rather than upon any clear supporting evidence that oxygen used for more than 15 hours per day (as in the two abovementioned studies) provides symptomatic relief of breathlessness. However, within the supportive care field, the focus of care is shifted away from prolonging survival to reducing symptoms and improving quality of life. Many guidelines recognize this and allow for prescription of 'palliative' oxygen therapy in patients with life-limiting disease who have refractory dyspnoea without severe hypoxaemia (3, 4). This is predicated upon the belief that oxygen therapy is a benign intervention and may relieve dyspnoea. Both of these beliefs are, however, challenged by the available evidence.

In this section we will examine the evidence for using oxygen in severe respiratory diseases and other conditions requiring palliation of dyspnoea, both at rest and with exercise. Much of the evidence is based upon studies in people with COPD and, until recently, most of these studies did not include dyspnoea as an outcome measure, centring rather on outcomes such as survival and effects on pulmonary haemodynamics, exercise capacity and quality of life. These studies are, however, used as a basis for currently available recommendations and provide a platform from which new research is being carried out.

Use of oxygen therapy in the patient dyspnoeic at rest

As described above, the survival benefit of oxygen therapy for those severely hypoxaemic at rest (PaO_2 <55mmHg) is widely accepted. However, its symptomatic benefit in those with dyspnoea from chronic respiratory diseases and other conditions requiring palliation of dyspnoea where resting PaO_2 >55mmHg is unclear. The main studies reporting the effect of oxygen therapy on dyspnoea are described in Table 8.1.

As shown in Table 8.1, until recently many of the studies have been small and focused on investigating the effect of oxygen on dyspnoea in the acute setting. These studies have shown similar findings, revealing there to be no consistent benefit of oxygen in relieving dyspnoea in a patient without severe hypoxaemia. They do, however, also show that there are small numbers of *individual* patients who may benefit or perceive a benefit from oxygen inhalation but that there are no predictive factors to determine who these patients are.

In the first large, international multicentre trial examining this question, Abernethy et al. (23) randomly allocated 239 patients with life-limiting disease, including COPD (64%) and cancer (16%), to receive oxygen or medical air. Both were delivered at 2L/min through nasal cannulae and via a concentrator for seven days. Primary outcomes were impact on breathlessness and quality of life (QoL). The study found that both medical gases induced small improvements in dyspnoea and quality of life and that most of the improvement occurred in the first 3 days. Whilst the overall benefit was small, it was most pronounced in the subgroup of patients with the most severe breathlessness. The conclusion was that palliative oxygen had no benefits over medical air for relieving dyspnoea or for improving QoL for the whole population and that there were small improvements with both arms of the treatment. A therapeutic trial of medical air or oxygen over 3–4 days was thus proposed as a way of assessing those dyspnoeic patients who would benefit from therapy.

It is thought that relief of breathlessness with either oxygen or air, as described in the abovementioned study, could be due to stimulation of nasal receptors by flow of a gas over them; however, the mechanism by which this occurs is not known. The role of air flow as an intervention has been explored in the past (13, 24), and cold air directed on the face has been shown to reduce breathlessness induced by inspiratory resistive loading and hypercapnia in normal subjects (51).

From both this theoretical basis, as well as from patient reports along with clinical observation, have arisen recommendations for the use of a hand-held fan in the breathless patient. Until recently such recommendations were not evidence-based; however, a recent

Table 8.1 Summary of studies using oxygen therapy in patients with COPD and cancer at rest

Author (year)	Disease	Number of patients	Intervention	Outcomes	Results
Abernethy (2010) (23)	COPD Cancer ILD Other	239	Double-blind randomized controlled trial. Oxygen or medical air via nasal cannulae at 2L/min for at least 15 hours per day for 7 days	Breathlessness (NRS— numerical rating scale) measured daily, McGill QoL Questionnaire	Dyspnoea and QoL improved slightly over 7-day period in both arms. Neither gas proved superior in relieving sensation of dyspnoea or improving QoL
O'Donnell (2001) (37)	COPD	11	Baseline test pre-exercise trial—60% oxygen vs. 21% while using mouth piece	Change in Borg	No difference in reported dyspnoea
Booth et al. (1996) (38)	Cancer (16 hypoxaemic)	38	Single-blind cross-over trial. Oxygen versus compressed air at 4L/min for 15min at rest via nasal cannulae	Change in VAS and Borg Score	Improvement with air and oxygen and no significant differences between the two gases
Bruera et al. (1993) (39)	Cancer (all hypoxaemic, SpO_2 <90%)	14	Double-blind cross-over trial. Oxygen versus air at 5L/min for 5min at rest via mask	Change in VAS	Less breathless on oxygen
Swinburn et al. (1991) (40)	COPD: 12 ILD: 10	22	Double-blind cross-over trial. Oxygen and air at 4L/min	Change in VAS and Borg scale	Improvement on air and oxygen and no significant difference between the two gases
Liss (1988) (24)	COPD (mostly hypoxaemic)	8	Single blind cross-over trial. Nasal prongs, zero flow, air then oxygen at 2L and 4L/min. This repeated after nasal mucosa anaesthetized.	Change in VAS	No change in dyspnoea until nasal mucosa anaesthetized and then dyspnoea increased

randomized cross-over trial of hand-held fan versus 'placebo' (fan onto thigh) in 49 patients by Galbraith et al. (54) suggested benefit from a hand-held fan improving dyspnoea. Whilst the results of this study are promising, further studies are required to confirm this benefit and to further explore the practicalities of the use of a hand-held fan.

As shown in Table 8.1, there are three studies which have looked at the benefits of oxygen therapy in treating dyspnoea in those with advanced cancer. These studies are important as the presence of dyspnoea in patients with advanced cancer has been estimated to be as high as 50–70% (25). LTOT is used widely in hypoxaemic cancer patients, but its perceived benefit has been extrapolated from data showing a survival benefit in COPD patients, and data in cancer patients are lacking. Data supporting its use in relieving dyspnoea are also limited. Meta-analyses of the above-mentioned studies by Uronis et al. (26) and by Ben-Aharon et al. (27) both acknowledge the limited number of studies and small populations used and confirm that oxygen was not effective in reducing dyspnoea in cancer patients who would not otherwise qualify for LTOT. The meta-analyses do, however, highlight the fact that there were a small number of individuals who did benefit from oxygen, although, once again, there were no factors predictive of the benefit.

Use of oxygen therapy for the patient who is dyspnoeic on exercise

International guidelines suggest that oxygen may be useful for those with stable chronic respiratory disease who desaturate during exercise (PaO$_2$ <55mmHg and SpO$_2$ <88%) and generally recommend that there be a demonstrable improvement in either dyspnoea or exercise capacity or both in order for patients to qualify to receive oxygen therapy. There is a lack of strong evidence for this practice. There have been numerous short-term in-laboratory studies of the effects of ambulatory oxygen therapy with exercise in chronic lung disease which have shown modest benefits in exercise capacity and reductions in dyspnoea. However, these studies have been limited by small numbers, the use of oxygen in the short term and a lack of consensus over what is a clinically important improvement in such exercise tests.

Determining the benefit a patient receives from oxygen will depend on our ability to measure such an improvement. This has traditionally been in the patient's walking distance and also in their dyspnoea score. With regards to breathlessness, it is uncertain how to determine what level of improvement will be meaningful for the patient. Similarly, there is debate as to what constitutes a useful improvement in walking distance in an individual.

One of the most commonly used tests of exercise capacity is the 6-minute walk test. The patient walks along a corridor of between 15–50m in length, with standardized encouragement, and the distance completed in 6min is recorded as the 6-min walk distance (6MWD). There has been much discussion about the minimal important difference (MID) in 6MWD, which is, in essence, the minimal improvement that patients can detect in a given outcome. In stable patients with COPD the 6MWD was reported as needing to change by 54m for the average patient to stop rating himself or herself as 'about the same' as other patients in a rehabilitation group (28). However, there is no consensus over this with a recent analysis of pooled data from nine prospective studies suggested a significant change was 35m or about 10% from baseline 6MWD (29) and a further recent study suggesting 25m as the MID in COPD (52). This distance may also vary between diseases (30). This lack of consensus is reflected in the fact that there is no guideline which recommends a specific MID for the 6MWD (53).

Moreover, little is known about the effectiveness of ambulatory oxygen therapy when used for longer periods and while the patient is at home during activities of daily living. Studies that have aimed to address the latter question are shown in Table 8.2.

Table 8.2 Selected studies using oxygen therapy for breathlessness in patients with COPD during exercise

Study	No. of patients	Hypoxaemic on exertion	Intervention	Outcome	Conclusion
Moore *et al.* (2010) (32)	153	Approximately one-third	12-week double blinded randomized trial of cylinder air versus cylinder oxygen provided at 6L/min intranasally for use during any activity provoking breathlessness	Chronic respiratory disease questionnaire and baseline/ transition dyspnoea index	Improvement in dyspnoea with both air and oxygen
O'Donnell (2001) (37)	11	Yes	Double-blind randomized controlled trial. Oxygen 60% versus oxygen 21% via mouth piece during exercise	Change in Borg	Increased endurance and reduced dyspnoea at isotime
Garrod *et al.* (2000) (41)	22		Single-blind randomized controlled trial over 6 weeks. Oxygen versus compressed air at 4L/ min during exercise via nasal cannulae	Change in Borg	Small decrease in dyspnoea
Rooyackers *et al.* (1997) (42)	24	$SaO_2 < 90\%$ at peak exercise	Non-blinded randomized controlled trial over 10 weeks. Oxygen 4L/ min versus room air during training	Change in Borg and chronic respiratory disease questionnaire	Rehabilitation programme improved dyspnoea, no increased benefit from supplemental oxygen during training
McDonald (1995) (43)	26	Yes	Double-blind cross-over study over 12 weeks. Oxygen and medical air at 4L/min via nasal cannulae during exercise	Change in Borg	Both oxygen and medical air improved QoL from baseline but did not affect sensation of breathlessness
Dean *et al.* (1992) (44)	12		Double-blind randomized controlled trial. 40% oxygen versus compressed air via mouth piece during exercise	Change in Borg	Increased endurance and reduced dyspnoea at isotime

As demonstrated, these studies have not consistently demonstrated a benefit of oxygen therapy over ambulatory air for relief of exercise-induced dyspnoea in a patient whose resting oxygen saturation is satisfactory but who may or may not desaturate with exertion. Eaton et al. (31) did demonstrate a small benefit in QoL in their randomized cross-over design trial of patients using ambulatory oxygen versus air over a 6-week trial at home, but the degree of improvement in health related quality of life was small.

The evidence also shows that while oxygen may prevent desaturation during exercise, it doesn't always relieve dyspnoea.

These findings were confirmed in a recent, large, randomized controlled study. Moore et al. (32) randomized breathless patients with COPD without severe hypoxaemia at rest (PaO$_2$ greater than 60mmHg at rest on room air) to use ambulatory oxygen or ambulatory air during exertion for 3 months at home. In results similar to those of the above-mentioned palliative oxygen study, there was a trend to improvement in both arms of treatment. However, there was no difference between supplemental air and supplemental oxygen used during exercise with regards to dyspnoea, QoL, or function. The presence of exertional desaturation was not predictive of outcome.

Practical considerations for prescribing oxygen in supportive care

Proposed guidelines for use of oxygen within supportive care

Despite the lack of evidence and numerous areas of uncertainty, use of palliative oxygen is widespread. Abernethy et al. (33) examined the oxygen prescribing practices of 214 palliative care specialists and respiratory physicians in Australia and New Zealand. They found that palliative oxygen is commonly prescribed with 58% of respondents believing that palliative oxygen was beneficial and 65% reporting refractory dyspnoea as being the most common reason for its prescription. A similar study of Canadian clinicians (34) showed similar practices, with 40% of patients in Canada receiving LTOT not meeting the current guidelines (35).

Due to the lack of evidence, developing guidelines for usage of palliative oxygen for refractory dyspnoea in the supportive care field is challenging. The Royal College of Physicians' 1999 guidelines for oxygen use are shown in Box 8.2. Over 10 years on, these guidelines are still widely used, due to a lack of robust evidence disproving their recommendations. Until recently, studies showing no consistent benefit for palliative oxygen in relieving refractory dyspnoea either at rest or on exercise have been small and have not changed practice. However, these findings have been recently confirmed in the two large studies by Abernethy et al. (23) and Moore et al. (32), which in both cases showed no consistent benefit of oxygen therapy over medical air in relieving dyspnoea in the patient without severe hypoxaemia, either at rest or on exercise. These studies once again support the findings from other smaller studies which have suggested that there are some patients who *do* benefit from oxygen therapy, although, again there are no individual factors to predict this benefit.

Box 8.2 Summary of the RCP recommendations on using different patterns of domiciliary oxygen therapy for palliative care

Long-term oxygen therapy (LTOT)

- Interstitial lung disease when PaO_2 is less than 8kPa (=60mmHg).

- Neuromuscular or skeletal disorders, either in combination with ventilatory support or alone. Assessment for LTOT in this situation requires referral to a physician with a special interest in these disorders.

- Cystic fibrosis where PaO_2 is less than 7.3kPa (=55mmHg) or when it is between 7.3–8kPa in presence of nocturnal hypoxaemia, secondary polycythaemia, pulmonary hypertension, or peripheral oedema.

- Pulmonary hypertension, without parenchymal lung involvement, when PaO_2 is less than 8kPa.

- Domiciliary oxygen therapy can be prescribed for palliation of dyspnoea in pulmonary malignancy and other causes of disabling dyspnoea due to terminal disease.

- Patients with heart failure can be prescribed LTOT if they have daytime hypoxaemia with a PaO_2 on air of less than 7.3kPa or nocturnal hypoxaemia (with SaO_2 below 90% for at least 30% of the night).

Indications for ambulatory oxygen therapy

- Patients with interstitial lung disease who show evidence of desaturation.

- Patients with cystic fibrosis who have chronic hypoxaemia requiring LTOT and when ambulation is required. Ambulatory oxygen therapy may also be prescribed to this group if they show evidence of exercise desaturation without chronic hypoxaemia (PaO_2 <7.3kPa).

- Ambulatory oxygen therapy should be considered in patients with chest wall and neuromuscular disorders who have exercise desaturation and are limited by dyspnoea.

- Ambulatory oxygen is not recommended in heart failure.

- Patients who are continuing to smoke cigarettes should not be prescribed ambulatory oxygen as the benefits are debatable in this situation and risk from burns is ever present.

- Despite extensive prescription of short-burst therapy; there is no adequate evidence available for firm recommendations; further research is required.

- Short burst oxygen should be considered for episodic breathlessness not relieved by other treatments in patients with severe COPD, interstitial lung disease, heart failure and those in palliative care.

- Short burst oxygen should only be prescribed if an improvement in breathlessness and/or exercise tolerance can be documented.

Results of these studies have yet to be translated into clinical practice. It remains to be seen whether or not they will change guidelines for use of palliative oxygen or for prescribing practices of oxygen therapy. They show that medical air and oxygen had some beneficial effects and thus that a trial of oxygen or medical air may be warranted. However, neither study contained a control arm where patients received neither gas, so it is also possible that these gases provide no more than placebo benefit. Currently medical air is as expensive as oxygen and it may be difficult to prescribe in many health systems.

Individual patient selection therefore remains the most important aspect of palliative oxygen prescription. At present there are no clearly delineated characteristics that are predictive of benefit and thus exactly how to assess individual patients remains unclear.

Patient preference and education

When prescribing oxygen therapy for palliation of breathlessness, patient preference and their preconceived notions of the potential benefits oxygen therapy may provide for them must be considered. Studies in COPD have shown that even patients who are shown to benefit from oxygen therapy do not always wish to receive it (31, 36). Oxygen is a therapy that needs to be extensively discussed with the patient and thorough education about its use must be provided. The 'mystique' of oxygen therapy should be exposed with education about the differences between oxygen aimed at prolonging life (for those who are significantly hypoxaemic) versus oxygen which may relieve hypoxaemia during exertion which may or may not at the same time improve dyspnoea. Oxygen should be discussed as just another form of treatment for the patient's respiratory or other condition (such as a bronchodilator or inhaled corticosteroid) which may or may not benefit them, and which may be ceased if no benefit is experienced. The potential cooling effects of air and oxygen and potentially also of a hand-held fan should also be pointed out (54). Furthermore, a discussion of the hazards of oxygen therapy (see below) should be undertaken, highlighting potential risks of oxygen therapy.

General work-up of patient for consideration of oxygen therapy

Any patient being considered for palliative oxygen therapy for refractory dyspnoea should undergo a full assessment to establish the cause of their breathlessness and to determine whether they are hypoxaemic. If they are hypoxaemic at rest, LTOT should be offered if hypoxaemia persists despite maximal treatment, as per the guidelines of the relevant health system. The presence of hypoxaemia should be confirmed by arterial blood gases, but in the palliative setting pulse oximetry may be adequate.

There are many causes of breathlessness in patients with respiratory disease or other conditions being palliated and therefore an extensive work-up for the cause of the dyspnoea is necessary. In the terminal setting (last hours or days of life) however, this may not be appropriate. The work-up should include a careful history and examination as well as investigations. Investigations include lung function tests, electrocardiogram (ECG), and echocardiogram (left and right heart function and estimation of pulmonary arterial pressures). A measurement estimation of the haemoglobin should also be obtained to exclude anaemia and to assess for polycythaemia.

Any chronic lung disease that is present must be stable and optimally managed before oxygen therapy should be considered and any reversible causes of hypoxaemia or dyspnoea need to be adequately treated.

It is essential that the patient is a non-smoker. Apart from the fire risk that smoking poses, it also inhibits the efficacy of oxygen therapy due to carbon monoxide binding with a higher affinity to the haemoglobin molecules. There are no clear recommendations to guide the duration for which the patient needs to have been abstinent from smoking. It is commonly set at 4–6 weeks. Arterial blood gases are helpful in assessing smoking status by measuring carboxyhaemoglobin, but smoking status may also be deduced using the less invasive measurements of urinary cotinine or breath carbon monoxide.

Assessing for oxygen use at rest in non-hypoxaemic patient

There are no firm guidelines for determining who will benefit from palliative oxygen at rest. Many guidelines advocate its use in the non-hypoxaemic breathless patient in the palliative setting. The recent large international study by Abernethy et al. (23) suggests there may be a small benefit from air or oxygen in this setting, which may not be more than a placebo effect. A short-term trial may be undertaken with the understanding that the treatment will not continue if the patient does not perceive a benefit. A trial of a fan also appears reasonable in this setting.

Assessing for oxygen use with exercise

If possible an exercise test should be performed to assess for any desaturation. If there is no desaturation, it is reasonable not to offer oxygen but to suggest that a hand-held fan may be useful when the patient stops to rest after walking when out of the house or at home if they become breathless. For those who desaturate and in whom there seems to be a benefit in terms of increased distance walked or improved breathlessness in a laboratory test (using a measure such as Borg, modified Borg, numerical rating scale (NRS), or visual analogue scale (VAS)) it may be reasonable to provide a trial of ambulatory oxygen for use during exertion for a pre-determined period (an example being 3 months). The patient and healthcare professional can review usage and any perceived benefit and determine whether or not the patient wishes to continue using the cylinders. This of course needs to be done in conjunction with extensive education about the uses of oxygen and its risks.

Oxygen in patients in the last stages of life

We do not suggest starting oxygen in this group for dyspnoea if the patient is not hypoxaemic. Many patients will, however, have already been started on oxygen and it is often perceived as inhumane to remove oxygen. If oxygen is to be continued it should be at low flows through nasal cannulae. These are more comfortable and less conspicuous than oxygen masks.

Hazards of oxygen therapy

The hazards of oxygen therapy are listed in Box 8.3. Much of the concern over oxygen therapy relates to improper administration with regards to fire risk and also in those with hypercapnia. This, however, fails to recognize the equally important adverse effects of: restriction of activities, discomfort, potential impairment of QoL, and occasional psychological dependence. Another potential hazard is accelerated oxidant injury to the airways.

- *Risk of oxidative injury:* the concept that oxygen, when used correctly, is a benign treatment has recently been challenged by papers demonstrating accelerated oxidative injury in the airways of people on LTOT (45). While this still remains a theoretical risk, the growing body of literature (46–48) and the fact that oxidative injury to the airways has been linked to COPD pathogenesis means this potential toxicity of LTOT needs further consideration if oxygen is prescribed for symptomatic reasons.

- *Fire risk:* oxygen in itself is not flammable, but it can increase the intensity and spread of a fire. Oxygen should not be used around open flames or fire sources and patients should be carefully educated about these risks. Serious and even life-threatening burns have resulted as a consequence of patients not appreciating this risk.

- *Use of oxygen in patients with hypercapnia:* caution must be used in prescribing oxygen in patients with hypercapnia. In a small proportion of hypercapnic patients excessive oxygen can result in hypoventilation and a rising carbon dioxide which can cause drowsiness, coma and even death. This results from a combination of mechanisms including suppression of hypoxic ventilatory drive and worsening of ventilation-perfusion mismatch due to attenuation of hypoxic pulmonary vasoconstriction. Despite the need for caution when using oxygen therapy in patients with hypercapnia, hypoxaemia must be corrected. The primary goal of therapy should be maintenance of SpO_2 88–93% or PaO_2 60–70mmHg. Increasing FiO_2 to achieve SpO_2 or PaO_2

Box 8.3 Adverse effects of oxygen therapy

- Fire hazard.
- Progressive hypercapnia.
- Restriction of activities.
- Psychological dependence.
- Impaired communication.
- Expense.
- Oxidative injury to airways.

above this level does not significantly improve the oxygen content of the blood but does increase the potential risk for more severe secondary hypercapnia in the very small subgroup of hypercapnic COPD patients.

◆ *Restriction of activities:* oxygen therapy with all of its attachments can severely restrict a patient's activities, both in moving around the house and also in outside activities.

◆ *Impaired communication between family and patient:* the presence of nasal cannulae or masks and the time attending to oxygen therapy can significantly impair both the ability of the patient to communicate with those around them and their willingness to do so.

◆ *Psychological addiction:* a small proportion of patients become 'addicted' to oxygen therapy and the presence of oxygen therapy can become a preoccupation and a great anxiety, significantly impacting on their quality of life. Within the supportive care setting this therefore negates the purpose of the oxygen use.

◆ *Discomfort:* there can be significant irritation to the nose and eyes associated with oxygen usage through nasal cannulae. Drying of the nasal mucosa can be painful and also associated with epistaxis.

◆ *Expense:* oxygen therapy is of considerable expense to the healthcare system. Many patients also may end up self-funding 'palliative oxygen' leading to a significant financial pressure.

Equipment

Concentrator

This is the most commonly dispensed device for home use. It is a machine that traps and removes nitrogen from room air to produce a mixture of 95% oxygen and 5% argon. There are two basic systems including a low-flow (1–6L/min) system and the more expensive high-flow system (1–10L/min). In general they are not portable and are provided with tubing of up to 10–15m for use around the house. Newer battery powered portable oxygen concentrators have been developed which weigh as little as 3kg, but at present their use is limited by expense.

Cylinders

Cylinders store oxygen either in a pressurized (see Table 8.3) or liquid form. Compressed gas cylinders are now made with lighter materials (compared with standard aluminium) that can withstand higher pressures, thus improving their portability. Liquid oxygen systems provide the highest efficiency in oxygen storage with decreased weight, and safe and easy filling but are more expensive to purchase and maintain. They do not require high pressure containers and 1L of liquid oxygen can be converted into 1000L of oxygen gas.

Oxygen-conserving devices

Devices are available to increase the efficacy of oxygen delivery systems.

Table 8.3 Oxygen cylinders and contents

Size	Volume (m³)	Duration of use at flow rate of 2L/min
Traveller	0.3–0.6	1–2 hours
C	0.55	3 hours
D	1.5	11 hours
E	3.8–5.2	30 hours
G	7.6–8.8	48 hours

Demand oxygen pulsing devices can increase oxygen efficiency by up to 500%. They deliver oxygen only during the early portion of inhalation, increasing the amount of oxygen actually delivered to the alveoli. They are available as stand alone modules or integrated into compressed gas systems, liquid oxygen systems, or portable oxygen concentrators. They do, however, make audible pulses which may be distracting, and some pulsing devices fail to adequately oxygenate patients during exertion.

Reservoir cannulae increase oxygen efficiency by storing oxygen during exhalation and making the oxygen available as a bolus upon onset of next inhalation. They are simple, reliable and inexpensive and can increase oxygen efficiency by up to 400% at low flow rates (e.g. 0.5L → 2L). As flow increases efficacy decreases and above 4L/min it tends to add approximately 2L/min. The reservoir that is used most commonly hangs in the form of a pendant on the chest. It is available as a reservoir that sits under the nose, but its use by patients is limited by its bulky appearance on the face.

Oxygen for air travel

With supportive care expanding to involve those with life-limiting chronic respiratory illnesses, the issue of air travel is an important one. Currently there is no indication for using oxygen on an airline for relief of breathlessness during flight. However, in a patient that may become hypoxaemic at altitude, oxygen therapy should be considered.

Worldwide, commercial airlines pressurize their cabins so that the maximum effective cabin pressure is equivalent to an altitude of 8000 feet. Although the FiO_2 does not change, the reduced barometric pressure means that the oxygen level experienced is equivalent to a FiO_2 of 0.15 at sea level (compared to the usual 0.21). Patients with a poor respiratory reserve may become significantly hypoxaemic during air travel and should be assessed for in-flight oxygen therapy. Room air saturations can guide this decision. If SpO_2 is <92% oxygen is necessary, while if SpO_2 is >95% oxygen will not be necessary. Where SpO_2 is 92–95% a high-altitude simulation test may be used to determine whether oxygen will be required. A flow rate of 2L/min is usually sufficient if supplementary oxygen is not normally required. If the patient is on LTOT, increasing the flow rate by 2L/min is usually sufficient.

Due to lack of standardization between airlines, patients and clinicians are advised to consult brochures and source documents for practical details about specific airline

Table 8.4 British Thoracic Society guidelines for in-flight oxygen assessment and recommendations (55). Reproduced from Thorax 57:289-304, 2002 with permission from BMJ Publishing Group Ltd.

Screening result (sea level)	Recommendation
SpO_2 >95%	Oxygen not required
SpO_2 92–95% and no risk factor	Oxygen not required
SpO_2 92–95% and risk factor	Hypoxic challenge test
SpO_2 <92%	In-flight oxygen
On LTOT	Increase by 2L/min at cruising altitude
Hypoxic challenge result	Recommendation
PaO_2 >55mmHg	Oxygen not required
PaO_2 50–55mmHg	Borderline, a walk test may be helpful
PaO_2 <50mmHg	In-flight oxygen (2L/min)

regulations and charges. A clinician letter documenting flow rate in litres per minute, duration, and underlying pulmonary condition is usually sufficient. Of note, for international flights there is a ban on the patient using their own oxygen cylinders or liquid oxygen on board. Some domestic airlines may allow a patient's own cylinder to be used. Most domestic and international airlines will allow a battery-powered portable oxygen concentrator to be used, but this needs to be approved beforehand by the airline. It is therefore very important to contact the individual airline well in advance of the flight regarding their regulations on oxygen use.

References

1. American Thoracic Society. Dyspnea: mechanisms, assessment, and management: a consensus statement. *Am J Respir Crit Care Med* 1999; **159**:321–40.
2. Edmonds P, Karlsen S, Khan S, Addington-Hall J. A comparison of the palliative care needs of patients dying from chronic respiratory diseases and lung cancer. *Palliat Med* 2001; **15**(4):287–95.
3. Wedzicha JA. Domiciliary oxygen therapy services: clinical guidelines and advice for prescribers. Summary of a report of the Royal College of Physicians. *J R Coll Phys London* 1999; **33**(5):445–7.
4. Rous RG. Long term oxygen therapy: Are we prescribing appropriately? *Int J COPD* 2008; **3**(2): 231–7.
5. Von Leopolt A, Balewski S, Petersen S, *et al.* Verbal descriptors of dyspnea in patients with COPD at different intensity levels of dyspnoea. *Chest* 2007; **131**:141–7.
6. Mahler D, Harver A, Lentine T, *et al.* Descriptors of breathlessness in cardiorespiratory diseases. *Am J Respir Crit Care Med* 1996; **154**:1357–63.
7. Killian KJ, Watson R, Otis J, *et al.* Symptom perception during acute bronchospasm. *Am J Respir Crit Care Med* 2000; **162**:490–6.
8. Binks AP, Moosavi SH, Banzett RB, *et al.* 'Tightness' sensation of asthma does not arise from the work of breathing. *Am J Respir Crit Care Med* 2002; **165**:78–82.

9. Elliot MW, Adams L, Cockcroft A, *et al.* The language of breathlessness: use of verbal descriptors by patients with cardiopulmonary disease. *Am Rev Respir Dis* 1991; **144**:826–32.

10. Smith J, Albert P, Bertella E, *et al.* Qualitative aspects of breathlessness in health and disease. *Thorax* 2009; **64**:713–18.

11. Harver A, Mahler DA, Schwartzstein RM, *et al.* Descriptors of breathlessness in healthy individuals: distinct and separable constructs. *Chest* 2000; **118**:679–90.

12. O'Driscoll BR. Short burst oxygen therapy in patients with COPD. *Monaldi Arch Chest Dis* 2008; **69**:70–4.

13. Tarpy S, Epstein S, Gottlieb D, *et al.* The effect of oxygen and air via nasal cannula on the oxygen cost of breathing in chronic airflow obstruction. *Am Rev Respir Dis* 1992; **145**:A646.

14. Cousser JI Jr, Make BJ. Transtracheal oxygen decreases inspired minute ventilation. *Am Rev Respir Dis* 1989; **139**:627–31.

15. Benditt J, Pollock M, Roa J, *et al.* Transtracheal delivery of gas decreases the oxygen cost of breathing. *Am Rev Respir Dis* 1993; **147**:1207–10.

16. Report of the Medical Research Council working party. Long term domiciliary oxygen in chronic hypoxaemic cor pulmonale complicating chronic bronchitis and emphysema. *Lancet* 1981; **1**:681–6.

17. Nocturnal Oxygen Therapy Trial Group. Continuous or nocturnal oxygen in hypoxaemia chronic obstructive lung disease. *Ann Int Med* 1980; **93**:391–8.

18. Gorecka D.K, Gorzelak P, Sliwinski M, *et al.* Effect of long term oxygen therapy on survival in patients with chronic obstructive pulmonary disease with moderate hypoxaemia. *Thorax* 1997; **52**:674–9.

19. Zielinski J, Tobiasz M, Hawrylkiewicz I, Sliwinski P, Palasiewicz G. Effects of long-term oxygen therapy on pulmonary haemodynamics in COPD patients. *Chest* 1998; **113**:65–70.

20. Weitzenblum E, Sartegeau A, Ehrhart M, Mammsser M, Pelletier A. Long term oxygen therapy can reverse the progression of pulmonary hypertension in patients with chronic obstructive pulmonary disease. *Am Rev Resp Dis* 1985; **131**:493–8.

21. Morrison DA, Stovall JR. Increased exercise capacity in hypoxaemic patients after long-term oxygen therapy. *Chest* 1992; **102**:542–50.

22. Heaton RK, Grant I, McSweeny AJ, *et al.* Psychological effects of continuous and nocturnal oxygen therapy in hypoxaemic chronic obstructive disease. *Arch Intern Med* 1983; **143**:1941–7.

23. Abernethy AP, McDonald CF, Frith PA, *et al.* Palliative oxygen versus medical air for relief of dyspnoea: an international, randomized controlled trial. *Respirology* 2009; **14** (Suppl.1):A29.

24. Liss HW, Grant BJ. The effect of nasal flow on breathlessness in patients with chronic obstructive pulmonary disease. *Am Rev Respir Dis* 1988; **137**:1285–8.

25. Bruera E, Schmitz B, Pither J, *et al.* The frequency and correlates of dyspnoea in patients with advanced cancer. *J Pain Symptom Manage* 2000; **19**:357–62.

26. Uronis HE, Currow DC, McCrory DC, *et al.* Oxygen for relief of dyspnoea in mildly or non-hypoxaemic patients with cancer: a systematic review and meta-analysis. *Br J Cancer* 2008; **98**(2):294–9.

27. Ben-Aharon I, Gafter-Gvili A, Paul M, *et al.* Interventions for alleviating cancer-related dyspnoea: a systematic review. *J Clin Oncol* 2008; **26**:2396–404.

28. Redelmeier D.A, Bayoumi A.M, Goldstein R.S, *et al.* Interpreting small differences in functional status: the six minute walk test in chronic lung disease patients. *Am J Respir Crit Care Med* 1997; **155**:1278–82.

29. Puhan MA, Mador MJ, Held U, Goldstein R, Guyatt GH, Schünemann HJ. Interpretation of treatment changes in 6-minute walk distance in patients with COPD. *Eur Respir J* 2008; **32**:637–43.

30. Holland AE, Hill CJ, Conron M, Munro P, McDonald CF. Short term improvement in exercise capacity and symptoms following exercise training in interstitial lung disease. *Thorax* 2008; **63**(6):549–54.

31. Eaton TC, Lewis P, Young Y, *et al.* Long-term oxygen therapy improves health-related quality of life. *Respir Med* 2004; **98**:285–93.

32. Moore RP, Berlowitz DJ, Denehy L, *et al. Double blind randomised trial of ambulatory oxygen versus air in COPD. Thorax* (in press)

33. Abernethy AP, Currow DC, Frith P, Fazekas B. Prescribing palliative oxygen: a clinician survey of expected benefit and patterns of use. *Palliat Med* 2005; **19**:168–70.

34. Stringer E, McParland C, Hernandez P. Physician practices for prescribing supplemental oxygen in the palliative care setting. *J Palliative Care* 2004; **20**:303–7.

35. Guyatt GH, McKim DA, Austin P, *et al.* Appropriateness of domiciliary oxygen therapy. *Chest* 2000; **118**:1303–8.

36. Currow DC, Fazekas B, Abernethy AP. Oxygen use–patients define symptomatic benefit discerningly. *J Pain Symptom Manage* 2007; **34**:113–14.

37. O'Donnell DE, D'Arsigny C, Webb KA. Effects of hyperoxia on ventilatory limitation during exercise in advanced chronic obstructive pulmonary disease. *Am J Respir Crit Care Med* 2001; **163**:892–8.

38. Booth S, Kelly MJ, Cox NP, Adams L, Guz A. Does oxygen help dyspnoea in patients with cancer. *Am J Respir Crit Care Med.* 1996; **153**:1515–18.

39. Bruera E, de Stoutz N, Velasco-Leiva A, Schoeller T, Hanson J. Effects of oxygen on dyspnoea in hypoxaemic terminal-cancer patients. *Lancet.* 1993; **342**:13–14.

40. Swinburn CR, Mould H, Stone TN, Corris PA, Gibson GJ. Symptomatic benefit of supplemental oxygen in hypoxaemic patients with chronic lung disease. *Am Rev Respir Dis* 1991; **143**:913–15.

41. Garrod R, Paul EA, Wedzicha JA. Supplemental oxygen during pulmonary rehabilitation in patients with COPD with exercise hypoxaemia. *Thorax* 2000; **55**(7):539–43.

42. Rooyacker JM, Dekhuijzen PN, Van Herwaarden CL, Folgering HT. Training with supplemental oxygen in patients with COPD and hypoxaemia at peak exercise. *Eur Respir J* 1997; **10**(6):1278–84.

43. McDonald CF, Blyth CM, Lazarus MD, Marchner I, Barter CE. Exertional oxygen of limited benefit in patients with chronic obstructive disease and mild hypoxaemia. *Am J Respir Crit Care Med* 1995; **152**:1616–19.

44. Dean NC, Brown JK, Himelman RB, *et al.* Oxygen may improve dyspnoea and endurance in patients with chronic obstructive pulmonary disease and only mild hypoxaemia. *Am Rev Respir Dis* 1992; **146**:941–5.

45. Crapagnano GE, Kharitonov SA, Foschino-Brabaro MP, *et al.* Supplementary oxygen in healthy subjects and those with COPD increases oxidative stress and airway inflammation. *Thorax* 2004; **59**:1016–19.

46. Mantell LL, Lee PJ. Signal transduction pathways in hyperoxia-induced lung cell death. *Mol Genet Metab* 2000; **71**:359–70.

47. Philips M, Cataneo RN, Greenberg J, *et al.* Effect of oxygen on breath markers of oxidative stress. *Eur Respir J* 2003; **21**:48–51.

48. Loiseaux-Meunier MN, Bedu M, Gentou C, *et al.* Oxygen toxicity: simultaneous measure of pentane and malondialdehyde in humans exposed to hyperoxia. *Biomed Pharmacother* 2001; **55**:163–9.

49. Dempsey JA, Wagner PD, Exercise-induced arterial hypoxemia. *J Appl Physiol* 1999; **87**(6): 1997–2006.

50. West JB. *Respiratory physiology: the essentials.* New York: Lippincott Williams & Wilkins, 2004.

51. Heaton RK, Grant I, McSweeny AJ, Adams KM, Petty TL. Psychologic effects of continuous and nocturnal oxygen therapy in hypoxemic chronic obstructive pulmonary disease. *Arch Intern Med* 1983; **143**:1941–7.

52. Shwartzstein RM, Lahive K, Pope A, *et al.* Cold facial stimulation reduces breathlessness induced in normal subjects. *Am Rev Respir Dis* **1987**; 136:68–1.

53. Holland AE, Hill CJ, Rasekaba T, *et al.* Updating the minimal important distance for 6 minute walk distance in patients with chronic obstructive pulmonary disease. *Arch Phys Rehabil* 2010; **91**:221–5.

54. Galbraith S, Fagan P, Perkins P, Lynch A, Booth S. Does use of a hand-held fan improve chronic dyspnoea? A randomized, controlled, cross-over trial. *J Pain Symptom Manage* 2010; **39**(5):831–8.

55. British Thoracic Society Standards of Care Committee. Managing passengers with respiratory disease planning air travel: British Thoracic Society recommendations. *Thorax* 2002; **57**:289–304.

Chapter 9

Occupational therapy, environmental modifications, and pulmonary rehabilitation

Sally Singh and Louise Sewell

Introduction

Occupational therapy concerns itself with an individual's ability to perform occupations or activities and thereby '. . . enables people to achieve as much as they can for themselves and get the most out of life'(1).

The philosophy of occupational therapy is based on two theoretical assumptions:

1. Occupation is fundamental to the basic well-being of a person. Enabling a person to regain their ability to complete daily activities or occupations can improve an individual's general health status.
2. Each individual is different, has differing roles, and so needs to be independent in a variety of activities. A holistic assessment is therefore required prior to commencing a treatment programme.

Occupational therapy and the breathless patient

Occupational therapy is applied to the breathless patient in a variety of settings, usually within acute hospitals or in community based social services. Typical examples of referrals to an occupational therapist may include:

- A man in his 70s, living alone who has been admitted to a medical ward following an acute exacerbation of his chronic obstructive pulmonary disease (COPD). He feels that he will be unable to manage personal care tasks on discharge from hospital.
- A woman in her 60s who has advanced interstitial lung disease and is unable to use the stairs at home.
- A woman in her 50s with bronchiectasis living with her husband who is anxious to maintain her ability to cope with household tasks.
- Regardless of the setting, the occupational therapy process is broadly similar and is summarized in Box 9.1. Specifically the stages of assessment, intervention, and evaluation will be examined.

Assessment

The precise nature of the assessment will depend on the location but regardless of this, information about the breathless patient's home environment and their current level of

---

Box 9.1 Steps in the occupational therapy process

- Receipt of referral and collection of relevant information.
- Initial assessment to identify presenting problems.
- Negotiate a treatment plan in conjunction with the patient.
- Initiate and complete intervention.
- Evaluate intervention.
- Discharge.

---

functioning is essential to enable a specific problem list to be formulated with the patient. Assessment methods vary but generally information is gathered by means of examination of medical records, observation, and interviews. Increasingly, standardized assessments are employed in order to evaluate both the therapist's input and the patient's progress through the intervention period. These will be discussed later.

An interview conducted in the patient's home allows the therapist to examine any physical, social and environmental barriers that are preventing the patient from achieving his or her optimal level of functional independence. Thus home visits are often arranged prior to discharge from hospital to allow a thorough assessment before discharge.

Assessment of functional status

Leidy (2) described functional status as: '. . . the ability to perform those activities people do in the normal course of their lives to meet basic needs, fulfil usual roles and maintain their life, health and well-being'.

Leidy (2) proposes that functional status comprises four dimensions. These are: functional capacity, functional performance, functional reserve, and functional capacity utilization. Functional capacity describes the individual's maximum potential to perform daily activities. Functional performance refers to the day-to-day activities that people actually do as part of their daily routine. Leidy states that these activities are the outcome of individual choice and are subject to limits imposed by functional capacity. Functional reserve is the difference between functional capacity and functional performance. Finally, functional capacity utilization describes the extent to which functional capacity is called on in the selected level of performance. This dimension can be used to illustrate why two patients with the same functional capacity can display different levels of performance.

Assessment of functional performance is essential in the occupational therapy assessment process and there are a variety of methods to measure it. These fall into three main groups: standardized functional status scales, individualized scales, and objective monitoring of daily activity.

Standardized functional status scales

These scales are normally completed by the patient and usually consist of a list of 'valid' daily activities against which the patient indicates how independent/breathless/tired they are when they complete these tasks. The 'valid' activities are usually identified after in depth discussion with the relevant patient group. Examples of functional status scales that have been developed for use with the breathless patient are listed in Box 9.2. These scales are usually quick and easy to complete and are easily scored by the therapist but can be limited if tasks are not relevant to the individual patient.

Individualized measures of functional status

These measures allow a patient to choose the daily tasks, which are important and relevant to them, against which they wish to be assessed. A limitation of these scales is that more time is needed to complete them when compared to the standardized scales, but they are helpful in identifying individualized treatment goals. One example of an individualized measure that has been used with the breathless patient is the Canadian Occupational Performance Measure (COPM) (9).

The COPM been shown to a reliable (10) and sensitive (11) measure in patients with chronic respiratory disease. It takes the form of a semi-structured interview and takes approximately 30min to complete. During the interview patients are asked to identify specific tasks that they are either unable to do or would like to do better. These problems will fall into the areas of self-care, productivity, and leisure. Patients then rate their performance and satisfaction in up to five of the most important of these problem areas. These scores are then reassessed following an agreed period of intervention. Patients need to have adequate cognitive skills to cope with the interview process but the authors have suggested that carers may be interviewed.

Objective monitoring of daily activity

Daily activity levels are difficult to measure and so activity monitors, that contain accelerometers, are increasingly being viewed as a valid and reliable tool to objectively measure physical activity levels in a patient's home environment. Movement detectors and, in particular, accelerometers have been shown to accurately measure activity in patients with chronic respiratory disease (12). These devices are usually lightweight and are worn by the patient for a number of days. More sophisticated monitors produce a plot of daily activity and this information could be useful in evaluating the need for and impact of energy conservation advice.

Box 9.2 Examples of standardized functional status scales

- The Pulmonary Functional Status Scale (3).
- Pulmonary Functional Status and Dyspnoea Questionnaire (4).
- Nottingham Extended Activities of Daily Living Index (NEADL) (5).
- Functional Performance Inventory–Short Form (FPI-SF) (6).
- London Chest Activity of Daily Living scale (LCADL) (7).
- The Manchester Respiratory Activities of Daily Living (MRADL) scale (8).

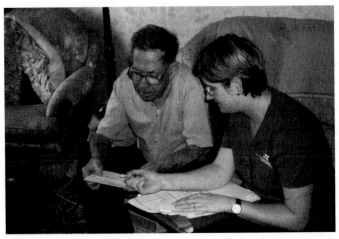

Fig. 9.1 A patient with COPD completes the Canadian Occupational Performance Measure with one of the authors.

Common problems in respiratory illness

Declining independence

Completion of daily tasks is commonly limited by increasing levels of breathlessness on exertion. This sensation is uncomfortable and frightening and so typically patients begin to reduce their overall level of activity (13). Common functional restrictions include decreased ability to climb stairs, walk outside, attend to personal care, and complete household tasks.

Fatigue

Breathless patients often report high levels of fatigue at differing times during the day which limit their ability to plan their day effectively. Previous studies have established that fatigue ranks second to breathlessness in patients with COPD, with one study citing that fatigue was reported as the worst or one of the worst symptoms in 51% of a sample of patients with COPD compared to only 27% of healthy controls (14). Kapella et al. (15) examined subjective fatigue in patients with COPD using self-reported measures. They concluded that fatigue in COPD is closely related to breathlessness during activity and is experienced more in the afternoon than morning. They also documented that fatigue had a negative effect on functional performance.

Loss of self-esteem and motivation

The respiratory disease process will often mean that individuals are forced to withdraw from their established roles. This could mean retirement from paid employment, curtailment of voluntary work, withdrawal from family roles, and decreased participation in sports and hobbies. This can often be measured in terms of self-reported symptoms of depression and self-efficacy.

Anxiety and depression

Anxiety and depression are often underdiagnosed in the breathless patient and prevalence has been difficult to determine (16). The measurement of anxiety and depression relies on the accuracy and honesty of self-reported symptoms and also on the level of sensitivity of the measure used, e.g. The Hospital Anxiety and Depression Scale (17). However, there can be no doubt that dyspnoea leads to raised anxiety levels in some patients. This anxiety often, if unaddressed, will go on to affect the patients' own management of their respiratory symptoms—they become anxious and so become more breathless.

Intervention

Energy conservation

The cumulative effect of limited exercise tolerance and increasing levels of fatigue mean that the breathless patient will have a limited capacity to take them through their day. The occupational therapist is well placed to assist patients to examine their current daily routine and then to offer advice on how they can gain the optimal level of productivity from their limited capacity. A key concept to explain to the patient is that each daily task has an 'oxygen' or 'energy' or 'vitality' cost. It is often a useful analogy to encourage patients to liken their energy levels to a daily monetary budget and to explain that some tasks are more 'expensive' than others. Tasks can increase or decrease in 'value' throughout the day. For instance, taking a bath in the evening may expend more energy for some patients than if they were to bathe in the morning. The therapist should encourage the patient to examine their own daily routine and begin to identify any patterns of fatigue during their day. Their objective is to budget their energy levels throughout the day. An understanding of managing energy levels can allow the patient to increase their overall level of independence and could lead to an improvement in levels of self-esteem and anxiety as patients regain their level of autonomy.

The efficacy of 'energy conservation' techniques has been examined by Velloso et al. (18). They were able to measure the effect of energy conservation techniques in four activities of daily living on oxygen consumption and ventilation. They demonstrated that energy conservation advice in patients with moderate to severe COPD decreased oxygen uptake and the perception of breathlessness (Box 9.3). This is the first study to use objective measures to establish the efficacy of energy conservation techniques in patients with COPD.

The individual points to consider are described in the following sections.

Pace activity

- Break activities down into small, manageable parts.
- When beginning new tasks, set small, achievable goals, rather than attempting to complete or master the whole task all at once.
- Pace overall levels of daily activity by alternating heavy tasks with light tasks.

Plan activity

- Allow ample time to complete tasks—do not squeeze too much into one day.
- Consider the times at which medication is taken—often more can be achieved after these times.
- Avoid too many trips up and down stairs—use written prompts to remember what needs to be done or brought down from upstairs.
- Organize the environment to cut down on wasting energy. Consider the layout of kitchens and any storage space.

Be energy efficient

- If objects need to be moved—push them rather than pull them.
- Use correct lifting techniques, keeping objects close to the body in order to use the larger muscle groups.
- Exhale during the most strenuous part of the activity, e.g. pulling the vacuum cleaner towards the body.
- Sit down to complete activities wherever possible.

Delegate

Consider who really needs to complete each task. Delegating one task could mean more energy to complete two other more enjoyable or essential tasks being completed.

Anxiety management

Management of anxiety is usually based on the cognitive behavioural school of psychology and often takes place in a group setting. The occupational therapist takes on the role of educator, using a structured course aiming to provide patients with the practical skills and knowledge to enable them to deal with episodes of anxiety or stress.

The content of an anxiety management programme often includes:

- Explanation of the physical and psychological processes that occur when a person experiences anxiety.
- Assertiveness skills.
- Discussions on how to recognize common, everyday stresses.
- Relaxation training.

Sometimes it may be necessary to provide this service on an individual basis.

Box 9.3 Important points in energy conservation

- Pace activity.
- Plan activity.
- Prioritize activity.
- Be energy efficient.
- Delegate.

Relaxation training

Relaxation training has its origins rooted in the behavioural approach to treating anxiety and techniques are taught on either an individual setting or, more commonly, in a group setting.

There are three main techniques employed by occupational therapists to treat both physical and psychological symptoms of anxiety. Patients may choose their preferred technique as there is no evidence for superiority of one over another.

◆ Progressive muscle relaxation: this approach teaches the patient to become aware of any tension in different muscle groups. The patient is then taught to release this tension, working their way down through the body.

◆ Autogenic training: this involves concentrating on each area of the body in turn and imagining this area becoming warm, heavy, and relaxed. The patient completes this process throughout the whole of their body continually concentrating on cue words such as 'warm', 'heavy', 'calm', and 'peaceful'.

◆ Visual imagery: this technique involves the patient being talked through a story, e.g. walking along a warm, sunny beach. Patients are encouraged to pay attention to what they may be able to hear, feel or smell. The aim is to divert any anxious thoughts and to replace them with calm, peaceful ones.

Whichever technique is used the therapist should always emphasize that relaxation is a skill that needs to be first learnt and then practised on a daily basis in order to obtain maximum benefit.

Other issues

Sexual dysfunction

Problems with sexual intercourse and intimacy, whilst often embarrassing to discuss, are important, especially as relationships could already be under strain due to the pressures of respiratory disease. Despite this, issues of sexual dysfunction are often poorly addressed (19). Limitations of physical function often lead to the erosion of roles within a relationship and loss of intimacy can only compound this process. Educational information should be presented just as any other information regarding activities of daily living. It is often helpful to link any advice regarding sexual positions and intimacy to other recommendations in relation to energy conservation and anxiety management.

The role of the carer

The pressures placed on the carer of a patient with respiratory disease can be immense. Carers face problems of exhaustion and increased levels of stress due to overwork. There can also be a loss of income that causes further problems and stresses.

The needs of the carer as well as the patient therefore form part of the assessment. Implications of any intervention for the carer must be considered before deciding on any treatment plan. Carers may find patient support groups helpful. Carers are able to attend locally run groups which offer information, support, and advice. Respite care may be appropriate in some cases and often coordinated by occupational therapists in liaison with the social workers.

Environmental modifications

A key role of occupational therapy is the assessment of the need for any major adaptations to the breathless patient's home environment. Referrals can be made by the patient themselves or their carers. One the most common problems to be addressed by the occupational therapist is that of access. This could be access into the property, to the first floor of the house, or to bathroom and toilet facilities. To address these problems adaptations commonly needed by patients with respiratory problems include:

+ Stair lifts.
+ Through-floor lifts.
+ Ground floor extensions to incorporate bathroom/bedroom and toilet facilities.
+ Installations of walk-in or level access showers with seats.

In the UK, the Disabled Facilities Grant is used to fund these adaptations. This is a means-tested grant and the occupational therapist will be involved throughout the whole process. To date, the maximum Disabled Facilities Grant is £30,000 in England, £36,000 in Wales, and £25,000 in Northern Ireland. The Disabled Facilities Grant does not affect any other benefits that the patient may be in receipt of. In addition, some adaptations works may be eligible for VAT relief.

There are also other agencies that can assist in smaller works that may help the breathless patient live independently in their own home. Home improvement agencies can provide advice and assistance to homeowners. 'Foundations' is the government body that includes many home improvement agencies England. These home improvement agencies are referred to as 'Care and Repair' schemes in Scotland and Wales. Their aim is to provide support for people to arrange minor housing improvement and maintenance works. They provide free advice and are able to arrange quotes from builders, architects, and surveyors.

Equipment provision

The occupational therapist will assess for and arrange provision of equipment that may increase the patient's ability to complete activities of daily living independently.

Equipment that is commonly found to be helpful by respiratory patients includes:

+ Perching stool (for use in kitchen and/or bathroom).
+ Chair/bed raisers.
+ Toilet seat raisers/toilet frame.
+ Bath board and bath seat.
+ Dressing aids, e.g. sock/tights gutter, dressing stick.
+ Helping hand or 'reacher'.

There is now potentially a wide range of equipment available from a variety of sources and patients may be able to purchase smaller pieces of equipment from an increasing number of local and national retail outlets. It is important to remember that whilst a piece of equipment may appear to improve function there are occasional difficulties in fitting or using it. Patients should seek the advice of an occupational therapist before purchasing equipment themselves.

In the UK, The Disabled Living Foundation is a national charity that provides impartial and expert advice on daily living aids. There is network of local Disabled Living Centres (run by Assist UK) that stock a wide range of equipment that the breathless patient may find useful. These centres will be able to demonstrate the equipment and offer the patient expert advice. Larger items of equipment are also often available on loan from social services departments. These can also be provided by occupational therapists who work in the hospital setting.

The funding of environmental modifications recommended as part of occupational therapy is highly variable world-wide. Modifications can be funded through a variety of government grants, through voluntary services and charities or via the private sector. The cost-effectiveness of these interventions has not been formally assessed, as for pulmonary rehabilitation (see below), but there is at least a theoretical argument that such interventions keep patients out of the costly in-patient environment.

(a) (b)

(c)

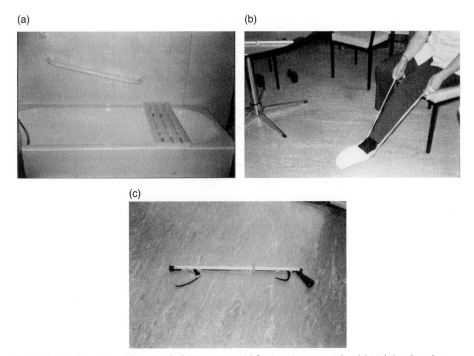

Fig. 9.2 (a) Bath seat and hand rail. (b) Dressing aid for putting on socks. (c) Helping hand or reacher for grabbing articles without bending.

Pulmonary rehabilitation

Pulmonary rehabilitation has become an established intervention for patients with chronic respiratory disease following the availability of increasing high quality evidence for efficacy. The majority of data involve patients with chronic obstructive pulmonary disease but there is a growing acknowledgement that the benefits may extend to most chronic respiratory diseases. Pulmonary rehabilitation has most recently been described in a COPD European Respiratory Society statement (20) as:

> . . . an evidence-based, multidisciplinary, and comprehensive intervention for patients with chronic respiratory diseases who are symptomatic and often have decreased daily life activities. Integrated into the individualised treatment of the patient, pulmonary rehabilitation is designed to reduce symptoms, optimise functional status, increase participation, and reduce healthcare costs through stabilising or reversing systemic manifestations of the disease.

One of the most important symptoms for patients with chronic respiratory disease is dyspnoea. Initially, this may be associated with strenuous activity but over time is increasingly associated with less demanding tasks, and it is sadly too often the point at which patients present to primary care teams. Interestingly, this reduction in task achievement is largely independent of absolute level of ventilator impairment as indicated by the patients' spirometry. Often patients become trapped in a vicious cycle of inactivity, initiated by breathlessness. Activities are avoided to reduce the impact of the sensation of breathlessness; inevitably, loss of fitness ensues, and patients become de-conditioned and activities of daily living become disproportionately difficult. In the extreme, individuals become depressed and socially isolated.

The consequence of this lack of activity is reflected in overall reduced exercise capacity and a decline in peripheral muscle strength. Recent work has demonstrated that this decline in both exercise capacity (21) and strength (22) may occur early in the disease process. It has also been suggested in independent studies that declining peak exercise performance is associated with increased mortality as is declining peripheral muscle strength (23). Importantly both reduced aerobic capacity and peripheral muscle strength are potentially modifiable, through a process of rehabilitation. A third piece of this complex jigsaw suggests that physical activity may also be an independent risk factor for mortality and hospital admission, inevitably this outcome must be linked to declining strength and exercise capacity. In a large cohort study, those with this very low level of activity were at a significantly increased risk of admission or death (24). The same research group had previously documented that readmission rates after initial hospitalization for an exacerbation of COPD were significantly higher for the following 12 months in patients who had not received rehabilitation (25) and likelihood of readmission was reduced if patients undertook regular activity accumulating more than 60min walking a day (26).

Independent of any patient-related outcomes there is an emerging health economic benefit to providing rehabilitation. This was confirmed in a large randomized trial that completed a full cost-effectiveness analysis (27).

Selection of patients for rehabilitation

Rehabilitation could be extended to all patients with chronic respiratory disease who have noticeable disability as a consequence of the systemic effects of the disease. This usually translates into the Medical Research Council (MRC) Dyspnoea grades 3–5, those individuals who are moderately affected by their disease through to those who have difficulty dressing or undressing, feel unable to leave the house due to breathlessness, or are breathless at rest. Selection should not be based on the level of respiratory impairment or age. Patients should not be included in the exercise component of rehabilitation if they have, for example, unstable angina or any of the other contraindications to exercise catalogued by the American College of Sports Medicine. It is quite likely that participants will present with other significant comorbidities but the impact of these should be assessed at the time of the initial assessment. There is some literature to indicate that rehabilitation can be equally successful in patients with less severe disability defined by their MRC grade and rehabilitation should perhaps be extended to those patients with milder disease (28).

The process of rehabilitation

The process of rehabilitation starts at the point of the initial assessment.

This assessment can include a number of the following observations:

◆ Basic demographics, past medical history, medication, spirometry, height, and weight.
◆ Exercise capacity (maximal and endurance, including the requirement for supplemental oxygen).
◆ Physical activity (barrier to exercise).
◆ Peripheral muscle strength (and muscle mass).
◆ Respiratory muscle strength.
◆ (Health-related) quality of life.
◆ Psychological well-being.
◆ Nutritional status.
◆ Patient goals.

Exercise tolerance

Classically this is defined using a laboratory-based exercise test; a great deal of physiological data can be acquired from this type of testing, including an evaluation of the limitation to exercise. In the past it has been suggested that those patients demonstrating a ventilatory limit may be less likely to achieve a positive outcome from rehabilitation (29) but this is not consistently demonstrated (30). More commonly a field-based exercise test is used as a surrogate marker of exercise capacity. The two most commonly employed are the 6-minute walking test (6MWT) (31) and the incremental shuttle walking test (ISWT) (32). Both have been reported in the literature. The incremental shuttle walking test is externally paced, and provokes a maximal performance with physiological variables following a similar trajectory to those recorded during a maximal laboratory based test (33).

The 6MWT is self-paced, although an 'encourage' test may result in a similar peak values the trajectory is different, patients seem to have an abrupt rise in heart rate and oxygen consumption that peaks by the third minute of the test and is sustained until completion (34). The endurance shuttle walking test, in principle is like the ISWT but has a constant pace, and may be a useful outcome measure for an exercise-based intervention (35). Step test are less frequently used in this setting. An exercise test is important to define the level of disability, observe the response to exercise and prescribe a training regimen that is unique to the individual patient. They do of course act as an important outcome measure. The utility of these field tests has been described in the context of rehabilitation, they are known to be sensitive to change and the minimum clinically important difference has been described for patients with COPD has been reported. As a mean change it has been estimated that patients need to walk 54m further on the 6MWT (36) and 48m (or five shuttles) on the ISWT (37). A comparable figure has not been identified for the ESWT. The reported response to rehabilitation is less pronounced for patients with interstitial lung disease, and it has therefore been suggested that the minimum clinically important difference may be reduced (38). The equivalent figure for the ESWT has not been published.

An exercise test is employed to identify important changes in oxygen saturation, usually using a pulse oximeter. Significant changes suggest that ambulatory oxygen should be used during the exercise programme, although the evidence to support this in patients who document a fall is not convincing (39).

Physical activity has become an increasingly important outcome measure for rehabilitation, and is believed to reflect a genuine change in behaviour. The utility and choice of outcome measures will be discussed elsewhere in this chapter.

Strength

The decline of peripheral muscle strength is an important systemic consequence of chronic respiratory disease, and is potentially modifiable through rehabilitation. The gold standard measure of strength is achieved on an isokinetic dynamometer, the measure reported most frequently is isometric strength (Nm). This equipment can be expensive and limited to research centres. Alternative equipment is commercially available and can range from simple hand-held dynamometers to strain gauges attached to a chair and calibrated with a dedicated software package allowing accurate recording of the peak and sustained force generated. The change in strength after a rehabilitation programme is in the region of 20% when a specific resistance training programme is offered as part of the regimen.

Respiratory muscle strength is usually estimated by measuring peak inspiratory pressure. It is important to identify respiratory muscle strength as a potential target for rehabilitation: it is suggested that those with reduced respiratory muscle strength are most likely to benefit from a programme incorporating inspiratory muscle training (IMT). Again there is a range of techniques and equipment to measure respiratory muscle strength, ranging from simple hand-held devices to sophisticated equipment that is able to differentiate the contribution made by the diaphragm and the intercostals muscle.

Health-related quality of life and measures of psychological well-being

Improvement of health-related quality of life is important to reflect the impact of the disease on the patient's well-being, and there are a number of questionnaires that could be employed including the St Georges Respiratory Questionnaire (SGRQ) (40) and the chronic respiratory questionnaire (CRQ) (41, 42) (See chapter 6). The questionnaires are mainly self-completed. They explore the effect of living with chronic respiratory disease in areas such as the symptoms experienced, the activity restriction, the emotional impact of the disease, the social impact of the disease, and the feeling of control. The minimum clinically important difference for the SGRQ and the CRQ have been defined—4 points and 0.5 per domain for the questionnaires respectively.

Nutritional status

The measurement of nutritional status is assumed to be reflected in BMI (body mass index), although this may not always reflect nutritional depletion. Historically it has been the underweight individuals that have been of most concern, as the prognosis of a patient with COPD is worse if the BMI is low. However, the effectiveness of nutritional supplementation has not been established in COPD.

The exercise programme

The cornerstone of rehabilitation has been endurance training although more recently the role of resistance training has been recognized.

Aerobic training provokes a change in muscle metabolism to support a greater level of endurance activity. Aerobic exercise is usually offered as a walking- or cycling-based programme and should be prescribed at a level corresponding to at least 60% of peak oxygen capacity (20). Although it is established that high intensity training may provoke a greater physiological response, some authors have suggested that compliance outside of the supervised environment may be more challenging for patients (43). The most accessible form of exercise is walking, and is the most important activity to patients with COPD (11). Initial assessment of walking capacity is imperative, this is an incremental exercise test that compares favourably with the physiological response provoked by a conventional laboratory-based exercise test. Because of this relationship it is straightforward to identify a training load that corresponds to between 60% and 85% of predicted peak performance. The individually prescribed speed of walking can be formally calibrated against the endurance shuttle walking test, which along with the ISWT forms a useful outcome measure. Cycle-based training is more easily controlled and progressed although this depends on the patient having this equipment at home for continuing exercise. Rowing and stepping, whilst constituting aerobic training, are seldom reported in this population.

Resistance training directly addresses the issue of peripheral muscle dysfunction. The degree of impairment is significant in the population attending rehabilitation. Both quality and quantity of muscle is disrupted in chronic lung disease and resistance training provokes both a change in muscle mass and the composition of the muscle. It is suggested in current guidelines that resistance training should be formalized and structured. The weights are set (after an initial assessment of strength) to allow the individual to repeat two to three sets of eight to ten repetitions. Once this can be completed the weight should be increased.

Of particular importance is general advice about a home exercise programme. The ultimate aim should be 30min of exercise/brisk walking for 5 days per week. Many patients never achieve this, but all participants should be encouraged to extend their walking times gradually.

Educational programme

The educational programme covers a number of topics including chest clearance, exacerbation management, relaxation advice, breathing control, tests and travelling, and managing physical activity. The agenda is to equip the individual with the knowledge and skills to self-manage their disease. It has recently been reported that the process of rehabilitation does indeed improve the individuals' knowledge. There is not one preferred definition of self-management, and the term is often used interchangeably with self-care. Fundamental to the terms is a process of knowledge acquisition that provokes important lifestyle changes, which is the aim of rehabilitation.

Duration of rehabilitation programme   The programme usually extends over 6–8 weeks, with two sessions per week of supervised exercise. Within the UK this is standard practice, although in some parts of Europe the programme may extend over 6 months (44). There is some evidence exploring the value of a shortened 4-week course of rehabilitation, suggesting that it may be comparable in the short term to a 7-week programme (45).

One of the challenges for rehabilitation services is to describe the optimal maintenance strategy. Various packages have been tested with no clear favourite. A number of approaches have been tested ranging from repeating courses of rehabilitation, regular maintenance exercise groups, to telephone follow-up. Unlike cardiac rehabilitation there is no mechanism to provide long-term maintenance in the community

Summary

Occupational therapy and pulmonary rehabilitation share common approaches towards delivery of supportive care. Occupational therapy aims firstly to establish what changes in functional performance would improve the breathless patient's quality of life and then set about formulating an effective treatment plan. Pulmonary rehabilitation is directed towards achieving specific improvements in functional capacity and thereby improvements in quality of life. Both of these components of supportive care include consideration of the physical and psychological needs of the breathless patient. It is important to recognize that the work may be usefully done in conjunction with a physiotherapist. For cancer patients, nurses also contribute significantly in this area.

Interventions may help the many practical problems caused by dyspnoea, fatigue, and limited muscle function, and the related problems of anxiety, depression, and demotivation. Standardized measures are available which can document clinically significant changes in the patient's functional performance. An occupational therapy assessment will provide the breathless patient with an opportunity to discuss their functional difficulties in detail and the specific intervention of pulmonary rehabilitation may serve to improve functional capacity. Both occupational therapy and pulmonary rehabilitation are important aspects of supportive care in patients with respiratory disease that can lead to significant improvements in quality of life.

Key points

- ◆ Occupational therapy aims to enable the breathless patient to attain optimal independence in activities of daily living.
- ◆ Standardized measures of function are now available which enable the occupational therapist to measure the clinical effectiveness of their intervention.
- ◆ Energy conservation techniques allow the breathless patient to make the most efficient use of their reduced level of exercise tolerance.
- ◆ Specific interventions such as anxiety management and relaxation training may be essential in helping the breathless patient to maintain some control over their condition.
- ◆ Pulmonary rehabilitation programmes need to be individually tailored after assessment.
- ◆ Pulmonary rehabilitation with endurance and resistance training improves functional capacity.
- ◆ Occupational therapy involves the provision of equipment that often enables the breathless patient to maintain their independence in activities of daily living as their respiratory condition deteriorates.

References

1. British Association of Occupational Therapists and College of Occupational Therapists. OT helps you [Internet, undated]. http://www.cot.co.uk/Homepage/About_Occupational_Therapy/Occupational_therapy_explained/
2. Leidy NK. Using functional status to assess treatment outcomes. *Chest* 1994; **106**:1645–6.
3. Weaver TE, Narsavage GL, Guilfoyle MJ. The development and psychometric evaluation of the Pulmonary Functional Status Scale: an instrument to assess functional status in pulmonary disease. *J Cardiopulm Rehabil* 1998; **18**:105–11.
4. Lareau SC, Meek PM, Roos PJ. Development and testing of the modified version of the Pulmonary Functional Status and Dyspnea Questionnaire (PFSDQ-M). *Heart and Lung* 1998; **27**:159–68.
5. Lincoln NB, Gladman, JRF. The Extended Activities of Daily Living scale: a further validation. *Disabil Rehabil* 1992; **14**:41–3.
6. Leidy NK, Knebel AR. Clinical validation of the Functional Performance Inventory in patients with chronic obstructive pulmonary disease. *Respir Care* 1999; **44**:932–9.
7. Garrod R, Bestall JC, Paul EA, Wedzicha JA, Jones PW. Development and validation of a standardized measure of activity of daily living in patients with severe COPD: the London Chest Activity of Daily Living scale (LCADL). *Respir Med* 2000; **94**:589–96.
8. Yohannes AM, Roomi J, Winn S, Connolly MJ. The Manchester Respiratory Activities of Daily Living questionnaire: development, reliability, validity and responsiveness to pulmonary rehabilitation. *J Am Geriatr Soc* 2000; **48**(11):1496–500.

9. Law M, Baptiste S, McColl MA, Opzoomer A, Polatajko, H, Pollock, N. The Canadian Occupational Performance Measure (3rd edn). Toronto: CAOT Publications, 1998.

10. Sewell L, Singh SJ. The reproducibility of the Canadian Occupational Performance Measure. *Br J Occup Ther* 2001; **64**(6):305–10.

11. Sewell L, Singh SJ, Williams JE, Collier R, Morgan MDL. Can individualised rehabilitation improve functional independence in elderly patients with COPD? *Chest* 2005; **128**:1194–1200.

12. Pitta F, Troosters T, Probst VS, *et al.* Quantifying physical activity in daily life with questionnaires and motion sensors in COPD. *Eur Resp J* 2006; **27**:1040–55.

13. Griffiths TL, Burr ML, Cambell IA, *et al.* Results at 1 year of outpatient multidisciplinary pulmonary rehabilitation: a randomised controlled trial. *Lancet* 2000; **355**:362–68.

14. Theander K, Jakobsson P, Torstensson O, *et al.* Severity of fatigue is related to functional limitation and health in patients with chronic obstructive pulmonary disease. *Int J Nurs Pract* 2008; **14**(6):455–62.

15. Kapella MC, Larson J, Patel MK, *et al.* Subjective fatigue, influencing variables and consequences in chronic obstructive pulmonary disease. *Nursing Research* 2006; **55**(1):10–17.

16. Chronic obstructive pulmonary disease. National clinical guideline on management of chronic obstructive pulmonary disease in adults in primary and secondary care. *Thorax* 2004; **59**(suppl 1):1–232.

17. Zigmond A, Snaith, RP. The Hospital Anxiety and Depression Scale. *Acta Psychiatri Scand* 1983; **67**:361–70.

18. Velloso M, Jardim JR. Study of energy expenditure during activities of daily living using and not using body position recommended by energy conservation techniques in patients with COPD. *Chest* 2006; **130**:126–132.

19. Vincent EE, Singh SJ. Addressing the sexual health of patients with COPD: the needs of the patient and implications for health care professionals. *Chronic Respir Dis* 2007; **4**:111–15.

20. Nici L, Donner C, Wouters E, *et al.* American Thoracic Society/European Respiratory Society statement on pulmonary rehabilitation *Am J Respir Crit Care Med* 2006; **173**:1390–413.

21. Watz H, Waschki B, Meyer T, Magnussen H. Physical activity in patients with COPD. *Eur Respir J* 2009; **33**:262–72.

22. Seymour JM, Spruit MA, Hopkinson NS, *et al.* The prevalence of quadriceps weakness in COPD and the relationship with disease severity. *Eur Respir J* 2009; **36**:81–8.

23. Swallow EB, Reyes D, Hopkinson NS, *et al.* Quadriceps strength predicts mortality in patients with moderate to severe chronic obstructive pulmonary disease. *Thorax* 2007; **62**:115–20.

24. Garcia-Aymerich J, Lange P, Benet M, Schnohr P, Anto JM. Regular physical activity reduces hospital admission and mortality in chronic obstructive pulmonary disease: a population based cohort study. *Thorax* 2006; **61**:772–8.

25. Garcia-Aymerich J, Farrero E, Félez MA, *et al.* Risk factors of readmission to hospital for a COPD exacerbation: a prospective study. *Thorax* 2003; **58**:100–5.

26. Garcia-Aymerich J, Barreiro E, Farrero E, Marrades RM, Morera J, Anto JM. Patients hospitalized for COPD have a high prevalence of modifiable risk factors for exacerbation (EFRAM study). *Eur Respir J* 2000; **16**:1037–42.

27. Griffiths TL, Phillips CJ, Davies S, Burr ML, Campbell IA. Cost effectiveness of an outpatient multidisciplinary pulmonary rehabilitation programme. *Thorax* 2001; **56**:779–84.

28. Evans RA, Singh SJ, Collier R, Williams JE, Morgan MD. Pulmonary rehabilitation is successful for COPD irrespective of MRC dyspnoea grade. *Respir Med* 2009; **103**:1070–5.

29. Troosters T, Gosselink R, Decramer M. Exercise training in COPD: how to distinguish responders from nonresponders. *J Cardiopulm Rehabil* 2001; **21**:10–17.

30. Calvert LD, Singh SJ, Greenhaff PL, Morgan MD, Steiner MC. The plasma ammonia response to cycle exercise in COPD. *Eur Respir J* 2008; **31**:751–8.

31. ATS. ATS statement: guidelines for the six-minute walk test. *Am J Respir Crit Care Med* 2002; **166**:111–17.

32. Singh SJ, Morgan MD, Scott S, Walters D, Hardman AE. Development of a shuttle walking test of disability in patients with chronic airways obstruction. *Thorax* 1992; **47**:1019–24.

33. Singh SJ, Morgan MD, Hardman AE, Rowe C, Bardsley PA. Comparison of oxygen uptake during a conventional treadmill test and the shuttle walking test in chronic airflow limitation. *Eur Respir J* 1994; **7**:2016–20.

34. Casas A, Vilaro J, Rabinovich R, *et al.* Encouraged 6-min walking test indicates maximum sustainable exercise in COPD patients. *Chest* 2005; **128**:55–61.

35. Revill SM, Morgan MD, Singh SJ, Williams J, Hardman AE. The endurance shuttle walk: a new field test for the assessment of endurance capacity in chronic obstructive pulmonary disease. *Thorax* 1999; **54**:213–22.

36. Redelmeier DA, Bayoumi AM, Goldstein RS, Guyatt GH. Interpreting small differences in functional status: the Six Minute Walk test in chronic lung disease patients. *Am J Respir Crit Care Med* 1997; **155**:1278–82.

37. Singh SJ, Jones PW, Evans R, Morgan MD. Minimum clinically important improvement for the incremental shuttle walking test. *Thorax* 2008; **63**:775–7.

38. Holland AE, Hill CJ, Conron M, Munro P, McDonald CF. Small changes in six-minute walk distance are important in diffuse parenchymal lung disease. *Respir Med* 2009; **103**:1430–5.

39. Bradley JM, Lasserson T, Elborn S, Macmahon J, O'Neill B. A systematic review of randomized controlled trials examining the short-term benefit of ambulatory oxygen in COPD. *Chest* 2007; **131**:278–85.

40. Jones PW, Quirk FH, Baveystock CM, Littlejohns P. A self-complete measure of health status for chronic airflow limitation. The St George's Respiratory Questionnaire. *Am Rev Respir Dis* 1992; **145**:1321–7.

41. Guyatt GH, Berman LB, Townsend M, Pugsley SO, Chambers L.W. A measure of quality of life for clinical trials in chronic lung disease. *Thorax* 1987; **42**:773–8.

42. Williams JE, Singh SJ, Sewell L, Guyatt GH, Morgan MD. Development of a self-reported Chronic Respiratory Questionnaire (CRQ-SR). *Thorax* 2001; **56**:954–9.

43. Normandin EA, McCusker C, Connors ML, *et al.* An evaluation of two approaches to exercise conditioning in pulmonary rehabilitation. *Chest* 2002; **121**:1085–91.

44. Troosters T, Gosselink R, Decramer, M. Short- and long-term effects of outpatient rehabilitation in patients with chronic obstructive pulmonary disease: a randomized trial. *Am J Med* 2000; **109**:207–12.

45. Sewell L, Singh SJ, Williams JE, Collier R, Morgan MD. How long should outpatient pulmonary rehabilitation be? A randomised controlled trial of 4 weeks versus 7 weeks. *Thorax* 2006; **61**:767–71.

Chapter 10

Non-pharmacological strategies for dyspnoea

Virginia Carrieri-Kohlman and DorAnne Donesky-Cuenco

Symptom prevalence of dyspnoea and comorbidities

Despite optimal medical therapy and rehabilitation, nearly 75% of individuals with moderate to severe chronic obstructive pulmonary disease (COPD; the dominant cause of chronic breathlessness in the community) continue to experience dyspnoea with daily activities (1–3). Dyspnoea causes social isolation, difficulty performing routine activities, and impairs sexual function. Less than 50% of patients with COPD experience relief from dyspnoea during the final 6 months of life (4). Dyspnoea is known as the symptom that is the 'least controlled' by traditional medical therapies (5).

Depression and anxiety often precipitate dyspnoea or are escalated by dyspnoea (6). In a systematic review that focused on patients with severe disease, the prevalence of anxiety was found to be 50–75%, with depression ranging from 37–71% (6). The anxiety–dyspnoea–anxiety cycle experienced by patients in clinical situations has been validated by patients in qualitative interviews (7). Anxiety was associated with more frequent symptom-based exacerbations and a longer hospital stay (8). Because dyspnoea is so strongly predictive of anxiety, it has been proposed that respiratory physiology may have an effect on the psychophysiological mechanisms in anxiety (9, 10).

Recently in a large sample of people with COPD living in China, after adjusting for disease severity, depression was significantly associated with a higher risk of exacerbations and hospitalizations with a dose–response trend (8). Both anxiety and depression increase a patient's symptom burden in the palliative care phase (11).

Dyspnoea as a multidimensional symptom

Non-pharmacological strategies discussed in this chapter are based on a multidimensional definition of dyspnoea as a symptom, accepted phases of symptom perception, evidence of strong relationships between malleable factors and dyspnoea intensity, and principles of biological, sociological, and cognitive-behavioural theory.

Dyspnoea derives from interactions between 'multiple physiological, psychological, social, and environmental factors, and may induce secondary physiological and behavioral responses' (12; p. 322). Dyspnoea is a consciously appreciated subjective experience reflecting changes in the biopsychosocial functioning, sensations, or cognition, resulting in the integration of multiple factors (13, 14).

Affective dimension

Both laboratory and clinical studies have recently shown that, like pain, dyspnoea has a sensation intensity, but also an affective unpleasantness or distress dimension (15, 16).

Functional magnetic resonance imaging (fMRI) has been used to examine the subcortical areas of the brain associated with rating the perceived intensity and the unpleasantness of dyspnoea. Neuroimaging studies have shown activation of the anterior insular cortex, anterior cingulate gyrus, and the amygdala during laboratory-induced air hunger (17, 18). These findings indicate that the affective dimension of dyspnoea is processed in areas of the brain that also are activated by the sensations of pain (19), thirst (20), hunger (21), and fear (22).

The magnitude and change of the two dimensions can be rated independently and are independently influenced by interventions (15, 16, 23–25). Healthy volunteers in the laboratory (26, 27), people with asthma and COPD (28), people with COPD during exercise (15, 29, 30), and patients with lung cancer (31) have differentiated the sensory from the affective dimension of dyspnoea. Both may be appropriate targets for therapy.

Phases of symptom perception

All theories of symptom perception acknowledge the phases of information input, the person's attention to the information, detection of the sensation as something different, attribution or assigning meaning, the multitude of factors that change the individual's perception of the symptom, and subsequent behaviour that results from this process (13, 32, 33).

In the study of dyspnoea it is proposed that a change of sufficient magnitude (threshold) in the respiratory sensory systems leads to the stimulation of receptors and the transmission of afferent information centrally resulting in the cognitive awareness of breathing. It is not merely the awareness of breathing, but the perception that the drive to breathe is not being matched by adequate pulmonary ventilation (34). Different physiological derangements lead to qualitatively different sensations including breathing effort, air hunger, or tightness (16, 35). These respiratory sensations are further modulated by attention, experience, learning, and the affective state of the individual (33).

Factors related to the intensity and distress of dyspnoea

Psychosocial factors that influence the perception of dyspnoea include personality (36), emotions including anxiety (37, 38) and depression (39–41), attention to the symptom (42), the meaning of the symptom for the person (32), and beliefs in the effectiveness of coping strategies (43, 44). Social-environmental influences, such as prior history with the symptom, the social context in which it is experienced (45), family conflict (46), and comorbidities such as fatigue, anxiety, and depression (47, 48) also influence the perception of shortness of breath. Bodily preoccupation, level of awareness, usual level of physical activity, body weight, state of nutrition, ethnicity (49), and medications may also influence the perception or rating of dyspnoea (50).

Cognitive-behavioural perspective

Most non-pharmacological strategies proposed in this chapter can be labelled cognitive-behavioural strategies or coping strategies that are targeted towards altering the patient's interpretation or meaning of the symptom. Cognitive-behavioural strategies suggest that individuals can be taught new patterns of thinking, feeling, and behaving to manage their symptoms (51). A major tenet of this approach is that symptoms occur in a social context and a patient's behaviour with dyspnoea is in part shaped by others, and influences the behaviour of others (52).

Increased perceived confidence for coping can reduce symptoms in several ways (53). For example, if a person believes he or she can cope with the amount of dyspnoea they will experience while climbing stairs, his or her anxiety about climbing stairs may be less. People who believe they can exercise control over their symptoms are more likely to tolerate unpleasant sensations than those who believe there is nothing they can do (53).

Illness trajectories

People with COPD are usually ill for many years with a slowly progressive illness that may be interrupted abruptly with acute exacerbations potentially requiring hospitalization. They often have social isolation and a low quality of life (54–56). Management strategies for shortness of breath should be taught in the early palliative phases of COPD with ongoing reinforcement. With the early introduction of a strategy, the patient and caregiver can test the effectiveness of the strategy for them and optimize ways to implement.

Assessment of dyspnoea

The most frequent measurement of dyspnoea is 'Mr Smith, are you short of breath?' This question typically brings a 'yes' or 'no' answer. The American College of Chest Physicians Position Statement on the management of dyspnoea in advanced disease (57) recommend that dyspnoea assessment should include a measure of intensity and the associated distress.

Strategies used in the early phases of stable chronic illness
Pulmonary rehabilitation programmes

Structured pulmonary rehabilitation (PR) is a comprehensive therapy for people with moderate COPD. PR is now also recognized as effective for patients with other pulmonary diseases, including interstitial lung disease (58–63).

In PR, it has been demonstrated that lower- and upper-extremity exercise training reduce dyspnoea, increase ability to perform exercise, and improve health-related quality of life (HRQL) (64, 65). PR also significantly reduces healthcare utilization and improves psychosocial outcomes, including anxiety and depression (57, 66). Some new evidence indicates that longer-term rehabilitation, maintenance strategies following rehabilitation, and the incorporation of strength training in pulmonary rehabilitation add benefits to an 8-week structured programme (57). Home-based PR programmes with nurse visits are an alternative to structured outpatient PR and have had equivalent improvements in dyspnoea, activities of daily living and function (68, 69). Home-based 'exercise only' programmes also have had positive outcomes reinforcing the need to include exercise as an integral part of any programme (70–72).

Exercise training

There is good evidence that exercise alone is one of the most successful non-pharmacological approaches for managing breathlessness (60, 73, 74). A major goal of exercise training is to transfer the improvement in performance and dyspnoea that is achieved with one form of exercise (e.g. treadmill walking, cycling) to activities of daily living (57, 75). A meta-analysis of 14 clinical trials strongly supported PR programmes with exercise training for at least 4 weeks for clinically and statistically significant improvements in dyspnoea (76). Exercise training alone also decreases dyspnoea (29, 77). Weight training of upper- and lower-limb muscles may also improve exercise performance and dyspnoea (78). Modalities that improve function (i.e. walking) are important because they can also enhance quality of life (79).

Self-management programmes

Support for collaborative self-management has been recognized as a vital component in chronic illness care (80, 81). Self-management is a primary focus in the Chronic Care Model (CCM) (82). The patient and family become partners in their every day care. Specifically, self-management requires that patients: 1) engage in activities that promote health and reduce the likelihood of adverse outcomes; 2) interact with healthcare providers and adhere to recommended treatment protocols; 3) monitor symptoms, exacerbations, and emotional status and make appropriate management decisions on the basis of the results of monitoring symptoms; and 4) manage the effects of their illness on emotions, self-esteem, relationships with others, and their ability to function in important roles (83–85). Although studies have shown self-management programmes to be effective for people with asthma (86), studies in COPD are inconsistent (87).

Studies have confirmed that education alone is not sufficient to bring about positive outcomes for patients with COPD (87, 88). Group or individual education sessions (1–26 hours) were the most common intervention. No positive effects were found on hospital admissions, emergency visits, days lost from work, or lung function.

A recent critical review of 14 trials comparing self-management programmes for patients with COPD to usual care found a statistically and clinically significant reduction in healthcare utilization and a small but significant improvement in dyspnoea; however, there were no effects on the number of exacerbations, lung function, or other symptoms (89).

Two studies that provided action plans and prescriptions for antibiotics and steroids had the greatest effect on healthcare utilization but no effect on symptoms (70, 90).

Adams and colleagues (91) reviewed programmes in COPD that contained the CCM components of self-management, delivery system design, decision support, and clinical information systems. The programme that had lower rates of hospitalizations and emergency room visits and shorter length of hospital stays compared with the control groups provided '. . . an extensive self-management programme with an individualized action plan, advanced access to care with a knowledgeable healthcare provider and guideline based therapy. . .' (91; p. 558) Interestingly, three of the RCTs demonstrated a statistically significant, but clinically insignificant improvement in dyspnoea using the Borg scale to measure dyspnoea (91).

A recent multicentre randomized trial (RCT) provided support for the positive effect of giving patients an action plan with ready access to medications. Rice and colleagues (92) implemented a simplified disease management (DM) programme in a multisite study in Veterans Administration hospitals. The DM programme included a single 1–1.5-hour group education session which included general information about COPD, direct observation of inhaler techniques, a review and adjustment of outpatient COPD medications, and smoking cessation counselling. All patients received an individualized written action plan that included self-treatment of exacerbations with refillable prescriptions for prednisone and an oral antibiotic, the telephone number of the 24-hour VA helpline, and encouragement to call a case manager, who followed up with monthly calls. Compared to usual care, the DM programme reduced the frequency of COPD hospitalizations and emergency visits by 41% and significantly improved self-reported health status.

An outpatient palliative medicine consultation team, improved outcomes in patients with COPD, cancer or congestive heart failure who had a prognosis of 1–5 years (93). This programme of multiple consultations by a palliative medicine team, advanced care planning, psychosocial support, and family caregiver training over a year was compared with a control group who received standard care in general medicine clinics. The patients who received intervention from the consultation team had significantly less dyspnoea and anxiety, and better sleep and spiritual well-being than the usual care group.

Three studies suggest that some educational interventions may reduce dyspnoea. One study in a group of patients with COPD received teaching and counselling by a nurse, compared with three other groups of patients (who underwent non-specific surveillance with psychotherapy, analytic psychotherapy from experienced psychotherapists, and supportive psychotherapy from experienced psychotherapists); the study found that the group treated by the nurse was the only one that experienced a 'sustained relief in breathlessness' (94). Eight interactive small-group education-only sessions significantly decreased dyspnoea with activity, measured by the CRQ, compared with untreated control subjects (95). A group with lung cancer, decreased their dyspnoea and dyspnoea-related distress more than a control group after completing a clinic-based programme on dyspnoea management strategies (31, 96).

One study included individualized education and demonstration of dyspnoea self-management strategies, an action plan, plus different doses of an individualized home walking prescription reinforced with biweekly nurse telephone calls. Patients who received 24 supervised exercise sessions had greater improvement in exercise performance and dyspnoea during laboratory exercise in the short term (97); however, at one year this group was no different in their improvements in dyspnoea with daily activities, physical functioning, or health-related quality of life than the patients who had four nurse-coached exercise sessions or those who only completed prescribed walks at home (75).

Technological advances in monitoring and communication provide an opportunity to expand self-management efforts. Patients with COPD access information and support groups via the internet. Many sites are available for patients and families to learn more about their disease and symptoms, and hear from others' strategies. A dyspnoea self-management programme (DSMP) has been modified for internet application to bring education about dyspnoea management strategies, peer support, symptom monitoring and reinforcement of exercise to patients with COPD in their homes. A pilot study with a small sample of COPD patients to determine the feasibility and preliminary efficacy of an Internet-based dyspnoea self-management programme (eDSMP) found that most of these elderly chronically ill patients were able to participate in the web-based programme and their confidence in managing their dyspnoea improved (98). After making content, functional, and process changes in the programme the eDSMP Internet programme was compared to a tested face-to-face programme and found that they were similar in their positive clinically meaningful short-term outcomes of dyspnoea with daily activities, physical functioning, self-efficacy for managing dyspnoea, and adherence to daily exercise (99).

Non-pharmacological strategies

The non-pharmacological treatments appropriate for teaching and practice when the patient is relatively well are listed in Box 10.1 as outlined by Booth (100).

Effective dyspnoea management strategies identified by adults with COPD

People with a chronic disease like COPD become 'symptom managers' and adopt the strategies that 'work for them'. Self-management relies heavily on knowledge and skills people with chronic illnesses already use (101). Five studies report descriptions of strategies used by patients to manage dyspnoea (46, 102–104, 123–125). Most patients develop and use 6–10 strategies to manage their dyspnoea (Box 10.2) (102, 103). Women tend to use distraction or diversion and prayer more than men and both genders use problem-focused more than emotion-focused strategies (102, 104).

Patients who received formal training in breath control techniques reported significantly more benefit compared to those who had not received formal training (103). It is important to ask the patient what has helped them in the past and build on that repertoire of dyspnoea management strategies.

Box 10.1 Non-pharmacological treatments to be taught and practiced when patient is relatively well

- Remind patient and caregiver to use the strategies they previously found effective.
- Facial cooling with a hand-held fan around the mouth, nose and surrounding cheeks).
- Keeping physically active: exercise programmes tailored to individual.
- Breathing retraining.
- Relaxation, music, and anxiety control techniques.
- Psychological support for both patient and caregiver.
- Addressing fears about breathlessness—'I will not let you suffer'.
- Education about strategies to manage symptoms of breathlessness, fatigue, and pain.
- Assessment for depression and active treatment.
- Support/respite for the family, e.g. hospice care.

Adapted from Booth S. End of life care for the breathless patient. *General Practice Update* 2009: 39–43. Copyright Elsevier (2009).

Box 10.2 Dyspnoea management strategies ranked by adults with COPD as most effective

1. Oxygen
2. Self control of medications
3. Get fresh air
4. Plan in advance
5. Inhaler use
6. Keep still
7. Move slower
8. Stop or modify activities to conserve energy
9. Assisted devices
10. Sit down
11. Relaxation
12. Pursed lips breathing/breathing exercises

Adapted from (102, 103).

Patient education

Although patient education alone does not seem to change outcomes significantly (87), it is a necessary component of PR and self-management programmes. Patient education must involve a combination of teaching, counselling, and behaviour modification techniques to promote self-management skills and self-efficacy (60).

Energy conservation

Dyspnoea and fatigue are strongly related to each other and are highly related to activity level (47, 48, 105, 106). A study of the energy spent with and without energy conservation techniques by patients with COPD during activities of daily living found that dyspnoea was significantly decreased by the use of energy conservation techniques (107).

Breathing retraining

Laboratory studies and recent clinical studies have shown that pursed lip breathing (PLB) promotes slow and deeper breathing (108), improves oxygen saturation (109, 110), and decreases dyspnoea (111, 112). People who are experiencing shortness of breath have a tendency to take shallow, rapid breaths (113–115). Therefore breathing strategies also include teaching the patient to adopt a slower and deeper breathing pattern (112, 116).

Investigators have shown that patients can change their rate and depth of breathing through biofeedback while exercising (117–119). Others have suggested that the traditional yoga technique of 4–4–8 can be modified for COPD patients to a 4–2–7–0 pattern, i.e. a count of 4 during inhalation, a count of 2 while holding the breath, a count of 7 for exhalation (120). The length of inhalation and exhalation can be modified to accommodate the patient's abilities. It is the focus on the breathing and the instructions that may help the patient ultimately develop a new breathing rhythm. Continual practice of a new breathing pattern may ultimately become unconscious and automatic for the patient.

In acute dyspnoea, breathing with the patient and counting expiration often supports the patient in slowing down their breathing pattern (121, 122). During acute episodes a position that is often helpful in reducing dyspnoea for patients is the head down and leaning forward position with arms supported either standing or sitting. This postural relief is thought to be due to an improvement in the mechanical efficiency of the diaphragm and optimal functioning of the accessory muscles (123). Patients should always be encouraged to assume the position that is most comfortable for them, even during acute exacerbations.

Inspiratory muscle training

The evidence for inspiratory muscle training (IMT) on dyspnoea (62) was that six investigations showed consistent improvements in inspiratory muscle function, increases in exercise performance, and reductions in dyspnoea. Collectively, the positive results of the six new studies supported the findings of a meta-analysis (124) that IMT by itself significantly increased inspiratory muscle strength and endurance, significantly improved dyspnoea related to ADLs and showed a non-significant trend for an increase in exercise capacity. The committee recommended that IMT be considered only in selected patients with COPD who have decreased inspiratory muscle strength and breathlessness despite receiving optimal medical therapy.

Non-invasive positive-pressure ventilation

The rationale for the use of non-invasive positive-pressure ventilation (NIPPV) as a non-pharmacological treatment for dyspnoea is the physiological unloading of the respiratory muscles that is expected to reduce the work of breathing and promote a reduction in dyspnoea. Three systematic reviews of NIPPV have concluded that patients' with advanced

COPD or acute respiratory failure have significantly reduced their level of dyspnoea with NIPPV (62, 125, 126). In four additional RCTs cited in the recent ACCP Consensus Statement on Dyspnoea in Advanced Disease (57), there was a significant improvement in dyspnoea (127–130). Two early small case studies are noteworthy for the reduction in dyspnoea and the preservation of patient autonomy in patients who declined invasive ventilator support (131, 132).

Neuromuscular stimulation

Several studies have tested the feasibility and efficacy of neuromuscular stimulation (NMES) of the lower extremities of patients to treat muscle weakness for those who suffer from severe disease and their incapacitating shortness of breath limits exercise training. NMES of quadriceps muscle, performed three times a week for 20min, for six weeks significantly improved both the quadriceps strength and hamstring muscle strength in the treated (n=9) and sham treated (n=9) patients with COPD, respectively (133). The improvement in muscle strength carried over to a significantly better performance in the shuttle walk test in the treated group. In another study (134), NMES was added to PR for one month in a randomized group and NMES significantly improved performance of daily tasks and dyspnoea during the tasks. In both studies, muscle stimulation was well tolerated by the patients. A recent Cochrane review of non-pharmacological therapies for dyspnoea reported that NMES is helpful in relieving breathlessness in patients with COPD (135).

Fresh air and fans

Patients with chronic dyspnoea have identified 'fresh air' or fans providing a stream of cold air to the face relieve dyspnoea (104). This clinical observation is supported by a laboratory study that investigated the effect of directing a flow of cold air against the cheek in normal subjects, causing a decrease in dyspnoea (136). A fan tested in an adequately powered cross-over trial showed a significant improvement in breathlessness (137) and the study of the effect of fans has gained favour with two clinical trials in progress (138, 139). A fan that allows the patient to breathe circulating cold air may be one of the most effective non-pharmacological strategies available for chronic dyspnoea or acute dyspnoea at end of life. This treatment is inexpensive, free of side effects, and can be applied almost anywhere (140).

Relaxation exercises

Strategies that decrease levels of distress might reduce dyspnoea. Relaxation may have a physiologic effect by reducing the respiratory rate and increasing tidal volume (VT), thus improving breathing efficiency (141). When a patient relaxes and is able to avert a panic situation by breathing more slowly and deeply, he or she most often reports less shortness of breath. However, the scientific evidence for the positive effect of relaxation on dyspnoea remains inadequate for recommendation in a recent published statement (57). Most relaxation methods include the use of a quiet environment, a comfortable position, loose clothing, some type of word or imagery repeated in a systematic fashion, slow abdominal breathing with deep breaths and slow expirations, and systematic tensing or relaxing of all muscles (142, 143).

One investigator studied the effect of relaxation on dyspnoea in ten patients with COPD compared with a control group that was instructed to relax but not given specific instructions. Although dyspnoea was significantly reduced for the relaxation group during treatment sessions, the scores were similar after 4 weeks (143). Relaxation techniques used by patients with COPD decreased state anxiety and the perception of dyspnoea at rest (142). Music and relaxation were compared in 82 hospitalized patients with COPD randomly assigned to two 30-min sessions (morning and afternoon) of selected music or a tape of progressive muscle relaxation (144). They found significant reductions for state anxiety, trait anxiety, dyspnoea, blood pressure, heart rate, and respiratory rate in the music group. Immediate decreases in dyspnoea did not persist outside the experimental session. These studies provide initial evidence that teaching a patient a programme of relaxation exercises to use when dyspnoea increases may prevent dyspnoea from escalating (145).

Complementary exercises: yoga, tai chi, and mindfulness meditation

'Eastern' exercises, such as yoga or tai-chi, may be alternatives to aerobic or endurance training for people who are limited by severe shortness of breath. With the focus of yoga on achieving slow and deeper breathing, improved breath control, and improved stress management and physical fitness, yoga would be expected to promote relaxation and reduction in dyspnoea or distress related to dyspnoea. Reductions in dyspnoea without physiological changes from greater 'aerobic fitness' have been attributed to patients' increased feeling of control over their breathing, a response shift in the perception of the symptom, or a decrease in anxiety, which often enhances dyspnoea (29, 146, 147). Two early investigators using a case study and a matched group design with male participants who had COPD or chronic bronchitis studied the effect of yoga breathing exercises over time on dyspnoea. In one study more participants in a yoga programme compared to a physiotherapy group stated that they had 'easier control' of their dyspnoea attacks (148). In another, there were significant reductions in dyspnoea measured with a VAS at week 4, but not at week 2 (149). Their findings provided preliminary evidence that light yoga may be an alternative exercise to relieve dyspnoea, especially in advanced disease.

Tai chi focusing on meditation and well-being appears to be associated with reduced stress, anxiety, depression and mood disturbance (150). A pilot study of tai chi for patients with COPD (n=10) found significant improvement in quality of life compared to usual care, excellent adherence to the study protocol, and indicated that a randomized clinical trial of tai chi would be feasible (151).

Mindfulness meditation (MM) is defined as paying total attention to the present moment with a non-judgemental awareness of the inner and outer experiences (151). A recent systematic review of MM (152) found that mindfulness-based stress reduction was efficacious for chronic conditions but study quality was poor. A study of an 8-week mindfulness-based breathing and relaxation response therapy course compared to a support group in 86 people with COPD found no significant differences in dyspnoea at the end of the 6-minute walk test (6MWT) (153).

Music

Music can be used as a management strategy that may help distract a patient from their shortness of breath during exercise. Thornby and colleagues (154) found that at every level of treadmill exercise, perceived 'respiratory effort' was lower and exercise achieved better in patients with COPD while listening to music than while listening to grey noise or silence. Another recent study investigated music on dyspnoea and anxiety during a home walking programme in 24 COPD patients (155). There was a significant decrease in dyspnoea and anxiety following the use of music as reported in the music diary at week 2 but this was not seen at week 5.

Other investigators used a crossover design to measure the effect of music on dyspnoea and anxiety experienced by 30 subjects with COPD while walking in their home (156). Dyspnoea was measured after a 6-min walk. Subjects then walked in random order for 10 min without music and for 10min while listening to music. There were no differences in the change in dyspnoea or anxiety before and after the intervention. Singh and colleagues (144) compared the effectiveness of a randomised study of music versus progressive muscle relaxation (PMR) in hospitalized COPD patients experiencing an acute exacerbation using two sessions within the same day. Both groups had significant reductions after each session for dyspnoea, heart and respiratory rates, and anxiety.

Acupuncture/acupressure

Theoretical mechanisms for the possible effects of acupuncture or acupressure on dyspnoea are unclear. One review of CAM therapies concluded that the use of acupuncture and acupressure to relieve dyspnoea in patients with moderate to severe COPD was supported by a number of RCTs (79). Jobs (157) hypothesized that the mechanism for the relief of dyspnoea may be a release of endogenous opiates and compared the effects of 'traditional' and 'sham' acupuncture for 13 sessions over 3 weeks in 24 patients with COPD who were matched for demographics, severity of breathlessness, and lung function. The acupuncture group improved their dyspnoea at the end of a 6MWT significantly more than the placebo group. Using an uncontrolled design with one group, Filshie (158) studied acupuncture with cancer-related breathlessness in 20 participants, who received four needles (two in the upper sternum and one in each hand). Needles were left in place for 90min. Seventy per cent of the participants reported significantly improved relief in breathlessness, anxiety, and relaxation that peaked at 90min and lasted up to 6 hours. Lewith (159) using a cross-over design, evaluated an acupuncture technique of two studs placed into sternal points in 36 participants with lung disease (predominantly COPD). Mock transcutaneous electrical nerve stimulation (TENS) applied on the same points where acupuncture is normally used was the placebo. Each participant received six treatments in two phases. Dyspnoea measured on a daily VAS at baseline, during the first treatment phase, at wash-out, and during the second treatment phase improved significantly with no significant differences between the groups.

Maa and colleagues conducted a single-blind cross-over design where acupressure treatment was added to a pulmonary rehabilitation programme. Thirty-one patients with COPD practised acupressure daily at home for 6 weeks, alternating with a 'sham' acupressure for 6 weeks. Dyspnoea, measured on a VAS, was significantly less during acupressure than during the sham (160). Later, these investigators randomly assigned 41 patients with asthma to: 1) 20 acupuncture treatments in addition to standard care; 2) self-administered acupressure and standard care; or 3) standard care alone for 8 weeks. All three groups had a slight improvement in dyspnoea measured by both the VAS and modified Borg Scale after 8 weeks; however, there were no significant differences within or between groups (161).

Acupuncture and acupressure were compared in a sample of cancer participants (162). A single session of acupuncture or placebo acupuncture was followed by true acupressure or placebo acupressure. Dyspnoea was measured on a NRS every 15min for 75min immediately before and one hour after acupuncture and acupressure with a daily diary for 7 days. Participants in both groups improved, but there were no differences between groups (162).

More positive results were found by a group of Taiwanese investigators (163) who matched and randomly assigned 44 patients with COPD to true or sham acupressure for five 16-min sessions per week for 4 weeks. The true acupressure group experienced significantly greater improvements in dyspnoea than did the sham group, as measured by the PFSDQ-M (164), 6MWT, state–trait anxiety inventory (165), and O_2 saturation.

Although the evidence remains inconclusive, acupuncture and acupressure are strategies available for patients to increase their repertoire of support.

Non-pharmacological strategies for anxiety and depression

The effect of pulmonary rehabilitation programmes on anxiety and depression is mixed. Although some outpatient pulmonary rehabilitation programmes have been found to improve psychological well-being and depression (66, 166–169), others have not (170). A dyspnoea self-management programme that included education about dyspnoea management strategies improved depression (171). Psychotherapy added to physical therapy and educational sessions (172) and an education programme with group cognitive behavioural therapy sessions also improved depression and anxiety (173). The literature to date appears to support the positive effects of pulmonary rehabilitation, and a combination of education and exercise training on anxiety and depressed mood for patients with COPD (174).

Cognitive-behavioural therapy (CBT) is often cited as a therapy for anxiety and depression; however, in patients with COPD the evidence is limited (175, 176). In one systematic review of CBT studies that showed a significant reduction in anxiety and/or depression, only RCTs were found to be of moderate to high quality and decrease mild-to-moderate depression and anxiety in patients with COPD. These effective CBT interventions were combined with exercise and education (177). One group-based multicomponent CBT programme found that when compared to education alone, brief CBT sessions can significantly improve anxiety and depression in patients with COPD (168)

End of life phase

Quality domains for patients and families

What factors are important at the end of life for patients, their families, and care providers? (178,179). The patients identified five domains that were important to them (180) including pain and management of other symptoms, and achieving a sense of control of their care at the end of life.

Adaptation of non-pharmacological strategies

It is during the end of life phase that the use of practised non-pharmacological strategies on a daily basis becomes paramount. Only 50% of patients with end-stage COPD benefit from any intervention and many live and hence die with constant overwhelming breathlessness (5, 181). There is also evidence that caregivers suffer (55, 182). It is difficult for patients and caregivers to learn new techniques during the end of life phase, so strategies for managing dyspnoea should begin early in the palliative phase. The most common approaches for modulating dyspnoea when patients are homebound and near the end of life are fans, energy conserving measures, breathing techniques, and relaxation strategies (183).

A 'ritual for a breathing crisis' can be taught and practised with patients and families. This 'ritual' might include strategies such as using a fan, reassurance, giving a simple hand or back massage, or medication given by the caregiver (100). Repeated use and practice of these strategies will increase the patient's and caregiver's self-efficacy or confidence in controlling their symptoms.

Conclusion and summary

There is increasing recognition that chronically ill people should be offered the opportunity to receive expert symptom control (100). Further research to support non-pharmacological strategies that can be used by providers, patients and caregivers to manage dyspnoea across the trajectory of illness is being undertaken and will further refine practice.

References

1. Lanken PN, Terry PB, Delisser HM, *et al.* An official American Thoracic Society clinical policy statement: palliative care for patients with respiratory diseases and critical illnesses. *Am J Respir Crit Care Med* 2008; **177**(8):912–27.
2. Uronis HE, Currow DC, Abernethy AP. Palliative management of refractory dyspnea in COPD. *Int J COPD* 2006; **1**(3):289–304.

3. Walke LM, Byers AL, Tinetti ME, Dubin JA, McCorkle R, Fried TR. Range and severity of symptoms over time among older adults with chronic obstructive pulmonary disease and heart failure. *Arch Intern Med* 2007; **167**(22):2503–8.

4. Hardin KA, Meyers F, Louie S. Integrating palliative care in severe chronic obstructive lung disease. *COPD* 2008; **5**(4):207–20.

5. Elkington H, White P, Addington-Hall J, Higgs R, Edmonds P. The healthcare needs of chronic obstructive pulmonary disease patients in the last year of life. *Palliat Med* 2005; **19**(6):485–491.

6. Maurer J, Rebbapragada V, Borson S, *et al.* Anxiety and depression in COPD: current understanding, unanswered questions, and research needs. *Chest* 2008; **134**(4 Suppl):43S–56S.

7. Bailey PH. The dyspnea-anxiety-dyspnea cycle—COPD patients' stories of breathlessness: 'It's scary/when you can't breathe'. *Qual Health Res* 2004; **14**(6):760–78.

8. Xu W, Collet JP, Shapiro S, *et al.* Independent effect of depression and anxiety on chronic obstructive pulmonary disease exacerbations and hospitalizations. *Am J Respir Crit Care Med* 2008; **178**(9):913–20.

9. Abelson JL, Khan S, Giardino N. HPA axis, respiration and the airways in stress-A review in search of intersections. *Biol Psychol* 2010; **84**(1):57–65.

10. Smoller JW, Pollack MH, Otto MW, Rosenbaum JF, Kradin RL. Panic anxiety, dyspnea, and respiratory disease. Theoretical and clinical considerations. *Am J Respir Crit Care Med* 1996; **154**(1):6–17.

11. Bausewein C, Booth S, Gysels M, Kuhnbach R, Haberland B, Higginson IJ. Understanding breathlessness: cross-sectional comparison of symptom burden and palliative care needs in chronic obstructive pulmonary disease and cancer. *J Palliat Med* 2010; **13**(9):1109–18.

12. American Thoracic Society. Dyspnea. Mechanisms, Assessment, and Aanagement: a consensus statement. American Thoracic Society. *Am J Respir Crit Care Med* 1999; **159**(1):321–40.

13. Dodd M, Janson S, Facione N, *et al.* Advancing the science of symptom management. *J Adv Nurs.* 2001; **33**(5):668–76.

14. Pennebaker JW. *The psychology of physical symptoms.* New York: Springer-Verlag; 1982.

15. Carrieri-Kohlman V, Donesky-Cuenco D, Park SK, Mackin L, Nguyen HQ, Paul SM. Additional evidence for the affective dimension of dyspnea in patients with COPD. *Res Nurs Health* 2010; **33**(1):4–19.

16. Lansing RW, Gracely RH, Banzett RB. The multiple dimensions of dyspnea: review and hypotheses. *Respir Physiol Neurobiol* 2009; **167**(1):53–60.

17. Evans KC, Banzett RB, Adams L, McKay L, Frackowiak RS, Corfield DR. BOLD fMRI identifies limbic, paralimbic, and cerebellar activation during air hunger. *J Neurophysiol* 2002; **88**:1500–11.

18. von Leupoldt A, Sommer T, Kegat S, *et al.* The unpleasantness of perceived dyspnea is processed in the anterior insula and amygdala. *Am J Respir Crit Care Med* 2008; **177**(9):1026–32.

19. Casey KL. Forebrain mechanisms of nociception and pain: analysis through imaging. *Proc Natl Acad Sci U S A* 1999; **96**(14):7668–74.

20. Parsons LM, Denton D, Egan G, *et al.* Neuroimaging evidence implicating cerebellum in support of sensory/cognitive processes associated with thirst. *Proc Natl Acad Sci U S A* 2000; **97**(5): 2332–6.

21. Del Parigi A, Gautier JF, Chen K, *et al.* Neuroimaging and obesity: mapping the brain responses to hunger and satiation in humans using positron emission tomography. *Ann N Y Acad Sci* 2002; **967**:389–97.

22. LeDoux J. The emotional brain, fear, and the amygdala. *Cell Mol Neurobiol* 2003; **23**(4–5): 727–38.

23. Price DD. Psychological and Neural Mechanisms of the Affective Dimension of Pain. *Science* 2000; **288**(5472):1769–72.

24. Wells N, Ridner SH. Examining pain-related distress in relation to pain intensity and psychological distress. *Res Nurs Health* 2008; **31**(1):52–62.

25. von Leupoldt A, Dahme B. Experimental comparison of dyspnea and pain. *Behav Res Methods* 2007; **39**(1):137–43.

26. Banzett RB, Pedersen SH, Schwartzstein RM, Lansing RW. The affective dimension of laboratory dyspnea: air hunger is more unpleasant than work/effort. *Am J Respir Crit Care Med* 2008; **177**(12):1384–90.

27. Banzett RB, Mulnier HE, Murphy K, Rosen SD, Wise RJ, Adams L. Breathlessness in humans activates insular cortex. *Neuroreport* 2000; **11**(10):2117–20.

28. Meek PM, Lareau SC, Hu J. Are self-reports of breathing effort and breathing distress stable and valid measures among persons with asthma, persons with COPD, and healthy persons? *Heart Lung* 2003; **32**(5):335–46.

29. Carrieri-Kohlman V, Gormley JM, Douglas MK, Paul SM, Stulbarg MS Exercise training decreases dyspnea and the distress and anxiety associated with it. Monitoring alone may be as effective as coaching. *Chest* 1996; **110**(6):1526–35.

30. Wilson RC, Jones PW. Differentiation between the intensity of breathlessness and the distress it evokes in normal subjects during exercise. *Clin Sci* 1991; **80**(1):65–70.

31. Bredin M, Corner J, Krishnasamy M, Plant H, Bailey C, A'Hern, R. Multicentre randomised controlled trial of nursing intervention for breathlessness in patients with lung cancer. *BMJ* 1999; **318**:901–4.

32. Cioffi D. Beyond attentional strategies: A cognitive-perceptual model of somatic interpretation. *Psychol Bull* 1991; **109**(1):25–41.

33. O'Donnell DE, Banzett RB, Carrieri-Kohlman V, *et al.* Pathophysiology of dyspnea in chronic obstructive pulmonary disease: a roundtable. *Proc Am Thorac Soc* 2007; **4**(2):145–168.

34. Banzett RB. Dynamic response characteristics of CO2-induced air hunger. *Respir Physiol* 1996; **105**(1–2):47–55.

35. Mahler DA, O'Donnell DE. *Dyspnea: mechanisms, measurement, and management,* Vol 208. Boca Raton, FL: Taylor & Francis, 2005.

36. Chetta A, Gerra G, Foresi A, *et al.* Personality profiles and breathlessness perception in outpatients with different gradings of asthma. *Am J Respir Crit Care Med* 1998; **157**(1):116–22.

37. Gift AG, Plaut SM, Jacox A. Psychologic and physiologic factors related to dyspnea in subjects with chronic obstructive pulmonary disease. *Heart Lung* 1986; **15**(6):595–601.

38. Dudley DL, Glaser, Jorgenson BN, Logan DL. Psychosocial concomitants to rehabilitation in chronic obstructive pulmonary disease. Part 1. Psychosocial and psychological considerations. *Chest* 1980; **77**:413–20.

39. Janson C, Bjornsson E, Hetta J, Boman G. Anxiety and depression in relation to respiratory symptoms and asthma. *Am J Respir Crit Care Med* 1994; **149**:930–4.

40. van Ede L, Yzermans CJ, Brouwer HJ. Prevalence of depression in patients with chronic obstructive pulmonary disease: a systematic review. *Thorax* 1999; **54**(8):688–92.

41. van Manen JG, Bindels PJ, Dekker FW, CJ IJ, van der Zee JS, Schade E. Risk of depression in patients with chronic obstructive pulmonary disease and its determinants. *Thorax.* May 2002; **57**(5): 412–16.

42. Meek PM. Influence of attention and judgement on perception of breathlessness in healthy individuals and patients with chronic obstructive pulmonary disease. *Nursing Research* 2000; **49**(1):11–19.

43. Davis AH, Carrieri-Kohlman V, Janson SL, Gold WM, Stulbarg MS. Effects of treatment on two types of self-efficacy in people with chronic obstructive pulmonary disease. *J Pain Symptom Manage* 2006; **32**(1):60–70.

44. Janson-Bjerklie S, Ferketich S, Benner P, Becker G. Clinical markers of asthma severity and risk: importance of subjective as well as objective factors. *Heart Lung* 1992; **21**(3):265–72.

45. Pennebaker JW. Psychological factors influencing the reporting of physical symptoms. In Stone AA, Turkkan JS, Bachrach CA, Jobe JB, Kurtzman HS, Cain VS (eds) *The science of self report: Implications for research and practice*, pp. 299–316. Mahwah, NJ: Lawrence Erlbaum Associates, 2000.

46. Brown ML, Carrieri V, Janson B, Dodd MJ. Lung cancer and dyspnea: the patient's perception. *Oncol Nurs Forum* 1986; **13**(5):19–24.

47. Janson-Bjerklie S, Kohlman-Carrieri V, Hudes M. The sensation of pulmonary dyspnea. *Nurse Res* 1986; **35**(3):154–9.

48. Kapella MC, Larson JL, Patel MK, Covey MK, Berry JK. Subjective fatigue, influencing variables, and consequences in chronic obstructive pulmonary disease. *Nurs Res* 2006; **55**(1):10–17.

49. Hardie GE, Janson S, Gold WM, Carrieri-Kohlman V, Boushey HA. Ethnic differences: word descriptors used by African-American and white asthma patients during induced bronchoconstriction. *Chest* 2000; **117**(4):935–43.

50. Stulbarg MS, Adams L. Dyspnea. In Mason RJ, Broaddus VC, Murray JF, Nadel JA (eds) *Murray and Nadel's textbook of respiratory medicine*, Vol 2, 4th edn, pp. 815–30. Philadelphia, PA: Saunders, 2005.

51. Turk DC, Rudy TE, Sorkin BA. Neglected topics in chronic pain treatment outcome studies: determination of success [see comments]. *Pain* 1993; **53**(1):3–16.

52. Keefe FJ, Dunsmore J, Burnett R. Behavioral and cognitive-behavioral approaches to chronic pain: recent advances and future directions. *J Consult Clin Psychol* 1992; **60**(4):528–36.

53. Bandura A. *Self Efficacy: The Exercise of Control*. New York: W.H. Freeman & Co, 1997.

54. Guthrie SJ, Hill KM, Muers ME. Living with severe COPD. A qualitative exploration of the experience of patients in Leeds. *Respir Med* 2001; **95**(3):196–204.

55. Seamark DA, Blake SD, Seamark CJ, Halpin DM. Living with severe chronic obstructive pulmonary disease (COPD): perceptions of patients and their carers. An interpretative phenomenological analysis. *Palliat Med* 2004; **18**(7):619–25.

56. Skilbeck J, Mott L, Page H, Smith D, Hjelmeland-Ahmedzai S, Clark D. Palliative care in chronic obstructive airways disease: a needs assessment. *Palliat Med* 1998; **12**(4):245–54.

57. Mahler DA, Selecky PA, Harrod CG, *et al.* American College of Chest Physicians consensus statement on the management of dyspnea in patients with advanced lung or heart disease. *Chest* 2010; **137**(3):674–91.

58. Casaburi R, ZuWallack R. Pulmonary rehabilitation for management of chronic obstructive pulmonary disease. *N Engl J Med* 2009; **360**:1329–35.

59. Celli BR, MacNee W. Standards for the diagnosis and treatment of patients with COPD: a summary of the ATS/ERS position paper. *Eur Respir J* 2004; **23**(6):932–46.

60. Nici L, Donner C, Wouters E, *et al.* American Thoracic Society/European Respiratory Society Statement on Pulmonary Rehabilitation. *Am J Respir Crit Care Med* 2006; **173**(12):1390–413.

61. Nici L, Raskin J, Rochester CL, *et al.* Pulmonary rehabilitation: What we know and what we need to know. *J Cardiopulm Rehabil Prev* 2009; **29**(3):141–51.

62. Ries AL, Bauldoff GS, Carlin BW, *et al.* Pulmonary Rehabilitation: Joint ACCP/AACVPR Evidence-Based Clinical Practice Guidelines. *Chest* 2007; **131**(5):4S-42S.

63. Ryerson CJ, Garvey C, Collard HR. Pulmonary rehabilitation for interstitial lung disease. *Chest* 2010; **138**(1):240–1.

64. Griffiths TL, Burr ML, Campbell IA, *et al.* Results at 1 year of outpatient multidisciplinary pulmonary rehabilitation: a randomised controlled trial. *Lancet* 2000; **355**(9201):362–8.

65. Troosters T, Gosselink R, Decramer M. Short- and long-term effects of outpatient rehabilitation in patients with chronic obstructive pulmonary disease: a randomized trial. *Am J Med* 2000; **109**(3):207–12.

66. Emery CF, Schein RL, Hauck ER, MacIntyre NR. Psychological and cognitive outcomes of a randomized trial of exercise among patients with chronic obstructive pulmonary disease. *Health Psychol* 1998; **17**(3):232–40.

67. Emery CF, Leatherman NE, Burker EJ, MacIntyre NR. Psychological outcomes of a pulmonary rehabilitation program. *Chest* 1991; **100**(3):613–17.

68. Boxall AM, Barclay L, Sayers A, Caplan GA. Managing chronic obstructive pulmonary disease in the community. A randomized controlled trial of home-based pulmonary rehabilitation for elderly housebound patients. *J Cardiopulm Rehabil* 2005; **25**(6):378–85.

69. Maltais F, Bourbeau J, Shapiro S, *et al.* Effects of home-based pulmonary rehabilitation in patients with chronic obstructive pulmonary disease: a randomized trial. *Ann Intern Med* 2008; **149**(12):869–78.

70. Bourbeau J, Julien M, Maltais F, *et al.* Reduction of hospital utilization in patients with chronic obstructive pulmonary disease: a disease-specific self-management intervention. *Arch Intern Med* 2003; **163**(5):585–91.

71. Hernández MT, Rubio TM, Ruiz FO, Riera HS, Gil RS, Gómez JC. Results of a home-based training program for patients with COPD. *Chest* 2000; **118**(1):106–14.

72. Puente-Maestu L, Sanz ML, Sanz P, Cubillo JM, Mayol J, Casaburi R. Comparison of effects of supervised versus self-monitored training programmes in patients with chronic obstructive pulmonary disease. *Eur Respir J* 2000; **15**(3):517–25.

73. Troosters T, Casaburi R, Gosselink R, Decramer M. Pulmonary Rehabilitation in Chronic Obstructive Pulmonary Disease. *Am J Respir Crit Care Med 2005* 2005; **172**(1):19–38.

74. ZuWallack R, Lareau SC, Meek PM. The Effect of Pulmonary Rehabilitation on Dyspnea. In: Mahler D, O'Donnell DE, eds *Dyspnea: Mechanisms, Measurement And Management*, Vol. 208, pp. 301–320. Boca Raton, FL: Taylor & Francis, 2005.

75. Carrieri-Kohlman V, Nguyen HQ, Donesky-Cuenco D, Demir-Deviren S, Neuhaus J, Stulbarg MS. Impact of brief or extended exercise training on the benefit of a dyspnea self-management program in COPD. *J Cardiopulm Rehabil* 2005; **25**(5):275–84.

76. Lacasse Y, Wong E, Guyatt GH, King D, Cook DJ, Goldstein RS. Meta-analysis of respiratory rehabilitation in chronic obstructive pulmonary disease [see comments]. *Lancet* 1996; **348**(9035):1115–19.

77. Lacasse Y, Goldstein R, Lasserson T, Martin S. Pulmonary rehabilitation for chronic obstructive pulmonary disease. *Cochrane Database Syst Rev* 2006(4):CD003793.

78. Clark CJ, Cochrane LM, Mackay E, Paton B. Skeletal muscle strength and endurance in patients with mild COPD and the effects of weight training. *Eur Respir* 2000; **15**(1):92–7.

79. Pan CX, Morrison S, Ness J, Fugh-Berman A, Leipzig R. Complementary and alternative medicine in the management of pain, dyspnea, and nausea and vomiting near the end of life: a systematic review. *J Pain Symptom Manage.* 2000; **20**(5):374–37.

80. Bodenheimer T, Lorig K, Holman H, Grumbach K. Patient self-management of chronic disease in primary care. *JAMA* 2002; **288**(19):2469–75.

81. Institute of Medicine. *Crossing the quality chasm: A new health system for the 21st century.* Washington, DC: National Academy Press, 2001.

82. Wagner EH, Austin BT, Von Korff M. Improving outcomes in chronic illness. *Manag Care Q* 1996; **4**(2):12–25.

83. Ryan P, Sawin KJ. The Individual and Family Self-Management Theory: background and perspectives on context, process, and outcomes. *Nurs Outlook* 2009; **57**(4):217–25 e6.

84. Tobin DL, Reynolds RVC, Holroyd KA, Creer TL. Self-management and social learning theory. In Holroyd KA, Creer TL (eds) *Self-Management of Chronic Disease*, pp. 29–58. Orlando, FL: Academic Press, 1986.

85. Von Korff M, Gruman J, Schaefer J, Curry SJ, Wagner EH. Collaborative management of chronic illness. *Ann Intern Med* 1997; **127**(12): 1097–1102.

86. Gibson P, Powell H, Couglan J, *et al.* Self-management education and regular practitioner review for adults with asthma (Cochrane Review). *The Cochrane Library* 1. Oxford: Update Software, 2003.

87. Monninkhof EM, Van Der Valk PD, Van Der Palen J, *et al.* Self-management education for chronic obstructive pulmonary disease (Cochrane Review). *Cochrane Database Syst Rev* 2003; 1:CD002990.

88. Harris M, Smith BJ, Veale A. Patient education programs—can they improve outcomes in COPD? *Int J Chron Obstruct Pulmon Dis* 2008; **3**(1):109–12.

89. Warsi A, Wang PS, LaValley MP, Avorn J, Solomon DH. Self-management education programs in chronic disease: a systematic review and methodological critique of the literature. *Arch Intern Med* 2004; **164**(15):1641–9.

90. Gallefoss F, Bakke PS. Cost-benefit and cost-effectiveness analysis of self-management in patients with COPD—a 1-year follow-up randomized, controlled trial. *Respir Med* 2002; **96**(6):424–31.

91. Adams SG, Smith PK, Allan PF, Anzueto A, Pugh JA, Cornell JE. Systematic review of the chronic care model in chronic obstructive pulmonary disease prevention and management. *Arch Intern Med* 2007; **167**(6):551–61.

92. Rice KL, Dewan N, Bloomfield HE, *et al.* Disease Management Program for Chronic Obstructive Pulmonary Disease: A Randomized Controlled Trial. *Am J Respir Crit Care Med* 2010; **182**:890–6.

93. Rabow MW, Dibble SL, Pantilat SZ, McPhee SJ. The comprehensive care team: a controlled trial of outpatient palliative medicine consultation. *Arch Intern Med* 2004; **164**(1):83–91.

94. Rosser R, Denford J, Heslop A, *et al.* Breathlessness and psychiatric morbidity in chronic bronchitis and emphysema: A study of psychotherapeutic management. *Psychol Med* 1983; **13**(1):93–110.

95. Ashikaga T, Vacek PM, Lewis SO. Evaluation of a community-based education program for individuals with chronic obstructive pulmonary disease. *J Rehabil* 1980; **46**(2):23–7.

96. Corner J, Plant H, A'Hern R, Bailey C. Non-pharmacological intervention for breathlessness in lung cancer. *Palliat Med* 1996; **10**:299–305.

97. Stulbarg MS, Carrieri-Kohlman V, Demir-Deviren S, *et al.* Exercise training improves outcomes of a dyspnea self-management program. *J Cardiopulm Rehabil* 2002; **22**(2):109–21.

98. Nguyen HQ, Carrieri-Kohlman V, Rankin SH, Slaughter R, Stulbarg MS Is Internet-based support for dyspnea self-management in patients with chronic obstructive pulmonary disease possible? Results of a pilot study. *Heart Lung* 2005; **34**(1):51–62.

99. Nguyen HQ, Donesky-Cuenco D, Wolpin S, *et al.* Randomized controlled trial of an internet-based versus face-to-face dyspnea self-management program for patients with chronic obstructive pulmonary disease: pilot study. *J Med Internet Res* 2008; **10**(2): e9.

100. Booth S. End of life care for the breathless patient. *General Practice Update* 2009:39–43.

101. Levin LS. Patient education and self-care: how do they differ? *Nurs Outlook* 1978; **26**(3): 170–5.

102. Thomas LA. Effective dyspnea management strategies identified by elders with end-stage chronic obstructive pulmonary disease. *Appl Nurs Res* 2009; **22**(2):79–85.

103. Christenbery TL. Dyspnea self-management strategies: use and effectiveness as reported by patients with chronic obstructive pulmonary disease. *Heart Lung* 2005; **34**(6):406–14.

104. Carrieri V, Janson-Bjerklie S. Strategies patients use to manage the sensation of dyspnea. *West J Nurs Res* 1986; **8**(3):284–305.

105. Gift AG, Pugh LC. Dyspnea and fatigue. *Nurs Clin North Am* 1993; **28**(2):373–84.

106. Ryerson CJ, Berkeley J, Carrieri-Kohlman VL, Pantilat SZ, Landefeld CS, Collard HR. Depression and functional status are strongly associated with dyspnea in interstitial lung disease. *Chest* 2011; **139**(3):609–16.

107. Velloso M, Jardim JR. Study of energy expenditure during activities of daily living using and not using body position recommended by energy conservation techniques in patients with COPD. *Chest* 2006; **130**(1):126–32.

108. Breslin EH. The pattern of respiratory muscle recruitment during pursed-lip breathing. *Chest*. 1992; **101**(1):75–8.

109. Faager G, Stahle A, Larsen FF. Influence of spontaneous pursed lips breathing on walking endurance and oxygen saturation in patients with moderate to severe chronic obstructive pulmonary disease. *Clin Rehabil* 2008; **22**(8):675–83.

110. Tiep BL, Burns M, Kao D, Madison R, Herrera J. Pursed lips breathing training using ear oximetry. *Chest* 1986; **90**(2):218–21.

111. Bianchi R, Gigliotti F, Romagnoli I, *et al.* Chest wall kinematics and breathlessness during pursed-lip breathing in patients with COPD. *Chest* 2004; **125**(2):459–65.

112. Nield MA, Soo Hoo GW, Roper JM, Santiago S. Efficacy of pursed-lips breathing: a breathing pattern retraining strategy for dyspnea reduction. *J Cardiopulm Rehabil Prev* 2007; **27**(4):237–44.

113. Javaheri S, Blum J, Kazemi H. Pattern of breathing and carbon dioxide retention in chronic obstructive lung disease. *Am J Med* 1981; **71**(2):228–34.

114. Otis AB, McKerrow CB, Bartlett RA, *et al.* Mechanical factors in distribution of pulmonary ventilation. *J Appl Physiol* 1956; **8**(4):427–43.

115. Parot S, Miara B, Milic-Emili J, Gautier H. Hypoxemia, hypercapnia, and breathing pattern in patients with chronic obstructive pulmonary disease. *Am Rev Respir Dis* 1982; **126**(5):882–6.

116. Spahija J, de Marchie M, Grassino A. Effects of imposed pursed-lips breathing on respiratory mechanics and dyspnea at rest and during exercise in COPD. *Chest* 2005; **128**(2):640–50.

117. Collins E, Fehr L, Bammert C, *et al.* Effect of ventilation-feedback training on endurance and perceived breathlessness during constant work-rate leg-cycle exercise in patients with COPD. *J Rehabil Res Develop* 2003; **40**(Suppl 2(5)):35–44.

118. Giardino ND, Chan L, Borson S. Combined heart rate variability and pulse oximetry biofeedback for chronic obstructive pulmonary disease: preliminary findings. *Appl Psychophysiol Biofeedback* 2004; **29**(2):121–33.

119. Ritz T, von Leupoldt A, Dahme B. Evaluation of a respiratory muscle biofeedback procedure-effects on heart rate and dyspnea. *Appl Psychophysiol Biofeedback* 2006; **31**(3):253–61.

120. Sharma V. personal communication; 2004.

121. Carrieri-Kohlman V. Dyspnea in the weaning patient: assessment and intervention. *Aacn Clin Issues Crit Care Nurs.* 1991; **2**(3):462–73.

122. Petty TL, Burns M, Tiep BL. *Essentials of Pulmonary Rehabilitation: A Do It Yourself Guide To Enjoying Life With Chronic Lung Disease*, 2nd edn, 2005. Available at: http://www.perf2ndwind.org/Essentials.html.

123. Sharp JT, Drutz WS, Moisan T, *et al.* Postural relief of dyspnea in severe chronic obstructive pulmonary disease. *Am Rev Respir Dis* 1980; **122**:201–13.

124. Lotters F, van Tol B, Kwakkel G, Gosslink R. Effects of controlled inspiratory muscle training in patients with chronic obstructive pulmonary disease: a meta-analysis. *Eur Respir J* 2002; **20**:570–6.

125. Curtis JR, Cook DJ, Sinuff T, *et al.* Noninvasive positive pressure ventilation in critical and palliative care settings: understanding the goals of therapy. *Crit Care Med* 2007; **35**(3):932–9.

126. Kolodziej MA, Jensen L, Rowe B, Sin D. Systematic review of noninvasive positive pressure ventilation in severe stable COPD. *Eur Respir J* 2007; **30**(2):293–306.

127. Casanova C, Celli BR, Tost L, *et al.* Long-term controlled trial of nocturnal nasal positive pressure ventilation in patients with severe COPD. *Chest* 2000; **118**(6):1582–90.

128. Clini E, Sturani C, Rossi A, *et al.* The Italian multicentre study on noninvasive ventilation in chronic obstructive pulmonary disease patients. *Eur Respir J* 2002; **20**(3):529–38.

129. Jolliet P, Tassaux D, Thouret JM, Chevrolet JC. Beneficial effects of helium: oxygen versus air: oxygen noninvasive pressure support in patients with decompensated chronic obstructive pulmonary disease. *Crit Care Med* 1999; **27**(11):2422–9.

130. Leung RS, Bradley TD. Long term treatment of refractory congestive heart failure by continuous positive airway pressure. *Can J Cardiol* 1999; **15**(9):1009–12.

131. Benhamou D, Girault C, Faure C, Portier F, Muir JF. Nasal mask ventilation in acute respiratory failure. Experience in elderly patients. *Chest* 1992; **102**(3):912–17.

132. Meduri GU, Fox RC, Abou-Shala N, Leeper KV, Wunderink RG. Noninvasive mechanical ventilation via face mask in patients with acute respiratory failure who refused endotracheal intubation. *Crit Care Med* 1994; **22**(10):1584–90.

133. Bourjeily-Habr G, Rochester CL, Palermo F, Snyder P, Mohsenin V. Randomised controlled trial of transcutaneous electrical muscle stimulation of the lower extremities in patients with chronic obstructive pulmonary disease. *Thorax* 2002; **57**(12):1045–9.

134. Vivodtzev I, Pepin JL, Vottero G, *et al.* Improvement in quadriceps strength and dyspnea in daily tasks after 1 month of electrical stimulation in severely deconditioned and malnourished COPD. *Chest* 2006; **129**(6):1540–48.

135. Bausewein C, Booth S, Gysels M, Higginson I. Non-pharmacological interventions for breathlessness in advanced stages of malignant and non-malignant diseases. *Cochrane Database Syst Rev* 16 2008(2):CD005623.

136. Schwartzstein RM, Lahive K, Pope A, Weinberger SE, Weiss JW. Cold facial stimulation reduces breathlessness induced in normal subjects. *Am Rev Respir Dis* 1987; **136**(1):58–61.

137. Galbraith S, Perkins P, Lynch A, Booth S. Does a handheld fan improve intractable breathlessness? Proceedings of the EAPC Research Forum, Trondheim, Norway, 2008.

138. Bausewein C. 'Effectiveness of a Hand-held Fan for Breathlessness.' King's College London. ClinicalTrials.gov Identifier: NCT01123902. Available at: http://www.clinicaltrials.gov.

139. Galbraith S, Booth S. 'The Use of a Handheld Fan to Manage Breathlessness – A Feasibility Study.' Cambridge University Hospitals. ClinicalTrials.gov Identifier: NCT00974558. Available at: http://www.clinicaltrials.gov.

140. Hansen-Flaschen J. Advanced lung disease: palliation and terminal care. *Clinics Chest Med* 1997; **18**(3):645–55.

141. Gosselink R. Controlled breathing and dyspnea in patients with chronic obstructive pulmonary disease (COPD). *J Rehabil Res Dev* 2003; **40**(5: Suppl 2):25–34.

142. Gift AG, Moore T, Soeken K. Relaxation to reduce dyspnea and anxiety in COPD patients. *Nurs Res* 1992; **41**(4):242–6.

143. Renfroe KL. Effect of progressive relaxation on dyspnea and state anxiety in patients with chronic obstructive pulmonary disease. *Heart Lung* 1988; **17**(4):408–13.

144. Singh VP, Rao V, Prem V, Sahoo RC, Keshav Pai K. Comparison of the effectiveness of music and progressive muscle relaxation for anxiety in COPD—A randomized controlled pilot study. *Chron Respir Dis* 2009; **6**(4):209–16.

145. McBride S, Graydon J, Sidani S, Hall L. The therapeutic use of music for dyspnea and anxiety in patients with COPD who live at home. *J Holistic Nurs* 1999(3):229–50.

146. Kidd P, Parshall MB, Wojcik S, Struttmann T. Assessing recalibration as a response-shift phenomenon. *Nurs Res* 2004; **53**(2):130–5.

147. Wilson IB. Clinical understanding and clinical implications of response shift. In Schwartz CE, Sprangers MAG (eds) *Adaptation to changing health: Response shift in quality-of-life research*, pp. 159–174. Washington DC: American Psychological Association, 2000.

148. Tandon MK. Adjunct treatment with yoga in chronic severe airways obstruction. *Thorax* 1978; **33**(4):514–17.

149. Behera D. Yoga therapy in chronic bronchitis. *J Assoc Physicians India* 1998; **46**(2):207–8.

150. Wang C, Bannuru R, Ramel J, Kupelnick B, Scott T, Schmid CH. Tai Chi on psychological well-being: systematic review and meta-analysis. *BMC: Altern Med* 2010; **10**:23.

151. Yeh GY, Roberts DH, Wayne PM, Davis RB, Quilty MT, Phillips RS. Tai chi exercise for patients with chronic obstructive pulmonary disease: a pilot study. *Respir Care* 2010; **55**(11):1475–82.

152. Chiesa A, Serretti A. Mindfulness based cognitive therapy for psychiatric disorders: A systematic review and meta-analysis. *Psychiatry Res* 2011; **187**(3):441–53.

153. Mularski RA, Munjas BA, Lorenz KA, *et al.* Randomized controlled trial of mindfulness-based therapy for dyspnea in chronic obstructive lung disease. *J Altern Complement Med* 2009; **15**(10):1083–90.

154. Thornby MA, Haas F, Axen K. Effect of distractive auditory stimuli on exercise tolerance in patients with COPD. *Chest* 1995; **107**(5):1213–17.

155. Bauldoff GS, Hoffman LA, Zullo TG, Sciurba FC. Exercise maintenance following pulmonary rehabilitation: effect of distractive stimuli. *Chest* 2002; **122**(3):948–54.

156. Brooks D, Sidani S, Graydon J, McBride S, Hall L, Weinacht K. Evaluating the effects of music on dyspnea during exercise in individuals with chronic obstructive pulmonary disease: A pilot study. *Rehabil Nurs* 2003; **28**(6):192–6.

157. Jobst K, Chen J, McPherson K, *et al.* Controlled trial of acupuncture for disabling breathlessness. *Lancet* 1986; **2**:1416–19.

158. Filshie J, Penn K, Ashley S, Davis C. Acupuncture for the relief of cancer-related breathlessness. *Palliat Med* 1996; **10**:1447–52.

159. Lewith GT, Prescott P, Davis CL. Can a standardized acupuncture technique palliate disabling breathlessness: a single-blind, placebo-controlled crossover study. *Chest* 2004; **125**(5):1783–90.

160. Maa SH, Gauthier D, Turner M. Acupressure as an adjunct to a pulmonary rehabilitation program. *J Cardiopulm Rehabil* 1997; **17**(4):268–76.

161. Maa SH, Sun M, Hsu KH, *et al.* Effect of acupuncture or acupressure on quality of life of patients with chronic obstructive asthma: a pilot study. *J Altern Complement Med* 2003; **9**(5):659–70.

162. Vickers AJ, Feinstein MB, Deng GE, Cassileth BR. Acupuncture for dyspnea in advanced cancer: a randomized, placebo-controlled pilot trial [ISRCTN89462491]. *BMC Palliat Care* 2005; **4**:5.

163. Wu HS, Wu SC, Lin JG, Lin LC. Effectiveness of acupressure in improving dyspnoea in chronic obstructive pulmonary disease. *J Adv Nurs* 2004; **45**(3):252–9.

164. Lareau SC, Meek PM, Roos PJ. Development and testing of the modified version of the pulmonary functional status and dyspnea questionnaire (PFSDQ-M). *Heart Lung* 1998; **27**(3):159–68.

165. Spielberger C, Gorsuch R, Lushene R, Vagg P, Jacobs G. *Manual for the State-Trait Anxiety Inventory (Form Y) ('Self-evaluation questionnaire')* Palo Alto, CA: Consulting Psychologist Press; 1989.

166. Dekhuijzen PN, Beek MM, Folgering HT, Van Herwaarden CL. Psychological changes during pulmonary rehabilitation and target-flow inspiratory muscle training in COPD patients with a ventilatory limitation during exercise. *Int J Rehabil Res* 1990; **13**(2):109–17.

167. Paz-Diaz H, Montes de Oca M, Lopez JM, Celli BR. Pulmonary rehabilitation improves depression, anxiety, dyspnea and health status in patients with COPD. *Am J Phys Med Rehabil* 2007; **86**(1):30–6.

168. Stanley MA, Veazy C, Hopko D, Diefenbach G, Kunik ME. Anxiety and depression in chronic obstructive pulmonary disease: A new intervention and case report. *Cogn Behav Pract* 2005; **12**:424–36.

169. White RJ, Rudkin ST, Ashley J, *et al.* Outpatient pulmonary rehabilitation in severe chronic obstructive pulmonary disease. *J R Coll Physicians Lond* 1997; **31**(5):541–5.

170. Toshima M, Blumberg E, Ries AL. Does rehabilitation reduce depression in patients with chronic obstructive pulmonary disease. *J Cardiopulm Rehabil* 1992; **12**:261–9.

171. Nguyen HQ, Carrieri-Kohlman V. Dyspnea Self-Management in Patients With Chronic Obstructive Pulmonary Disease: Moderating Effects of Depressed Mood. *Psychosomatics* 2005; **46**(5):402–10.

172. de Godoy DV, de Godoy RF. A randomized controlled trial of the effect of psychotherapy on anxiety and depression in chronic obstructive pulmonary disease. *Arch Phys Med Rehabil* 2003; **84**(8):1154–7.

173. Kunik ME, Veazey C, Cully JA, *et al.* COPD education and cognitive behavioral therapy group treatment for clinically significant symptoms of depression and anxiety in COPD patients: a randomized controlled trial. *Psychol Med* 2008; **38**(3):385–396.

174. Hill K, Geist R, Goldstein RS, Lacasse Y. Anxiety and depression in end-stage COPD. *Eur Respir J* 2008; **31**(3):667–77.

175. Baraniak A, Sheffield D. The efficacy of psychologically based interventions to improve anxiety, depression and quality of life in COPD: A systematic review and meta-analysis. *Patient Educ Couns* 2011; **83**(1):29–36.

176. Rose C, Wallace L, Dickson R, *et al.* The most effective psychologically-based treatments to reduce anxiety and panic in patients with chronic obstructive pulmonary disease (COPD): a systematic review. *Patient Educ Couns* 2002; **47**(4):311–18.

177. Coventry PA, Gellatly JL. Improving outcomes for COPD patients with mild-to-moderate anxiety and depression: a systematic review of cognitive behavioural therapy. *Br J Health Psychol* 2008; **13**(Pt 3):381–400.

178. Clarke EB, Curtis JR, Luce JM, *et al.* Quality indicators for end-of-life care in the intensive care unit. *Crit Care Med* 2003; **31**(9):2255–62.

179. Steinhauser KE, Christakis NA, Clipp EC, McNeilly M, McIntyre L, Tulsky JA. Factors considered important at the end of life by patients, family, physicians, and other care providers. *JAMA* 2000; **284**(19):2476–82.

180. Singer PA, Martin DK, Kelner M. Quality end-of-life care: patients' perspectives. *JAMA* 1999; **281**(2):163–8.

181. Elkington H, White P, Addington-Hall J, Higgs R, Pettinari C. The last year of life of COPD: a qualitative study of symptoms and services. *Respir Med* 2004; **98**(5):439–45.

182. Booth S, Silvester S, Todd C. Breathlessness in cancer and chronic obstructive pulmonary disease: using a qualitative approach to describe the experience of patients and carers. *Palliat Support Care* 2003; **1**(4):337–44.

183. Spathis A, Booth S. End of life care in chronic obstructive pulmonary disease: in search of a good death. *Int J Chron Obstruct Pulmon Dis* 2008; **3**(1):11–29.

Chapter 11

Nutrition and cachexia

Josep M. Argilés, Sílvia Busquets, Mireia Olivan, and Francisco J. López-Soriano

Summary

The cachexia syndrome, characterized by a marked weight loss, anorexia, asthenia, and anaemia, leads to a malnutrition status due to the induction of anorexia or decreased food intake. In addition, metabolic disturbances (alterations in carbohydrate, lipid, and protein metabolism) lead to a decreased energy efficiency which accounts for weight loss. Muscle catabolism and wasting is one of the most prominent trends of the syndrome. Although the search for the cachectic factor(s) that triggers these metabolic alterations started a long time ago, and although many scientific and economic efforts have been devoted to its discovery, we are still a long way from knowing the whole truth. This chapter is focused on the role of nutrition in the treatment of cachexia, associated with both cancer and non-malignant respiratory diseases. The main aim is to summarize and evaluate the different approaches used in the past and to project trends for future nutritional interventions.

The cachexia syndrome: definition

Perhaps the most common manifestation of severe disease, such as acquired immuno-deficiency syndrome (AIDS), chronic heart failure (CHF), chronic obstructive respira-tory disease (COPD), and cancer, is the development of cachexia. Indeed, cachexia occurs in the majority of cancer patients before death and it is responsible for the deaths of at least 30% of cancer patients. Interestingly, in studies performed before the era of highly active antiretroviral therapy, estimates of prevalence of wasting as the first AIDS-defining diagnosis ranged up to 31%. Fatigue, as a result of muscle wasting, is an extremely com-mon symptom in cardiac cachexia and COPD patients. Cachexia is a term which origi-nally comes from the Greek: 'kakos' and 'hexis' meaning 'bad condition'. The cachectic state is observed in many pathological conditions such as cancer, sepsis, and chronic heart disease. The Washington DC Consensus Group recently defined cachexia as 'a com-plex metabolic syndrome associated with underlying illness and characterized by loss of muscle with or without loss of fat mass. The prominent clinical feature of cachexia is weight loss in adults (*corrected for fluid retention*) or growth failure in children (*excluding endocrine disorders*). Anorexia, inflammation, insulin resistance and increased muscle protein breakdown are frequently associated with wasting disease. Wasting disease is distinct from starvation, age-related loss of muscle mass, primary depression, malabsorption and hyperthyroidism and is associated with increased morbidity' (1).

Cancer cachexia

In the case of malignant diseases, cachexia is a complex syndrome that describes the progressive muscle wasting and weakness in many cancer patients. Muscle wasting reduces the ability of affected patients to perform the tasks of daily living, leading to a reduction in quality of life. Cancer cachexia is also associated with severe fatigue, which affects 70–100% of cancer patients. Fatigue related to cancer cachexia is a distressing symptom that negatively impacts on physical function and can lead to affected patients changing their employment status and reducing their overall quality of life. Cachexia is more common in children and in the elderly and becomes more pronounced as the cancer progresses (2). Cachexia is present in up to 80% of patients with advanced cancer, including cancers of the breast, sarcoma, lung, colon, prostate, pancreas and gastrointestinal tract. It is also present early in the disease progression with 85% of patients with gastrointestinal cancers, 83% of patients with pancreatic cancer and 60% of patients with lung cancer presenting with cachexia upon diagnosis (2). Cachexia is associated with reduced mobility, increased risk of complications in surgery, impaired response to chemo/radio-therapy and increased psychological distress, leading to an overall reduction in quality of life (2). The pathogenesis of cancer cachexia is multifactorial and includes anorexia (3), inflammation, metabolic disturbances, and enhanced muscle proteolysis, and each of these presents as a potential therapeutic target for ameliorating cancer cachexia. It is a multiorgan syndrome affecting not just skeletal muscle and adipose but also the gut, brain, and the immune system.

Nutritional approaches

The treatment of cancer cachexia has involved many different approaches using both nutritional and pharmacological strategies. Concerning the use of drugs, basically, existing therapies have focused on treating conditions secondary to the tumour. However, these approaches are limited and there are currently no drugs that are approved by the US Food and Drug Administration (FDA) for the treatment of cancer cachexia. Several factors have complicated the development of effective therapies for cancer cachexia, including the multifactorial pathogenesis of the syndrome. Another complication has been little consensus on the primary endpoint for clinical trials, which has hampered assessment of the efficacy of treatments. Anti-inflammatory treatments have also been used, but their efficacy has been limited and adverse side effects have restricted their use over prolonged periods. Most therapies using nutritional approaches have focused on reducing anorexia through pharmacological modulation, but such strategies do not influence, in general, lean body mass.

Nutritional support

The importance of nutritional counselling in cancer patients is supported by the studies of Ravasco et al. (4), which show that simple individualized nutritional counselling may help to preserve body weight in cancer patients. Enteral nutrition is a reasonable option as an alternative to the oral route in patients with a functional bowel. From this point of view, it can be useful in some patients with advanced head and neck tumours or oesophageal carcinoma who are not able to swallow properly, but still have an appetite and a good performance status.

Total parenteral nutrition has been used extensively in malnourished cancer patients who were unable to receive either oral or enteral nutrition. Its clinical use, however, has been subject to conflicting results. Although some studies have reported beneficial effects from this type of nutritional therapy (including wound healing, reduction in sepsis, and increased responsiveness to chemotherapy), others, after evaluating the influence of total parenteral nutrition following treatment sequelae, have concluded that these benefits are limited to improvements of operative mortality and major surgical complications. Short-term parenteral nutrition is, however, commonly accepted in patients with acute gastro-intestinal complications from chemotherapy and radiotherapy, whereas long-term (home) parenteral nutrition may represent a life-saving strategy in patients with sub acute/chronic radiation enteropathy.

Concerning the potential differences between the two types of nutritional support, it has to be pointed out that enteral feeding is above all more economical, and randomized trials with patients undergoing major surgery indicate that they lead to similar results concerning nitrogen balance, plasma proteins, body cell mass, or body weight. Altogether, the nutritional strategies represent tools for the treatment of anorexia and cachexia, and in combination with a pharmacological approach may lead to interesting and promising results in the near future.

Enhancing food intake

Different drugs have been used for increasing the appetite of cancer patients and therefore, their food intake. Megestrol acetate (MEGACE) and medroxyprogesterone (MPA) are synthetic, orally active derivatives of the naturally occurring hormone, progesterone. In humans, these compounds have been found to improve appetite, caloric intake and nutritional status in several clinical trials (5). In the case of MEGACE, the reason for the associated weight gain is mostly unknown, although it has been postulated that the effect is partially mediated by neuropeptide Y, a potent central appetite stimulant. In contrast, MPA has been shown to reduce the *in vitro* production of serotonin and cytokines (interleukin-1-β (IL-1), interleukin-6 (IL-6) and TNF-alpha) by peripheral blood mononuclear cells of cancer patients (6). All of these humoural factors have been implicated in the cachectic–anorectic response. Oral suspension of the progestational agent may be particularly useful in patients with far advanced disease, where taking larger amount of pills may lead to the decrease of patient compliance. Recent data by Tomíska et al. (7) showed that an oral MEGACE suspension given to patients with far advanced cancer suffering from anorexia and weight loss resulted in an improvement of appetite and quality of life.

The orexigenic mediator, ghrelin—a novel endogenous ligand for the growth hormone (GH) secretagogue receptor—has recently been reported as having a key role in increasing appetite and, therefore, food intake. In addition to increasing food intake, an experimental study has shown that repeated administration of ghrelin improves cardiac structure and function and attenuates the development of cardiac cachexia in CHF. These results suggest that ghrelin has cardiovascular effects and regulates energy metabolism through GH-dependent and GH-independent mechanisms. Thus, administration of ghrelin may be a new therapeutic strategy for the treatment of severe CHF. A phase II randomized, placebo-controlled, double-blind study using an oral ghrelin mimetic demonstrated an improvement in lean body mass, total body mass and hand grip strength in cachectic cancer patients (8).

Cannabinoids, which are present in marijuana, have a definitive effect on weight gain and, bearing this in mind, have been used to increase food intake in cancer patients. The mechanism by which cannabinoids exert their effects has yet to be clarified. It was postulated that they may act via endorphin receptors, or by inhibiting prostaglandin synthesis. Other reports suggest that the marijuana derivative may act by inhibiting cytokine production and/or secretion (9). A recent clinical trial, however, has shown very little efficacy of either orally administered cannabinoid extract or delta-9-tetrahydrocannabinol in treating patients with cancer-related anorexia–cachexia syndrome (10).

Melanocortin antagonists are also potential candidates for the treatment of cancer anorexia. Indeed, melanocortin (MC4) receptor is involved in the anorexigenic cascade leading to a decrease in neuropeptide Y and, therefore, a decrease in food intake. The use of MC4 antagonists has been proven to be effective in preventing anorexia, loss of lean body mass and basal energy expenditure in experimental animals suffering from cachexia (11). However, no data on human subjects are available and therefore, future clinical trials are awaited to prove the efficacy of this type of antagonist in the treatment of human cachexia.

Though nutritional support—or pharmacological strategies directed to increasing food intake—alone can improve energy intake to a variable extent and for a variable period of time, they will not address the underlying catabolic metabolism and are thus likely to be of limited efficacy if attempts to attenuate the tumour-induced catabolic response are not carried out at the same time. It is therefore, very desirable to combine nutrition with other compounds that are able to moderate the catabolic response. Among these compounds, we find different nutraceuticals.

Nutraceuticals

Omega-3-polyunsaturated fatty acids (PUFA), present in large amounts in fish oil, have been proposed as very active in reducing either tumour growth or the associated tissue wasting, particularly that of the adipose mass. In fact, the interest in omega-3-PUFA originated from the observation that populations consuming a diet rich in such constituents showed the lowest incidence of certain types of cancer. An improvement in the lean body mass and quality of life was observed in a randomized double-blind trial using a protein and energy dense omega-3-fatty acid-enriched oral supplement (12), provided that its consumption was equal to or in excess of 2.2g eicosapentaenoic acid (EPA)/day. However, other data, arising from a large multicentre double-blind placebo-controlled trial, indicate that EPA administration alone is not successful in the treatment of weight losing patients with advanced gastrointestinal or lung cancer (13). In addition, comparisons of EPA combined with a protein energy supplementation versus a protein energy supplementation (without EPA) in the presence of an appetite stimulant (MEGACE) provided no evidence that EPA improves symptoms associated with the cachexia syndrome often seen in patients with advanced cancer. Moreover, a meta-analysis based on several trials concluded that there were insufficient data to establish whether oral EPA was better than placebo (14).

More recent data on fish oil are more encouraging. Thus, Read et al. (15) reported in a phase II clinical trial involving patients under chemotherapy for advanced colorectal cancer an improvement in weight, quality of life, and a reduction in the inflammatory response in patients receiving an EPA-containing supplement. Similar results were obtained in another double-blind, randomized, placebo-controlled study involving non-small cell lung carcinoma patients (16).

Peripheral muscle proteolysis, which occurs in cancer cachexia, serves to mobilize amino acids required for the synthesis of liver and tumour protein. Therefore, the administration of exogenous amino acids may theoretically serve as a protein-sparing metabolic fuel by providing substrates for both muscle metabolism and gluconeogenesis. Based on this, branched chain amino acids (BCAA: leucine, isoleucine, and valine) have been used in parenteral nutrition with the aim of improving nitrogen balance and, particularly, muscle protein metabolism. Tayek et al. (17), in a prospective, randomized, crossover trial involving patients with advanced intra-abdominal adenocarcinoma, concluded that BCAA-enriched total parenteral nutrition resulted in an improved protein accretion and albumin synthesis. Cangiano et al. (18) have proposed that BCAA administration would also serve to counteract the anorexia associated with tumour growth. The authors postulated that increased hypothalamic serotonergic activity is one of the pathogenic mechanisms leading to the development of cancer anorexia. In fact, free tryptophan (the precursor of brain serotonin) is increased during cancer, and BCAA may act by competing for the same transport system as tryptophan across the blood-brain barrier. This hypothesis has been tested in anorectic cancer patients receiving an oral supplementation of BCAA with encouraging results since the treatment decreased the severity of the anorexia in the treated patients (18).

In a more recent study by Van Norren et al. (19), supplementating the diet of cachectic tumour-bearing mice with a combination of high protein, leucine and fish oil significantly reduced loss of carcass, muscle and fat mass loss and improved muscle performance. In addition, total daily activity became normalized after intervention with the specific nutritional combination, concluding that nutritional combination of high protein, leucine, and fish oil reduced cachectic symptoms and improved functional performance in cancer cachectic mice. Glutamine-enriched solutions have also been used in total parenteral nutrition with the aim of enhancing immunoregulation of tumour growth, and compensating for the uptake of the amino acid by the tumour. Indeed, tumour cells are major glutamine consumers (for both protein synthesis and oxidation) (3), and therefore lead to host glutamine depletion, which results in a decreased host immune response and gastrointestinal mucosal integrity. In patients undergoing bone marrow transplantation for haematological malignancies, glutamine supplementation was found to be beneficial, improving nitrogen balance and diminishing the incidence of clinical infection as compared to the standard parenteral nutrition therapy (20). It could be argued that glutamine supplementation may facilitate tumour growth since it is one of the preferred substrates for fast-growing tumours. However, evidence obtained in experimental models demonstrates that glutamine supplementation improves the tumoricidal effectiveness of methotrexate while reducing its toxicity. This could be due to the glutamine-induced increased number of tumour cells in S-phase, a cell cycle phase during which they are more susceptible to chemotherapy.

β-hydroxy-β-methylbutyrate (HMB) has been used to prevent body weight loss, to reduce skeletal muscle damage, to increase skeletal muscle mass and strength, and to decrease skeletal muscle protein breakdown (21). The mechanism of action involved in this process is unclear, but it is assumed that HMB acts like an anticatabolic agent. It is a leucine metabolite formed by transamination to α-ketoisocaproate in muscle, followed by oxidation of the α-ketoisocaproate in the cytosol of hepatic cells in liver, and perhaps in other tissues, resulting in HMB. Both leucine and α-ketoisocaproate have been suggested to decrease nitrogen and protein loss, and such effects seem to demand production of HMB. Cancer patients experiencing weight loss (stage IV) who are supplemented with a mixture of HMB, arginine, and glutamine show increased body weight. A few years ago, a direct action of HMB was reported in the ubiquitin-proteasome-ATP-dependent system component expression and activation, which could explain the antiproteolytic action of HMB. These actions occur due to inhibition of the nuclear factor-κB (NF-κB) pathway. Recently, a specific role of NF-κB activation in tumour development has been demonstrated using several animal models.

Non-malignant cachexia related to the respiratory system: potential for nutritional support

The causes of cachexia in patients with COPD are multifactorial and include decreased oral intake, the effect of increased work of breathing due to abnormal respiratory mechanics, and the effect of chronic systemic inflammation. It is clear that weight loss is a poor prognostic sign in COPD. Undernutrition is, at least in part, associated with the severity of airflow obstruction. While both weight and body mass index are useful screening tools in the initial nutritional evaluation, fat-free mass (FFM) may be a better marker of undernutrition in patients with COPD. Wilson et al. (22) succeeded in increasing body weight in six underweight patients with COPD. They calculated the basal metabolic rate (BMR), and caloric goals were set at 150% of the BMR. If the subject did not reach that goal with daily diet, a nutritional supplement was given. Patients gained 3kg in the 4-week study period on average and demonstrated an increase in the maximal inspiratory mouth (MIP) and transdiaphragmatic pressures, suggesting improved respiratory muscle function. No significant change occurred in lung function.

Efthimiou et al. (23) randomized 14 underweight patients with COPD into a control and a nutritional supplementation group. Subjects were followed for 9 months. The intervention group received 3 months of 'build-up' diet, increasing their daily calorie intake to 2300–2500 kcal/day and protein intake to 80–90g/day. Nutritional repletion increased body weight by 4kg and resulted in improved respiratory muscle function. General sense of well being, breathlessness, and 6-minute walk were improved during the build-up diet. Following return to regular diet, well-being and breathlessness remained improved. However, the 6-minute walk returned to the pre-intervention levels.

Because single-centre trials appeared promising, Ferreira et al. (24) performed a meta-analysis of nutritional support in COPD on 277 patients from nine randomized, placebo-controlled trials. Unfortunately, the meta-analysis could not identify clinically significant consistent improvements in weight, arm muscle circumference, triceps skin fold thickness, 6-minute walk distance, FEV_1 (forced expiratory volume in 1s), or maximum inspiratory and expiratory mouth pressure. Ferreira et al. (24) concluded that nutritional supplementation has not yet been demonstrated to be effective in COPD. Of course, all meta-analyses suffer from inconsistencies in study design, inclusion and exclusion criteria, and outcomes that make interpretation at this early stage difficult.

The specific type of nutritional supplement might also be an important factor. Vermeeren et al. (25) examined the differences between a fat-rich versus carbohydrate-rich diet on exercise performance in COPD. They hypothesized that a fat-rich diet would be better tolerated than a carbohydrate-rich diet due to a lower respiratory quotient and thus lower carbon dioxide production. Unexpectedly, they found that the fat-rich diet was associated with increased dyspnoea. The authors attributed these findings to the fact that glucose is rapidly available and easily oxidized. Patients with COPD have lower oxidative capacity in respiratory muscles, which may make it more difficult to extract ATP from fats, since they require greater oxidative capacity and energy input before entry into the Krebs cycle. Combining nutritional supplementation with pulmonary rehabilitation, Steiner et al. (26) found that a carbohydrate-rich dietary supplement of 570kcal failed to improve exercise performance in patients with COPD. However, this program prevented weight loss, whereas the placebo group did lose weight. Interestingly, the subgroup of patients in the nutritional supplement group who had a normal body mass index on entry did have significantly improved exercise performance.

Combination of the nutritional support with exercise is an ideal aim that not only increases body weight but also results in significant improvement in fat free mass and respiratory muscle strength, as shown by Schols et al. (27). In the studies of this investigator, the clinical relevance of the response to treatment was shown in a post-hoc survival analysis, which demonstrated that weight gain and increased respiratory muscle strength were associated with increased survival rates.

Overall, it would appear that a carefully planned nutrition program can reverse under-nutrition in patients with COPD, at least over the short term. Successful nutritional repletion in these patients can lead to improvement in exercise performance and respiratory muscle function. In patients with COPD a combination of nutritional support and exercise as an anabolic stimulus appears to be the best approach to obtaining functional improvement, patients responding to this type of combination having even a decreased mortality.

Conclusion: combined approaches

In the opinion of the authors, nutritional strategies are not sufficient to reverse the cachectic syndrome. Indeed, patients on total parenteral nutrition are still subject to significant wasting, therefore emphasizing the role of the metabolic abnormalities in cachexia. It is perhaps for this reason that any therapeutic approach based on increasing food intake has to be combined with a pharmacological strategy to counteract metabolic changes. Moreover, timing is very important and has to be considered seriously when designing the therapeutic approach. A very important aspect to be taken into consideration when treating cancer patients is that any nutritional/metabolic/pharmacological support should be started early in the course of the disease, before severe weight loss occurs. The loss of muscle mass is a hallmark of cancer cachexia, and it is essentially caused by an increase of myofibrillar protein (especially myosin heavy-chain degradation), sometimes accompanied by a decrease in protein synthesis. The enhanced protein degradation is caused by an activation of the ubiquitin-dependent proteolytic system. Therefore, therapeutic approaches based on the neutralization of the enhanced myofibrillar protein degradation should be encouraged.

Another important problem associated with the design of the ideal therapeutic approach is that no unique mediators of cachexia have been identified as yet. Since the therapy against wasting during cachexia has concentrated on either increasing food intake or normalizing the persistent metabolic alterations that take place in the patient, it is difficult to apply a therapeutic approach based on the neutralization of the potential mediators involved in muscle wasting (i.e. TNF-alpha IL-6, IFN-gamma, proteolysis-inducing factor (PIF)) because many of them are involved at the same time in promoting the metabolic alterations and the anorexia present in the cancer patients. Bearing this in mind, it is obvious that a good understanding of the molecular mechanisms involved in the signalling of these mediators may be very helpful in the design of therapeutic strategies. This is especially relevant because different mediators may be sharing the same signalling pathways. At the moment there are few studies describing the role of cytokines and tumour factors in the signalling associated with muscle wasting.

In conclusion, both tumoral and humoral (mainly cytokines) factors that trigger cachexia may share common signalling pathways and therefore, it is very unlikely that a single drug will block the complex processes involved in cachexia. In addition, some of the mediators proposed for the wasting syndrome also play a role in the regulation of body weight in absolutely opposite states such as obesity. The future treatment of the cachectic syndrome will no doubt combine different nutritional support and nutraceuticals with pharmacological approaches to efficiently reverse the metabolic changes described above and, at the same time, ameliorate the anorexia of the patients. Defining this therapeutic combination is an exciting project that will stimulate many scientific efforts.

References

1. Evans WJ, Morley JE, Argilés J, *et al.* Cachexia: a new definition. *Clin Nutr* 2008; **27**:793–9.

2. Bruera E. ABC of palliative care. Anorexia, cachexia, and nutrition. *BMJ* 1997; **315**:1219–22.

3. Rivera S, Azcón-Bieto J, López-Soriano FJ, Miralpeix M, Argilés JM. Amino acid metabolism in tumour-bearing mice. *Biochem J* 1988; **249**:443–9.

4. Ravasco P, Monteiro Grillo I, Camilo M. Cancer wasting and quality of life react to early individualized nutritional counselling! *Clin Nutr* 2007; **26**:7–15.

5. Loprinzi CL, Michalak JC, Schaid DJ, *et al.* Phase III evaluation of four doses of megestrol acetate as therapy for patients with cancer anorexia and/or cachexia. *J Clin Oncol* 1993; **11**:762–7.

6. Mantovani G, Macciò, A, Esu S, *et al.* Medroxyprogesterone acetate reduces the *in vitro* production of cytokines and serotonin involved in anorexia/cachexia and emesis by peripheral blood mononuclear cells of cancer patients. *Eur J Cancer* 1997; **33**:602–7.

7. Tomíska M, Tomisková M, Salajka F, Adam Z, Vorlícek J. Palliative treatment of cancer anorexia with oral suspension of megestrol acetate. *Neoplasma* 2003; **50**:227–33.

8. Garcia J, Boccia RV, Graham C, Kumor K, Polvino W. A phase II randomized, placebo-controlled, double-blind study of the efficacy and safety of RC-1291 (RC) for the treatment of cancer cachexia. *J Clin Oncol, ASCO Annual Meeting Proceedings Part I* 2007; **25**:9133.

9. Facchinetti F, Del Giudice E, Furegato S, Passarotto M, Leon A. Cannabinoids ablate release of TNFalpha in rat microglial cells stimulated with lypopolysaccharide. *Glia* 2003; **41**:161–8.

10. Strasser, F, Luftner D, Possinger K, *et al.* Comparison of orally administered cannabis extract and delta-9-tetrahydrocannabinol in treating patients with cancer-related anorexia-cachexia syndrome: a multicenter, phase III, randomized, double-blind, placebo-controlled clinical trial from the Cannabis-In-Cachexia-Study-Group. *J Clin Oncol* 2006; **24**:3394–400.

11. DeBoer MD, Marks DL. Therapy insight: Use of melanocortin antagonists in the treatment of cachexia in chronic disease. *Nat Clin Pract Endocrinol Metab* 2006; **2**:459–66.

12. Fearon KC, Von Meyenfeldt MF, Moses AG, *et al.* Effect of a protein and energy dense N-3 fatty acid enriched oral supplement on loss of weight and lean tissue in cancer cachexia: a randomised double blind trial. *Gut* 2003; **52**:1479–86.

13. Fearon KC, Barber MD, Moses AG, *et al.* Double-blind, placebo-controlled, randomized study of eicosapentaenoic acid diester in patients with cancer cachexia. *J Clin Oncol* 2006; **24**:3401–7.

14. Dewey A, Baughan C, Dean T, Higgins B, Johnson I. Eicosapentaenoic acid (EPA, an omega-3 fatty acid from fish oils) for the treatment of cancer cachexia. *Cochrane Database Syst Rev* 2007; **24**:CD004597.

15. Read JA, Beale PJ, Volker DH, Smith N, Child A, Clarke SJ. Nutrition intervention using an eicosapentaenoic acid (EPA)-containing supplement in patients with advanced colorectal cancer. Effects on nutritional and inflammatory status: a phase II trial. *Support Care Cancer* 2007; **15**:301–7.

16. Van der Meij BS, Languis JA, Van Adrichem V, Spreeuwenberg MD, Smit EF, Van Leeuwen PA. A double blind randomized controlled trial on oral nutritional supplementation of omega-3 fatty acids in non-small cell lung carcinoma. *Clin Nutr Suppl* 2008; **3**:111.

17. Tayek JA, Bistrian BR, Hehir DJ, Martin R, Moldawer LL. Blackburn, G.L. Improved protein kinetics and albumin synthesis by branched chain amino acid-enriched total parenteral nutrition in cancer cachexia. A prospective randomized crossover trial. *Cancer* 1986; **58**:147–57.

18. Cangiano C, Laviano A, Meguid, MM, *et al.* Effects of administration of oral branched-chain amino acids on anorexia and caloric intake in cancer patients. *J Natl Cancer Inst* 1996; **88**:550–2.

19. Van Norren K, Kegler D, Argilés JM, *et al.* Dietary supplementation with a specific combination of high protein, leucine, and fish oil improves muscle function and daily activity in tumour-bearing cachectic mice. *Br J Cancer* 2009; **100**:713–22.

20. Ziegler TR, Young LS, Benfell K, *et al.* Clinical and metabolic efficacy of glutamine-supplemented parenteral nutrition after bone marrow transplantation. A randomized, double-blind, controlled study. *Ann Intern Med* 1992; **116**:821–8.
21. Gallagher PM, Carrithers JA, Godard MP, Schulze KE, Trappe SW. Beta-hydroxy-beta-methylbutyrate ingestion, Part I: effects on strength and fat free mass. *Med Sci Sports Exerc* 2000; **32**:2109–15.
22. Wilson DO, Rogers RM, Sanders MH, Pennock BE, Reilly JJ. Nutritional intervention in malnourished patients with emphysema. *Am Rev Respir Dis* 1986; **134**:672–7.
23. Efthimiou J, Fleming J, Gomes C, Spiro SG. The effect of supplementary oral nutrition in poorly nourished patients with chronic obstructive pulmonary disease. *Am Rev Respir Dis* 1988; **137**:1075–82.
24. Ferreira IM, Brooks D, Lacasse Y. Goldstein, R.S. Nutritional support for individuals with COPD: a meta-analysis. *Chest* 2000; **117**:672–8.
25. Vermeeren MA, Wouters EF, Nelissen LH, Van Lier A, Hofman Z, Schols AM. Acute effects of different nutritional supplements on symptoms and functional capacity in patients with chronic obstructive pulmonary disease. *Am J Clin Nutr* 2001; **73**:295–301.
26. Steiner MC, Barton RL, Singh SJ, Morgan MD. Nutritional enhancement of exercise performance in chronic obstructive pulmonary disease: a randomised controlled trial. *Thorax* 2003; **58**:745–51.
27. Schols AM, Soeters PB, Dingemans AM, Mostert R, Frantzen PJ, Wouters EF. Prevalence and characteristics of nutritional depletion in patients with stable COPD eligible for pulmonary rehabilitation. *Am Rev Respir Dis* 1993; **147**:1151–6.

Part 4

Dyspnoea in special situations

Chapter 12

Diffuse airflow obstruction and 'restrictive' lung disease

Mary McGregor and David R. Baldwin

In this chapter we consider how supportive care can relieve symptoms due to chronic diffuse airflow obstruction and pulmonary or pleural disease that causes lung restriction. Together these conditions are responsible for the largest number of respiratory patients who may need supportive care.

The first part of this chapter considers the diseases causing chronic diffuse airflow obstruction and briefly discusses their pathophysiology and prognosis. It then looks at the measures available for supportive care and briefly summarizes the evidence for each of these.

There is far less evidence available for supportive care in restrictive lung disease but we consider that available in the same way as for chronic airflow obstruction.

Chronic diffuse airflow obstruction

By far the commonest cause of chronic airflow obstruction is chronic obstructive pulmonary disease (COPD). This disease is prevalent throughout the world and is currently the fourth leading cause of death in the US and Europe (1). Prevalence of COPD varies, partly because of inconsistent diagnostic methods, especially in early stages of the disease. However, data suggest that approximately 6% of US adults aged over 25 years have mild disease and a further 6% have moderate COPD (2). The disease is defined as 'a preventable and treatable disease state that is characterized by airflow limitation that is not fully reversible' (2). Airflow obstruction has been defined by the UK National Institute for Health and Clinical Excellence (NICE) as an FEV_1 (forced expiratory volume in 1s) less than 80%, or an FEV_1/FVC (forced expiratory volume) less than 0.7 (3). It is progressive, primarily caused by cigarette smoking and has systemic consequences (Figure 12.1).

The pathophysiology of COPD is determined by changes within the different areas of the lungs. In the central airways, mucus gland hypertrophy occurs causing simple bronchitis. More peripherally, bronchiolitis develops, leading to fibrosis and narrowing of the small airways. In the lung parenchyma destruction of the bronchioles causes emphysema, which leads to airway collapse and the formation of bullae. Finally, changes within the pulmonary vasculature can eventually result in pulmonary hypertension and cor pulmonale, (right-sided ventricular dysfunction).

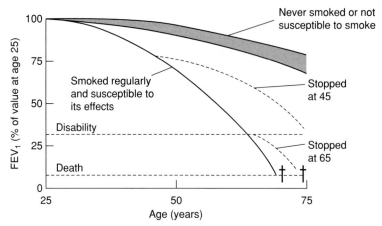

Fig. 12.1 The relationship between lung function (FEV_1) and ageing in patients who never smoke or who are not susceptible to it (hatched area) and patients who smoke regularly and who are susceptible. It can be seen that there is an inexorable acceleration of the natural loss of lung function with age in susceptible smokers. The decline resumes the natural track if smoking cessation occurs at any stage. Disability is usual when the FEV_1 falls to about 30% of young adult value. Adapted by permission from BMJ Publishing Group Limited. Thorax, Jones, P.W. Quality of life measurement for patients with diseases of the airways. Volume 46: 676–82, 1991.

The hallmark of COPD is airways obstruction best demonstrated as a low FEV_1 (see Chapter 2, this volume). With normal ageing the FEV_1 progressively but slowly falls during adult life due to an attrition of elastic tissue in the lung (Figure 12.1). In susceptible individuals smoking, or exposure to other lung toxins, causes an acceleration of this loss. This, if unchecked, causes impairment and disability, usually in late middle age. Premature death due to respiratory failure follows in severe cases. Severe disease may be associated with a number of complications such as abnormal blood gases, cor pulmonale, and others (Box 12.1). The commonest symptom in COPD is dyspnoea (breathlessness) initially on exertion but eventually progressing to occur at rest.

Other diseases in which diffuse chronic airflow obstruction may occur include asthma, bronchiectasis, cystic fibrosis, and some cases of TB and sarcoidosis.

The Scottish Intercollegiate Guidelines Network (SIGN) and British Thoracic Society (BTS) guidelines on the management of asthma indicate that there is no consensus on the definition of asthma. However, all definitions include the presence of key symptoms (two or more of wheeze, breathlessness, chest tightness, and cough) in association with variable airflow obstruction (4). It is only in a small minority of patients that irreversible airway narrowing is sufficiently severe to cause a permanent disability. This form of asthma is included within the definition of COPD because the clinical features are similar, although respiratory failure and cor pulmonale are less common. The long-term prognosis is usually much better than smoking-related COPD, with the patient often showing little decline in function over many years.

Bronchiectasis is similar to asthma is that there is a chronic inflammatory state but it differs in that this results in permanent bronchial dilatation. The inflammation is often secondary to ongoing infection that is the result of impaired mucociliary clearance of

---

Box 12.1 Possible complications of COPD

Direct

- Respiratory failure: chronic and acute as part of an exacerbation, type 1 or type 2.
- Acute exacerbations: often due to infection.
- Cor pulmonale: fluid retention, raised pulmonary artery pressure and right heart hypertrophy.
- Secondary polycythaemia.
- Susceptibility to pneumothorax.
- Increased risk of lung cancer.
- Skeletal muscle deconditioning.
- Malnutrition, loss of weight.

Indirect

- Loss of work capacity.
- Loss of independence.
- Depression and anxiety.
- Panic attacks.
- Increased impact of comorbidity.

---

pathogens from the airways. The main symptoms are a productive cough, dyspnoea, and frequent lower respiratory tract infections (depending on severity). Cystic fibrosis affects the lungs in the same way but generally produces more severe bronchiectasis and some fibrosis as well as other features caused by increased viscosity of secretions.

Occasionally sarcoidosis and TB may heal and cause bilateral upper lobe fibrosis and contraction. This leads to distortion and traction of the bronchi which is often severe and fixed. The result is obstructive lung disease, which is fixed and not responsive to bronchodilators. Complications are rare unless a secondary pathology is involved such as a mycetoma. Sarcoidosis more commonly causes a combined obstructive and restrictive ventilator pattern due to granulomatous inflammation that is distributed both in the lung parenchyma and airways.

Assessment of disease severity

The full assessment of a patient with COPD requires a multidisciplinary approach to elicit the physical, psychological, and social effects that the disease might be having on the patient and their carers. At this point both the disease modifying treatments can be offered as well as the supportive care options (see Table 1.5, Chapter 1). Although it does not necessarily follow that impairment can predict disability, it is an easy way of structuring the approach and treatment options available at each stage of the disease.

COPD is classified into three stages: mild, moderate, and severe. Below are the classes as defined by the British Thoracic Society (3).

◆ Mild disease: patients with an FEV_1 50–80% predicted.

◆ Moderate disease: patients with an FEV_1 30–50% predicted.

◆ Severe disease: patients with an FEV1 <30% predicted.

Decreasing FEV_1 correlates with increasing exacerbations and mortality but it does not accurately predict the level of symptoms and disability that a patient might have. Assessing body mass index and symptoms of breathlessness will also help categorize their disease stage (2).

The role of supportive care

Most illnesses that cause restrictive and obstructive lung disease do not have a cure so treatments are primarily designed to control and relieve symptoms. In this way they could all be considered 'supportive'. The only treatment proven to lengthen survival is long-term oxygen therapy (LTOT), and this is currently only available for those with severe disease. However, both obstructive and restrictive lung diseases have systemic effects and this chapter focuses on those therapies, both pharmacological and non-pharmacological, that address the aspects of the disease not treated by the standard drug therapies (Figure 12.2) They are designed to run in parallel with the disease-modifying treatments such as those listed for COPD in Box 12.2 and complement them. Unlike in the traditional model of palliative care, these options can be offered at any stage of the disease, long before the patient reaches the terminal phase.

In mild disease there should be little impairment on a day-to-day basis so often there is little need for regular medical or supportive therapy. What is important at this stage is to address risk factors such as smoking and put in place preventative measures such as the pneumococcal vaccine and the seasonal influenza vaccine.

As the disease progresses to moderate impairment, symptoms start to have a more disruptive effect on activities of daily living. At this point a formal assessment of supportive care needs would be appropriate. Options such as pulmonary rehabilitation, respiratory

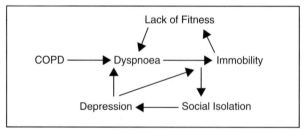

Fig. 12.2 The cycle of physical, social, and psychosocial consequences of COPD. Reproduced from (1) with permission.

Box 12.2 Disease-modifying treatments for COPD

- Treatment of acute exacerbation
- Inhaled and oral bronchodilators
- Inhaled and oral corticosteroids
- Antibiotics
- Treatment of cor pulmonale
- Treatment of secondary polycythaemia
- Mechanical ventilation
- Long-term oxygen therapy

muscle training, breath control techniques, and self-management education can be combined with advice on employment, housing, and benefits.

In severe disease all of the support offered in mild and moderate disease is appropriate as well as considering suitability for LTOT, assessing for concurrent anxiety or depression and, if appropriate, discussing end of life planning.

The evidence for the above options is now presented, however many of the therapies discussed have been covered in much more detail in other chapters. A list of the possible modalities of supportive care available for obstructive and restrictive lung disease can be found in Table 12.1. The most commonly needed modalities are listed first, and then it moves onto those needed in severe and end stage disease. This indicates in which chapter a more extensive review of these treatments can be found.

Assessment of supportive care needs

The assessment can be undertaken in a variety of settings, according to where the patient is in their pathway. Thus primary healthcare professionals or secondary care (respiratory physician, specialist nurses) may be involved. The main symptom of advancing respiratory disease is breathlessness and this can be notoriously difficult to assess objectively. Levels of assessment may be summarized as:

- Usual clinical history and examination.
- A simple questionnaire assessing exercise capacity such as the Medical Research Council (MRC) scale (see Table 12.2) (6).
- A questionnaire incorporating a patient's perception of effort of doing various things, e.g. the baseline dyspnoea index (BDI) (7).
- A questionnaire which evaluates the impact of dyspnoea on a patient's quality of life, e.g. the St George's respiratory questionnaire (SGRQ) (8).

Alongside assessment of the physical symptoms, social and psychological assessments should also be carried out. Often this is performed by another member of the health

Table 12.1 Possible supportive care measures in COPD

	See Chapter
Smoking cessation assistance	12
Exercise rehabilitation	9,10
Disease education	1,6,10,11
Social work advice (patient and carers)	9
Energy conservation and physical needs advice	9
Posture and breathing technique	9,10
Respiratory muscle training	9,10
Cognitive-behavioural therapy (CBT)	10
Stress and panic management	10
Drug treatment of anxiety and depression	6,10
Nutrition advice and prescription	11
Burst oxygen to relieve dyspnoea	10
Facial airflow to relieve dyspnoea	10
Self-help groups	6,9,10
Mucolytics	16
Drugs for severe breathlessness and terminal anxiety	7
End of life planning	10

Table 12.2 MRC dyspnoea scale

Grade	Degree of breathlessness related to activities
1	Not troubled by breathlessness except on strenuous exercise
2	Short of breath when hurrying or walking up a slight hill
3	Walks slower than contemporaries on level ground because of breathlessness, or has to stop for breath when walking at own pace
4	Stops for breath after walking about 100m or after a few minutes on level ground
5	Too breathless to leave house, or breathless when dressing or undressing

care team. In the UK it is often a respiratory nurse specialist, whereas within the US respiratory therapists with a background in physiotherapy have taken this role.

Pulmonary rehabilitation

Pulmonary rehabilitation (PR) is becoming the mainstay of supportive care for respiratory disease. This intervention is recognized worldwide, albeit with varying availability, and has an increasing body of evidence to support its benefits. This can be found in any respiratory disease that results in reduced functional capacity (9), although the majority of the studies have been carried out in patients with COPD. Meta-analyses have shown that a comprehensive rehabilitation programme encompassing exercise training, education, nutritional therapy, and psychosocial/behavioural interventions improves health-related quality of life. It can also have positive effects on exercise capacity, the perception of dyspnoea, and the frequency and duration of hospital admissions (10). Finally, it increases the sense of control patients have over their condition (11), something which is important in the management of all chronic diseases. This is despite the fact that it does not seem to have any sustained positive effect on pulmonary function (2).

Current evidence suggests that those with severe dyspnoea or very limited exercise tolerance do not seem to benefit from physical rehabilitation programmes, which makes referral at an earlier stage of the disease even more important. However, this is not to say that they will not benefit from the other aspects of supportive care within a formal PR programme. They should therefore not be completely excluded. There are no specific referral criteria, although it should be considered in all those with moderate to severe disease.

A programme should, at the minimum, contain exercise training which should ideally be supplemented by dietary assessment, disease education, and psychosocial support. In this way PR can introduce many of the therapies identified within this book as 'supportive care' within one setting.

The exercise training helps address the loss of peripheral muscle mass that occurs in chronic respiratory disease. This loss is suspected to be caused by a combination of corticosteroid use, hypoxia, inactivity, and chronic systemic inflammation. A programme of resistance and endurance training that involves both the upper and lower limb muscles has been shown to have enduring positive benefits on functional ability (12) and quality of life. There is currently no consensus of the length of the training but it seems that, generally, the longer the better (13).

An interesting recent development is the research suggesting that a mixture of helium and oxygen inspired during exercise increases the efficacy of rehabilitation. This is thought to be due to the finding that patients could achieve greater maximal exercise when breathing the Heliox mix (14).

An alternative to physical exercise programmes are ones that involve neuromuscular electrical stimulation. This helps train weight-bearing muscles without the limitation of exertional breathlessness. Several recent studies have found that this can improve muscle strength and, consequently, help relieve breathlessness and improve quality of life (15, 16).

Posture, breathing technique training, and respiratory muscle training

As an adjunct to PR, or as an alternative in those unable to manage physical activity, posture and breathing technique training can help relieve dyspnoea. Most patients spontaneously adopt the pursed lip breathing and a forward leaning posture with shoulder girdle support. This provides positive end-expiratory pressure which, intuitively, allows more complete emptying of the lungs. So far, research into the positive benefits of this technique has been limited but there is no proof of a sustained, positive effect (17).

Self-management

Programmes that educate a patient about their disease and how to manage an exacerbation have been shown to improve quality of life and reduce emergency hospital admissions. A recent Cochrane review (18) found that intervention could incorporate written educational material or more formal teaching in groups. There was no effect on exercise capacity or lung function.

Dietary support

Weight loss is a significant problem in patients with airflow obstruction. Mortality rates in underweight and normal weight patients are consistently higher than in those with raised body mass indexes (19). Weight loss itself is also associated with a higher mortality in patients with COPD, regardless of the base weight they start from (20). In any case, poor appetite and weight loss are themselves distressing symptoms for the patients and can become areas of conflict between them and their carers. Studies have been done on the benefits of nutritional advice and seem to show positive results (21). Having advice at an early stage helps to postpone the cycle of weight loss, reduced exercise capacity, and reduced muscle size. It is also much easier to give simple advice early on as opposed to intensive support at a later stage. Using strategies such as those outlined in the MacMillan Durham Cachexia pack (22) might help in targeting those who would benefit from this support.

A Cochrane review in 2005 (23) showed that there was no evidence at present that nutritional supplements changed outcomes in COPD but it recommended more research be done. At this stage, therefore, it seems that simple dietary advice has better and more long lasting benefits than oral supplements.

Smoking cessation

Whilst this obviously has disease-modifying consequences as well, smoking cessation is an important part of symptom management in any respiratory disease. Over the last 10 years more pharmacological approaches have become available, but it has also been recognized that those with a strong support network are better placed to stay cigarette free (24).

The mainstays of pharmacological assistance in quitting are the nicotine replacement therapies (NRT), such as patches, lozenges, or gum. These are readily available in pharmacies and so do not require a prescription or visit to a health professional. Bupropion and varenicline are prescription-only drugs that can be offered if NRT has not been effective and the motivation to stop smoking is strong. Studies have shown that all of the above options are more effective than placebo (25).

Psychological support

Both anxiety and depression have higher incidences in patients who have chronic disease, and COPD is no exception. Studies have shown the prevalence of both anxiety and depressive disorders can be well over 50% (26), and that this rises when looking at patients who have just had an acute exacerbation (27). It, however, remains relatively underdiagnosed in populations outside of research trials. This may be because many of the symptoms of anxiety or depression may well be attributed to the disease itself. As it appears that depression can contribute to the frequency of hospitalizations and lengthen the recovery time from exacerbations (28), it remains an important goal to recognize it and treat it.

Unfortunately there is no consensus as to how best to treat either anxiety or depression in the setting of chronic respiratory disease. There have been trials that have suggested both tricyclic antidepressants and selective serotonin reuptake inhibitors can be useful. However these have not yet been conclusive. Non-pharmacological therapies such as cognitive-behavioural therapy and psychotherapy also seem to be helpful (29). These can be structured into a pulmonary rehabilitation programme if resources allow.

Supplementary oxygen

Since the Nocturnal Oxygen Treatment Trial (NOTT) trial in the early 1980s, home LTOT has been prescribed as one of the few life prolonging treatments available in hypoxemic lung disease. The criteria are shown in Box 12.3.

Aside from the above criteria, oxygen is also prescribed for short bursts to help relieve the feelings of dyspnoea that ensue after exertion. There is however, little evidence that this makes any difference to how quickly the symptoms resolve (30). Ambulatory oxygen does appear to have some positive benefits on the length and intensity of exertion that a patient with COPD can achieve. There have been several recent reviews of the literature confirming this (31, 32) but all conclude that more research into the long-term effects of this therapy needs to be done. There is a risk of increased oxidative stress on the lungs which, in the long term, could do more damage. There are guidelines available from the Royal College of Physicians detailing when ambulatory oxygen should be considered (33).

Box 12.3 Criteria for long-term oxygen therapy

- Chronic hypoxaemia, PaO_2 <7.3kPa when breathing air during a period of stability (5 weeks or more without exacerbations).
- Chronic hypoxaemia, PaO_2 7.3–8kPa, during a period of stability, with the presence of one of the following:
  - Secondary polycythaemia.
  - Clinical and or echocardiographic evidence of pulmonary hypertension.

Surgical options

Lung volume reduction surgery has been shown to be effective at reducing symptoms of breathlessness and improving exercise capacity in a specific subset of patients with severe dyspnoea due to COPD. Those who have predominantly upper lobe disease seem to derive the most benefit from the operation. In other groups the risk of the surgery and postoperative complications outweigh the benefits gained (34, 35).

Drugs for severe breathlessness

There are misconceptions that managing breathlessness and anxiety in the final stages of respiratory disease is different to managing the same symptoms in malignant disease. In fact, the same medications are as useful despite the underlying pathology causing the breathlessness. After all, how many patients with lung cancer also have an element of obstructive airways disease contributing to their symptoms? Once reversible causes have been addressed and non-drug therapies have been tried, then both opiates and benzodiazepines have a role to play.

There have been many studies investigating the pharmacology of why opiates relieve breathlessness. It is thought that they have an effect both on the respiratory centre in the brain as well as on opioid receptors in the bronchial tree itself. However, whatever their route of action, opiates have been found to be effective at controlling breathlessness at rest without changing the respiratory rate or adversely affecting oxygenation (36). With this in mind, immediate-release morphine sulphate preparations could be trialled. Starting with a low dose would help manage any anxieties about respiratory depression as well as avoid unpleasant side effects that might prevent further use (37). If successful and needed more than twice in 24 hours a long-acting opiate can be given and the dose titrated up in the same way it would be for pain (38).

Advance care planning

Research done by numerous bodies over the last 10 years has highlighted that many people are not dying in the place or manner which they would choose. Only 18% of terminally ill people die at home in the UK, whereas surveys suggest that over 50% would wish to (39). The NHS End of Life Care Strategy (40) was launched in England and Wales in 2008 as a way of addressing the issues around providing satisfactory end of life care in both the primary and secondary sectors.

The first point of the strategy guarantees patients access to discussions with their health professionals about end of life decisions. It recognizes that, difficult as these conversations can be, they are an integral part of care for anyone with a life-limiting condition such as COPD or pulmonary fibrosis. Often the most challenging part of initiating these discussions is deciding when a person is approaching the final stages of their disease. With chronic illnesses such as those discussed above there may be many acute exacerbations that can be successfully treated with intensive interventions. The Gold Standards Framework (41) used in within the NHS has some useful guidance on identifying when people are likely to be within the last 6–12 months of life in non-malignant diseases (Box 12.4). These could be the trigger for discussions with patients and their families, as well as communication between the different healthcare organizations involved.

Initiating these discussions should be done in an appropriate setting and with ongoing support available for the people involved. There are numerous guidelines as to how this can be done sensitively and effectively (42–44). However, as communication skills training has only recently become a mandatory part of the medical undergraduate curriculum many healthcare professionals may not feel adequately trained. Within the UK there is a programme of advanced communication skills training being made available to all senior healthcare professionals involved in care of terminally ill patients. There will be similar courses available in other countries.

Within the context of respiratory disease the aims of such a discussion would be as follows:

◆ To establish the patient's understanding of their disease stage and how they perceive its progression.

◆ To explore their wishes regarding invasive and non-invasive ventilatory support during acute exacerbations. This could also extend to their wishes about further intensive care admissions if these are failing to aid recovery.

◆ To determine both the patient's and their carer's choices regarding end of life care.

Advance directives

Within the UK the passing of the Mental Capacity Act in 2005 (45) meant that written advance directives are legally binding if they met certain strict criteria. Within the context of supportive care, as part of a discussion about end of life care a patient may express wishes about refusing treatment in the event of them losing capacity. Obviously their wishes should be recorded in their health record, but it is something which they feel strongly about then they should be made aware about the criteria to be fulfilled to ensure the advance directive is legal.

Box 12.4 Clinical prognostic indicators in COPD

◆ Disease assessed to be severe (FEV_1 <30% predicted).

◆ Recurrent hospital admissions (>3 admissions in 12 months with COPD exacerbations).

◆ Fulfils long-term oxygen therapy.

◆ MRC grade 4/5: shortness of breath after 100m or confined to the house through breathlessness.

◆ Signs and symptoms of right heart failure.

◆ Combination of other factors, e.g. anorexia, depression, previous ITU/NIV/ resistant organism.

Non-obstructive/restrictive lung disease

Non-obstructive lung diseases are less understood and often more severe than obstructive airways disease. In the UK at 2008, compared with the 25,000 patients dying of COPD, the annual mortality of interstitial lung disease (CFA) was about 6500 (46). Probably for this reason, supportive care needs of patients like this are less studied (Table 12.3).

Diffuse parenchymal lung diseases (DPLD) comprise a large number of disparate and relatively rare disorders, which affect the interstitium. Essentially they cause inflammation and subsequent destruction and scarring of the lung parenchyma, comprising alveolus, respiratory bronchioles, vasculature, and interstitium (see Chapter 2, this volume). Gas exchange is impeded by inflammation, scarring, and distortion, but airway function is normal. With the onset of fibrosis, the lungs shrink, and become stiff with low lung compliance. Lung function test consequently show an increase in the ratio of FEV_1 to FVC (due to increased elastic recoil pressure) and marked diminution in tests of gas diffusion (DLCO and KCO) (due to alveolar inflammation and ventilation/perfusion defects) Patients usually report a gradual onset of exertional dyspnoea, which is the cardinal clinical feature. This often progresses inexorably to dyspnoea at rest with a fast

Table 12.3 Examples of non-obstructive lung disease which may require supportive care

Diffuse parenchymal lung disease	Pulmonary fibrosis	Idiopathic pulmonary fibrosis (IPF
		Usual interstitial pneumonia (UIP)
		Non-specific interstitial pneumonia (NSIP)
		Lymphocytic interstitial pneumonia (LIP)
		Desquamative interstitial pneumonia (DIP)
		Hypersensitivity pneumonitis (HSP)
		Occupational
		Drug induced
		Radiation
		Systemic vasculitis
	Pneumoconiosis	Coal workers pneumoconiosis
		Silicosis
	Postinflammatory	ARDS
		Tuberculosis, sarcoidosis
Post-pneumonectomy		
Diffuse pleural thickening		Asbestos induced (benign)
		Drug induced (bromocriptine)
		Mesothelioma
Pulmonary vascular disease		Primary pulmonary hypertension
		Recurrent pulmonary emboli

resting respiratory rate, a low tidal volume, and persisting and severe hypoxaemia. Some patients are troubled by a persistent dry cough that may occur at a relatively early stage of the illness when dyspnoea is not a major feature. The PCO_2 is normal or low until the disease is at an advanced stage. Complications include persistent cough, secondary infection, cor pulmonale, pulmonary embolism, and adenocarcinoma of the lung.

The pneumoconioses are lung disease caused by occupational exposure to dusts. The most important are silicosis, progressive massive fibrosis, and asbestosis. Silicosis is caused by exposure to silica and was common in pottery workers and other silica industry workers. The chronic form is similar in presentation and disease progression to idiopathic pulmonary fibrosis (IPF). Progressive massive fibrosis is characterized by enlarging conglomerate masses and progresses more slowly than IPF. Asbestosis results from asbestos exposure and is most strongly related to total inhaled dose of asbestos fibre and type of fibre. The incidence of lung cancer is increased. These conditions may present and progress long after dust exposure has ceased.

Patients surviving ARDS may be left with residual scarring, although often the damage will clear over months. Pneumonectomy patients can occasionally become extremely disabled by breathlessness after surgery. This is often out of proportion to their residual lung function. This may be because of the activation of chest wall mechanoreceptors on the operated side causing a marked disparity between respiratory effort and achieved ventilation. The same phenomenon is seen in mesothelioma and unilateral pleural thickening due to asbestos.

Patients with chronic pulmonary vascular disease have normal lung architecture and mechanics but are breathless because of a very abnormal gas exchange. Active treatment is sometimes possible—e.g. embolectomy, prostacycline, and vasodilators—but if these patients are not transplanted they usually progress to disabling breathlessness comparatively rapidly.

Assessment and treatment

The approach to the symptomatic patient with non-obstructive lung disease should probably be the same as for those with COPD:

- The physician should ensure an accurate diagnosis, treat the underlying disease where possible, recognize and treat any complications, and assess and treat any comorbidity.

- The physician should also ensure that the supportive care needs of these patients are assessed and met by a multiprofessional approach.

There are no published guidelines suggesting appropriate timing of referral or selection of these patients for a comprehensive supportive care assessment. However, by analogy with COPD, it would seem sensible to consider patients for this when they have troublesome limitation and/or breathlessness with activities of work, pleasure, and daily living, or they are suffering anxieties with these, or are losing previous independence.

The pitfall with this is that patients appear to be referred at a very late stage of disease. For example, in a review of the only 32 patients of 350 referred to their lung rehabilitation centre with non-obstructive lung disease, Foster and Thomas found a mean 6-min walk distance of only 276 feet (84m) on admission, which is likely to be only about 15% of predicted (47). Given the poor prognosis of many of these patients, a much earlier referral for assessment by a nurse-led team seems sensible.

Supportive care likely to be helpful in non-obstructive lung disease

Smoking cessation

Hypoxia leads to a reduction in tissue oxygenation and smoking diminishes the oxygen-carrying capacity of haemoglobin by 10% or more by producing carboxyhaemoglobin. Although no change in prognosis is to be expected, advice on smoking cessation is an important point in recent guidelines. Most significantly, patients with interstitial lung disease have a 5 times greater risk of lung cancer, before the risk of smoking is added (49). As with any one trying to stop smoking, specialist support should be offered and pharmacological therapy prescribed if appropriate.

Pulmonary rehabilitation

Recent research has confirmed what has been intuitively felt to be true, in that exercise training does help patients with non-obstructive lung disease. Improvements were seen after 12 weeks and this improved further after 24 weeks. As with obstructive airways disease, the longer the patients can participate in the rehabilitation programme, the better (48).

General measures

Many of the same measures applied to COPD may also be appropriate in those who have restrictive lung disease too. Advice on energy conservation, disease education, social work advice, stress management, and recognition of psychological issues such as depression should be given. There is no evidence that patients become nutritionally depleted before they become very ill, although this would not be unexpected given the high metabolic demands of an increased respiratory workload. Weight loss should therefore be assessed as in COPD. Many of these patients are treated with relatively high doses of oral corticosteroids. Issues surrounding bone density and steroid-induced myopathy also need to be considered.

Oxygen therapy

Unlike in obstructive lung diseases, there is no evidence that oxygen prolongs survival in restrictive lung disease. Short-burst oxygen is recommended in patients who desaturate on exertion to less than 90%, as long as the therapy is shown to increase exercise tolerance. Long-term oxygen is recommended for those who have a persistent resting hypoxemia, PaO_2 <7.3kPa, or those who have a PaO_2 <8kPa with evidence of pulmonary hypertension (33).

Drug treatment of severe dyspnoea

Opiates should be used as with COPD but there is much less risk of carbon dioxide retention. High doses of drugs may be needed to desensitize patients to their difficult combination of high respiratory drive and hypoxemia. A reduction in respiratory rate is likely to worsen hypoxemia and should be particularly allowed for.

Lung transplantation

This is more often considered than within patients with obstructive lung disease, because they are often younger and usually do not have other smoking-related disorders. Difficulties that then arise are

- There may be along delay (perhaps up to 2 years in the UK) between acceptance on a programme and any surgery. There is a risk that any deterioration in the mean time is overlooked as the definitive treatment is being awaited. Referring for supportive care assessment would still be appropriate at this point.

- Many patients are turned down for transplantation. This naturally leads to increased distress and sometimes bitterness that needs to be recognized and addressed.

It has been noted that those patients that do receive transplants often do not return to a level of exercise capacity predicted by their new lung and cardiorespiratory function. This seems to be due to persistent peripheral skeletal muscle abnormalities which are due principally to the previous underlying disease and perhaps immobility and anti-inflammatory treatment. This particular problem highlights the importance of pulmonary rehabilitation and continuing exercise in patients awaiting transplantation.

Medicolegal issues

Some restrictive lung diseases are occupationally induced. It is part of supportive care, and usually the physician's responsibility to ensure the patient and their family receive timely advice about their statutory rights to compensation and whether they should seek legal advice.

Advance care planning

As previously mentioned, acknowledging continued deterioration and the difficulties in predicting prognosis is an important part of supportive care. Patients with severe respiratory failure and increasing breathlessness should not normally be mechanically ventilated as there is virtually no possibility of improvement. Therefore, it is an advantage if this is discussed with patients and their carers in good time. They can then have the opportunity to express their wishes about management in their final stages of the disease.

References

1. Global Initiative for Chronic Obstructive Lung Disease (GOLD). *Global Strategy for the Diagnosis, Management and Prevention of COPD*, 2010. Available at: http://www.goldcopd.org.

2. American Thoracic Society &European Respiratory Society Task Force. *Standards for the Diagnosis and Management of Patients with COPD [Internet]. Version 1.2.* New York: American Thoracic Society, 2004 [updated 8 September 2005]. Available at: http://www.thoracic.org/go/copd.

3. National Collaborating centre for chronic conditions. Chronic obstructive pulmonary disease. National clinical guideline on the management of chronic obstructive pulmonary disease in primary and secondary care. *Thorax* 2004; **59**(S1):1–232.

4. Scottish Intercollegiate Guidelines Network and British Thoracic Society. *British guideline on the management of asthma: a national clinical guideline (revised 2009).* Edinburgh: SIGN and BTS, 2009.

5. King P. The pathophysiology of bronchiectasis. *Int J COPD* 2009; **4**:411–19.

6. Fletcher CM, Elms PC, Wood CH. The significance of respiratory symptoms and the diagnosis of chronic bronchitis in the working population. *BMJ* 1995; **1**:257–66.

7. Mahler D, Weinberg D, Wells C, Fienstine A. The measurement of dyspnoea: Inter-observer and physiologic correlates of two new clinical indexes. *Chest* 1984; **85**:751–8.

8. Guyatt G, Berman L, Townend M, Pugsley S, Chambers L. A measure of quality of life for clinical trials in chronic lung disease. *Thorax* 1987; **42**:733–78.

9. Nici L, Donner C, Wouters E, *et al.* American Thoracic Society/European Respiratory Society statement on pulmonary rehabilitation. *Am J Respir Crit Care Med* 2006; **173**:1390–413.

10. Trikalinos TA, Raman G, Kupelnick B, Chew PW, Lau J. *Pulmonary Rehabilitation for COPD and other lung diseases.* Rockville, MD: Agency for Healthcare Research and Quality (AHRQ). Technology Assessment, 2006

11. Lacasse Y, Goldstein R, Lasserson TJ, Martin S. Pulmonary rehabilitation for chronic obstructive pulmonary disease. *Cochrane Database Syst Rev* 2002; **3**:CD003793.

12. Carone M, Patessio A, Ambrosino N, *et al.* Effect of pulmonary rehabilitation in chronic respiratory failure (CRF) due to chronic obstructive pulmonary disease (COPD): the Maugeri Study. *Respiratory Medicine* 2007; **101**:2447–53.

13. Rossi G, Florini F, Romagnoli N, *et al.* Length and clinical effectiveness of pulmonary rehabilitation in out patients with chronic airway obstruction. *Chest* 2005; **127**:105–9.

14. Eves ND, Sandmeyer LC, Wong EY, *et al.* Helium-hyperoxia: a novel intervention to improve the benefits of pulmonary rehabilitation for patient with COPD. *Chest* 2009; **135**:609–18.

15. Bauswein C, Booth S, Gysels M, Higginson I. Non-pharmacological interventions for breathlessness in advanced stages of malignant and non-malignant diseases. *Cochrane Database Syst Rev* 2008; **2**:CD005623.

16. Sillen MJ, Speksnijder CM, Eterman RM, *et al.* Effects of neuromuscular electrical stimulation of muscles of ambulation in patients with chronic heart failure or COPD: a systematic review of the English language literature. *Chest* 2009; **136**:44–61.

17. Olsen A, Westerdahl E. Positive expiratory pressure in patients with chronic obstructive pulmonary disease: A systematic review. *Respiration* 2009; **77**:110–18.

18. Effing T, Monninkhof EEM, van der Valk PP, *et al.* Self management education for patients with chronic obstructive pulmonary disease (review). *Cochrane Collaboration* 2009; **4**.

19. Hallin R, Gudmundsson G, Suppli U, *et al.* Nutritional status and long term mortality in hospitalised patients with chronic obstructive pulmonary disease. *Respir Med* 2007; **101**: 1954–60.

20. Prescott E, Amdal T, Mikkelsen K, *et al.* Prognostic value of weight change in chronic obstructive pulmonary disease: results from the Copenhagen City heart study. *Eur Respir J* 2002; **20**:539–44.

21. Weekes C, Emery P, Elia M. Dietary counselling and food fortification in stable COPD: a randomised trial. *Thorax* 2009; **64**:326–31.

22. MacMillan Durham Cachexia Pack. Available at: http://www.learnzone.macmillan.org.uk.

23. Ferreria IM, Brooks D, Lacasse Y, *et al.* Nutritional supplementation for stable chronic obstructive pulmonary disease. *Cochrane Database Syst Rev* 2005; **2**:CD000998.

24. National Institute for Health and Clinical Excellence. *Brief interventions and referral for smoking cessation: guidance.* London: NICE, 2006.

25. Eisenberg M, Fillon K, Yavin D, *et al.* Pharmacotherapies for smoking -cessation:a meta-analysis of random controlled trials. *CMAJ* 2008; **172**:135–44.

26. Yohannes AM, Willgoss TG, Baldwin R, Connolly MJ. Depression and anxiety in chronic heart failure and chronic obstructive pulmonary disease: prevalence, relevance, clinical implications and management principles. *Int J Geriatr Psychiatry* 2010; **25**(12):1209–21.

27. Hill K, Geist R, Goldstein RS, Lacasse Y. Anxiety and depression in end stage COPD. *Eur Respir J* 2008; **31**: 667–77.

28. Maurer J, Rebbapragrada V, Borson S, *et al.* Anxiety and depression in COPD. Current understanding, unanswered questions and research needs. *Chest* 2008; **134**(4 Suppl):43S–56S.

29. Kunic M, Veazey C, Cully J, *et al.* COPD education and cognitive behavioural therapy group treatment for clinically significant symptoms of depression and anxiety in COPD patients: an randomized controlled trial. *Psychol Med* 2008; **38**:385–96.

30. Stevenson M, Calverley P. Effect of oxygen on maximal recovery from exercise in patients with chronic obstructive pulmonary disease. *Thorax* 2004; **59**:668–72.

31. Bradley J, O'Neill B. Short term ambulatory oxygen for chronic obstructive disease. *Cochrane Database Syst Rev* 2005; **4**:CD004356.

32. Bradley J, LassersonT, Elborn S, *et al.* A systematic review of randomized controlled trails examining the short term benefit of ambulatory oxygen in COPD. *Chest* 2007; **131**:278–85.

33. Royal College of Physicians of London. *Domiciliary oxygen therapy services: Clinical guidelines and advice for prescribers.* London: RCP, 1999.

34. Trow TK. Lung volume reduction surgery for severe emphysema: appraisal of its current status. *Curr Opin Pulmon Med* 2004; **10**:128–32.

35. Shah AA, D'Amico TA. Lung volume reduction surgery for the management of refractory dyspnoea in chronic obstructive pulmonary disease. *Curr Opin Support Palliat Care* 2009; **3**:107–11.

36. Jennings AL, Davies AN, Higgins JPT, *et al.* A systematic review of the use of opioids in the management of dyspnoea. *Thorax* 2002; **57**:939–44.

37. Rocker G, Horton R, Currow, *et al.* Palliation of dyspnoea in advanced COPD: revisiting a role for opioids. *Thorax* 2009; **64**:910–15.

38. Twycross R, Wilcock A, Stark Toller C. *Symptom Management in Advanced Cancer,* 4th edn. Oxford: Radcliffe Medical Press, 2009.

39. The King's Fund. *End of Life Care,* 2009. Available at: http://www.kingsfund.org.uk/research/topics/endoflife_care/

40. Department of Health. *End of life care strategy – promoting high quality care for all adults at the end of life.* London: Department of Health, 2008.

41. The Gold Standards Framework. *Prognostic Indicator Guidance,* 2008 Available at: http://www.goldstandardsframework.nhs.uk/Resources/Gold%20Standards%20Framework/PIG_Paper_Final_revised_v5_Sept08.pdf.

42. www.patient.co.uk/doctor/Breaking-Bad-News.htm (accessed 13 December 2011).

43. Department of Health, Social Services and Public Safety. *Breaking Bad News . . . Regional Guidelines,* 2003. Available at: http://www.dhsspsni.gov.uk/breaking_bad_news.pdf.

44. Buckman R. *Breaking Bad News: A Guide for Healthcare Professionals.* Baltimore: Johns Hopkins University Press, 1992.

45. *Mental capacity Act 2005.* Available at: http://www.opsi.gov.uk.

46. Foster S, Thomas HM. Pulmonary rehabilitation in lung disease other than chronic obstructive pulmonary disease. *Am Rev Respir Dis* 1990; **141**:601–4.

47. Salhi T, Troosters B, Behaegel M, *et al.* Effects of pulmonary rehabilitation in patients with restrictive lung disease. *Chest* 2010; **137**:273–9.

48. Wells AU, Hirani N. Interstitial lung disease guideline: The British Thoracic Society in collaboration with the Thoracic Society of Australia and New Zealand and the Irish Thoracic Society. *Thorax* 2008; **63**(Suppl V):v1–53.

49. Le Jeune I, Gribbin J, West J , Smith C, Cullinan P, Hubbard R. The incidence of cancer in patients with idiopathic pulmonary fibrosis. *Respiratory Medicine* 2007; **101**:2534–2540.

Neuromuscular and skeletal diseases, and obstructive sleep apnoea

John Shneerson

Neuromuscular and skeletal disorders affecting respiratory function may cause a variety of symptoms, of which breathlessness is the most prominent. Respiratory insufficiency usually occurs during sleep before it is apparent in wakefulness and can lead to episodes of breathlessness during sleep, early morning headaches due to carbon dioxide retention, and excessive daytime sleepiness due to fragmentation of sleep. This chapter focuses on the symptom of breathlessness, emphasizes the importance of the analysis of the factors contributing to this symptom, and describes the modern methods of supportive care.

Most of the symptoms of obstructive sleep apnoea (OSA) respond to treatment of the closure of the airway during sleep, particularly continuous positive airway pressure (CPAP) treatment. Occasionally, however, there are residual symptoms despite control of the apnoeas themselves and the treatment of these will be addressed in this chapter.

Neuromuscular and skeletal diseases

Clinical features

The quality of life of patients with neuromuscular and skeletal disorders does not correlate closely with the severity of the objective physical impairment or the need for non-invasive ventilation (1). Symptoms such as breathlessness and weakness are probably more important (2), as well as the psychological reaction to the illness (3), and the presence or absence of depression (4) or a partner (5).

Mild shortness of breath on exertion is common in many chronic neuromuscular and skeletal disorders. Patients usually adapt their activities to cope with this and rarely complain specifically about breathlessness unless it changes. This may be the result of an intercurrent illness, such as a chest infection, or the development of related disorders, such as left ventricular failure. This may be due to a cardiomyopathy associated with the skeletal muscle disorder as in Friedreich's ataxia and dystrophia myotonica. Cardiac dysrhythmias may also cause temporary breathlessness and are a feature of dystrophia myotonica and Duchenne muscular dystrophy.

Worsening of breathlessness over weeks or months in an otherwise stable disorder such as a thoracic scoliosis or following a thoracoplasty should raise the suspicion that respiratory failure is developing. This may arise after many years of clinical stability and is often associated with other symptoms such as ankle swelling. Breathlessness is more severe if hypercapnia leads to a rapid respiratory rate with relative little increase in tidal volume (6).

Breathlessness may also appear at night rather than during the day. The sensation of waking with shortness of breath is usually related to arousal at the end of a central sleep apnoea (i.e. a temporary cessation of central drive to breathing), or hypopnoea, or linked to Cheyne–Stokes respiration. Repeated arousals from sleep cause sleep fragmentation which leads to the sensation of waking unrefreshed in the mornings and increasing daytime sleepiness. Occasionally neuromuscular disorders cause weakness of the upper airway dilator muscles and predispose to obstructive sleep apnoeas. These cause snoring or snoring-like noises. Arousal at the end of the apnoea may simply lead to the awareness of waking suddenly, to awareness of a snoring noise, or to an inability to breathe if the airway remains closed at the moment of arousal. This combination of nocturnal breathlessness and choking should be distinguished clinically from gastro-oesophageal reflux, asthma, and left ventricular failure. Vocal cord adduction during sleep is a feature of motor neuron disease and multisystem atrophy, and presents with stridorous noises associated with breathlessness which may occur either at night or during the day.

The pattern of respiratory muscle weakness also influences the clinical presentation. Diaphragm paralysis out of proportion to weakness of the other respiratory muscles causes breathlessness on exertion and when swimming or wading in water up to the level of the lower ribcage. It also causes *orthopnoea*, and when weakness is severe, it is apparent within the first few breaths on assuming the supine position, but if it is milder breathlessness may take a few minutes to develop. Patients with this condition rarely sleep lying flat, but may adopt either an unusual sleeping position or prefer to sleep sitting up in a chair. Sleep fragmentation is common and thus daytime sleepiness is a feature. Conversely, weakness of the abdominal muscles with preservation of diaphragmatic function causes *platypnoea*, in which breathlessness is worse when sitting up. This arises, for instance, in low cervical spinal cord injuries (where diaphragm function is preserved).

Physical examination will confirm the nature of any skeletal abnormality and reveal specific features of neuromuscular disorders (Figure 13.1). The pattern of respiratory muscle weakness should be identified. For example, weakness and atrophy of the sterno-mastoid muscles is an early sign of dystrophia myotonica, whereas in Duchenne muscular dystrophy respiratory muscle weakness is global. Respiration should be observed in both the sitting and the supine position. The presence of diaphragm weakness is confirmed by observing paradoxical inward inspiratory abdominal movement in the supine position. Unilateral diaphragm weakness is hard to diagnose with certainty, but similar findings may be found unilaterally.

Hypoxia may be revealed by the finding of central cyanosis. This clinical sign is only reliable when the oxygen saturation falls below around 80%, which is equivalent to a PO_2 of less than around 6.7kPa. Hypercapnia causes a variety of cardiovascular and central nervous system physical signs (Box 13.1)

It should be remembered that breathlessness in these patients may also be due to unrelated additional causes such as asthma, or to cardiac diseases.

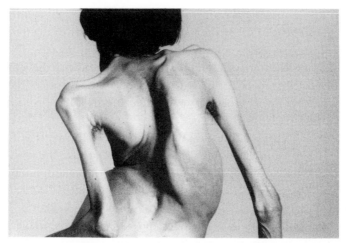

Fig. 13.1 Severe thoracic scoliosis associated with intercostal muscle atrophy due to previous poliomyelitis.

Box 13.1 Physical signs that may be detected in hypercapnia

Tachycardia	Papilloedema
Large volume pulse	Flapping tremor (asterixis)
Peripheral venous dilatation	Loss of tendon reflexes
Confusion*	Coma (carbon dioxide narcosis)*

* In severe hypercapnia

Pathophysiology

Breathlessness in neuromuscular and skeletal disorders may have a variety of causes as described in the following sections.

Weakness of chest wall muscles

Each of the chronic neurological disorders has its own characteristic pattern of muscle weakness. It is also important to be aware of whether the disorder is stable, slowly progressive, or rapidly progressive. In some conditions the sequence of respiratory muscle involvement is unpredictable. This is particularly the case with motor neuron disease, and careful analysis of the pattern of weakness at each stage of the illness is essential in planning treatment.

The relationship of breathlessness to the severity of the chest wall muscle weakness is variable because of individual differences in awareness of the symptom of breathlessness and of reporting it (7). Breathlessness is, in general, related to the percentage of the maximal force that can be generated by the chest wall muscles which is actually developed in these patients. The implication of this is that if the muscles are weak, the maximal force is reduced and a level of work of breathing that would not in normal circumstances cause breathlessness, will now do so. As the muscles become weaker or the thorax becomes more deformed, the threshold for becoming breathless gradually falls. The moment at which breathlessness is experienced and reported also depends on the level of physical activity. Breathlessness is much less likely to be a problem if the patient is confined to a wheelchair or bed because of other aspects of the neuromuscular disorder, than if the limb muscles are relatively spared.

The most important chest wall muscle is the diaphragm (8). Unilateral weakness reduces the tidal volume and the mechanical efficiency of breathing since the affected hemidiaphragm moves upwards (paradoxically) into the thorax during inspiration, instead of descending. This is worse in the supine position when the weight of the abdominal contents pushes the paralysed hemidiaphragm even further into the thorax. In effect, the diaphragm is fixed ('splinted') in an expiratory position. When the whole diaphragm is paralysed bilaterally, it moves paradoxically during both inspiration and expiration and the intrapleural pressure changes are transmitted across it so that the abdominal pressure falls during inspiration and the anterior abdominal wall moves inwards.

Symptoms usually appear when the maximum transdiaphragmatic pressure falls to around $25 cmH_2O$ (2.45kPa) compared to a normal value of $70 cmH_2O$ (6.86kPa). When the diaphragm is completely paralysed, the vital capacity falls by 50% in moving from the sitting to the supine position. Ventilation is reduced, particularly at the bases of the lungs when supine, with shunting of blood past the alveoli, so that the arterial PO_2 falls.

Breathlessness in skeletal disorders without any involvement of the muscles also has a variety of causes. In scoliosis, for instance, the compliance of the ribcage is reduced, as is also the compliance of the lungs, primarily because of their small volume. The ribcage distortion puts the inspiratory muscles at a mechanical disadvantage on the convexity of the scoliosis. They become shortened and on the concavity they are lengthened. Diaphragmatic function is impaired, as shown by low transdiaphragmatic pressures and a fall in the vital capacity when changing from the sitting to the supine position. Exercise ability and breathlessness on exertion are linked to the reduction of vital capacity. The tidal volume increases initially, then remains constant and the respiratory frequency rises as exercise becomes more intense. The rise in pulmonary artery pressure on exertion, which is related to the severity of the restrictive defect, may also limit the cardiac output and contribute to breathlessness.

Upper airway muscles

Weakness of the upper airway muscles may cause obstructive sleep apnoeas and stridor as described above. Bulbar impairment may also cause dysarthria, dysphagia, and impaired coughing and swallowing, and can lead to aspiration of material into the tracheobronchial tree. This may cause sudden severe major airway obstruction, an intermittent cough which is worse during meals, or recurrent episodes of pneumonia. Weakness of the chest wall muscles, particularly the expiratory muscles, may significantly impair the ability to clear tracheobronchial secretions, and can thus lead to pneumonia.

Sleep

Normal sleep is associated with loss of the voluntary respiratory drive and a reduction in the reflex drive in response to hypoxia, hypercapnia, and other stimuli (9). Muscle activity is reduced and whereas in non-rapid eye movement sleep (NREM) this affects all the respiratory muscles to an equal extent, in rapid eye movement sleep (REM) diaphragmatic activity is selectively retained. Relaxation of the other respiratory muscles is more intense than during NREM sleep and loss of activity in the upper airway dilator muscles increases the upper airway resistance and the work of the chest wall muscles. These changes during sleep are particularly important in scoliosis where the diaphragm is attached to an asymmetrical ribcage and where the respiratory pump often has little reserve (10). The effects of sleep are accentuated in neuromuscular disorders causing scoliosis because of the presence of muscle weakness in addition to the skeletal deformities. A reduction in tidal volume and increase in respiratory frequency may result in alveolar hypoventilation and an increase in the deadspace ventilation. Arousals from sleep occur initially in REM, which becomes fragmented, and at a later stage in NREM sleep, particularly with loss of stages 3 and 4. Sleep fragmentation itself further reduces the respiratory drive and impairs the strength and probably the endurance of the respiratory muscles, promoting a vicious circle in which there are progressively more respiratory-induced arousals and a deterioration in respiratory drive and muscle function. Central apnoeas and hypopnoeas are seen and hypercapnia then develops during the day as well as at night.

Abnormalities of respiratory drive

The respiratory centre in the medulla functions normally in most neuromuscular and skeletal disorders, with the exception of central alveolar hypoventilation in which it is reduced or absent. Breathlessness is correspondingly diminished and these subjects may, for instance, be able to swim for prolonged episodes under water, and take physical exercise without being aware of any breathlessness, despite becoming intensely centrally cyanosed. Reversible impairment of the respiratory centres may arise because of chronic hypercapnia, sleep deprivation, or a metabolic alkalosis and these situations may be associated with less breathlessness, despite the severity of the underlying respiratory failure and muscle weakness.

Treatment

Most of the chronic neuromuscular and skeletal disorders are not amenable to curative treatment, but there is a wide range of supportive measures which can reduce breathlessness and other symptoms and improve the quality of life. Most of these have been inadequately evaluated. It is important to assess each individual's needs carefully before planning any type of rehabilitation or palliative treatment (11).

Energy conservation and physiotherapy

The physiotherapist should recognize inefficient patterns of movement and teach the patient how to correct them. Coordination of limb and other muscles can be improved by exercise training so that, for instance, walking can be performed with a lower oxygen consumption and less breathlessness. Coordination of the respiratory movements with those of the arms and legs may be helpful. The muscles of the upper arm may be used both as accessory muscles of respiration and in arm functioning, and coordination of these two activities can easily be disrupted. Synchronization of respiratory and leg movements during walking is often helpful.

It is important that the speed of movement, particularly walking, is adjusted to the patient's respiratory capacity. It is common for patients to walk too fast, and the increased oxygen consumption exacerbates their breathlessness. Breathlessness may be less severe while, for instance, standing leaning forward, or resting the arms on a surface so that the accessory muscles of respiration can be used. Energy can be conserved by the use of physical aids such as a walking stick or handrail. Modification of everyday activities to conserve energy such as sitting on a stool while washing up and arranging for frequently used objects to be at a convenient height, help to reduce breathlessness.

The physiotherapist should also try to improve the patient's confidence and aid relaxation, which reduces oxygen uptake by the skeletal muscles. Advice about taking periods of rest between exercise, and stopping exercise before becoming breathless, may help.

Breathing techniques

A range of breathing exercises has been developed to try to reduce breathlessness and to improve the respiratory pattern both at rest and during physical exertion. *Pursed-lip breathing*, which is useful in emphysema, has been little studied in neuromuscular and skeletal disorders, but in myotonic dystrophy it can reduce breathlessness and increase both the tidal volume and oxygen saturation (12).

Diaphragmatic breathing is an inaccurate term since the diaphragm cannot be selectively activated, but this type of breathing technique does encourage abdominal expansion during inspiration. Nevertheless in one study in motor neuron disease diaphragmatic breathing training did not have any benefit (13).

Deep breathing manoeuvres, including sighing, open distal airways and prevent sub-segmental lung collapse. They thereby increase lung compliance, and reduce the work of breathing and the degree of breathlessness. This technique, and diaphragmatic breathing, also reduces the respiratory rate, which can help to reduce breathlessness. The increase in the range of movement of what would otherwise be a hypomobile respiratory system may be particularly important in children since the growth of the rib cage depends on the mechanical forces generated during respiration. In myotonic dystrophy, deep breathing exercises have been linked to an increase in oxygen saturation and thoraco-abdominal movement when they were combined with proprioceptive neuromuscular facilitation (PNF) (14).

Frog breathing is a technique which utilizes the upper airway muscles (15). Air is pushed through the open larynx into the trachea under pressure generated by the oral muscles. This requires coordination of the upper airway muscles so that the soft palate seals off the nasopharynx while the glottis remains open at the time that air is gulped from the mouth downwards into the pharynx. The glottis then closes to trap air in the lungs until the next frog breath, which further inflates the lungs. Frog breaths of around 50–80mL are common, and 10–20 gulps can be taken before expiration occurs. This type of breathing is completely independent of chest wall and abdominal muscles and is of particular value in those with tetraplegia, poliomyelitis, Duchenne muscular dystrophy, and similar disorders (16). It can be used whenever the patient has retained bulbar muscle function and is able to increase the vital capacity significantly (17, 18). It can increase the time off ventilatory support whether this is provided non-invasively or through a tracheostomy.

Exercise training

This has been widely used in chronic obstructive pulmonary disease (COPD) (see Chapter 10, this volume), but there is little evidence about its effectiveness in neuromuscular and skeletal disorders. Programmes involving leg exercises, combined with educational programmes, have been used and may be of benefit, but in muscular dystrophies and myopathies the diseased muscles have a limited capacity to be improved by training. (19). One recent study, however, showed that in a group with primarily neuromuscular and skeletal disorders their exercise capacity and quality of life improved with 12 and 24 weeks of a multidisciplinary rehabilitation programme including cardiovascular exercise training (20).

Specific respiratory muscle training programmes have been attempted. These have been most effective in cervical spinal cord lesions where it is the spared normal muscles that are capable of being trained (21, 22). They may increase the vital capacity and the effectiveness of coughing. However, in muscular dystrophies such as Duchenne muscular dystrophy the results have been disappointing and improvements have been noticed only in mildly affected subjects who have least to gain from the training programme (23–25). In general, respiratory muscle training is ineffective in Duchenne muscular dystrophy if the vital capacity is less than 25–30% of the predicted value or if there is hypercapnia (26–28). The addition of an inspiratory resistance is also potentially dangerous in these patients with limited respiratory muscle reserve (29). There is, however, one report in myasthenia gravis in which inspiratory muscle training improved respiratory muscle strength and endurance, and unlike the other studies of inspiratory muscle training this report included a control group (30).

A separate type of training in neuromuscular disorders is aimed at improving upper airway function during and after intubation for episodes of respiratory failure. Coordination between the respiratory and swallowing related function of the larynx may be lost, with an increased risk of aspiration and of breathlessness during weaning (31). Deflation of the cuff on the tracheostomy or endotracheal tube so that air passes through the upper airway and enables speech to resume helps to coordinate the muscles and improve the likelihood of successful weaning.

Cough assistance

Weakness of the cough mechanism may lead to aspiration of material from the pharynx into the tracheobronchial tree or failure to expectorate tracheobronchial secretions. These problems may lead to worsening breathlessness because the material retained within the airways partially obstructs them and increases the work of breathing.

A normal cough requires a deep inspiration, closure of the glottis, and then a rapid forceful expiration as the glottis opens (see Chapter 15, this volume). In Duchenne muscular dystrophy, the inspiratory muscle weakness is a major factor. In motor neuron disease glottic function is often impaired and spinal cord lesions reduce expiratory muscle strength (32). In normal subjects a peak cough expiratory flow rate (PCEF) of 5–12L per second can be generated by an inspiration of around 1–1.5L. A PCEF of this rate is required to mobilize airway secretions (33), but this is often unable to be achieved in neuromuscular disorders. If the vital capacity is less than 1.5L the peak cough expiratory flow rate may need to be increased by techniques for assisting inspiration so that the maximum insufflation capacity (MIC) becomes greater than 1.5L.

The PCEF can be increased in several ways (34). Firstly, conventional ventilators or intermittent positive pressure breathing (IPPB) apparatus can be used to breath stack (35). An alternative is to use a conventional ventilator to breath stack. The depth of inspiration can also be increased by frog breathing and by specially designed cough assistance machines, which provide an approximately square wave of positive pressure which inflates the lungs. They can then be switched, either automatically or manually, to generate a sudden negative pressure. This assists exhalation of air with sputum and other material which is in the airways. Cough assist machines have been shown to be effective in children with stable neuromuscular disorders (36), motor neuron disease (37, 38), spinal cord injuries (39), and postoperatively (40).

Assistance to expiration can also be provided either manually through thoracic or abdominal compression, or by functional electrical stimulation of the abdominal muscles (41). This technique increases intra-abdominal pressure by producing a coordinated activation of the abdominal muscles by multiple cutaneous electrodes.

A combination of inspiratory and expiratory cough assistance may be more effective than either alone (42–44), but cough assistance techniques are ineffective if there is upper airway obstruction or bulbar muscle weakness.

Psychotherapy

Anxiety and depression are common in those with neuromuscular and skeletal disorders, especially in people who live alone or who have developed poor coping strategies (45). Antidepressants may be of value, but encouragement to develop new behaviours may help, including a positive approach to problems and the ability to feel in control of situations rather than attributing events to external forces or feeling a victim of these. Self-confidence can be increased; education, motivation, and encouragement to retain or develop social contacts, can all improve the quality of life and reduce awareness of breathlessness (46). Reassurance and encouragement from healthcare professionals is important, and support from family, carers, and friends is often a vital factor.

Nutrition

Adequate nutrition is important in optimizing respiratory and peripheral muscle strength. Several factors combine to increase risk of malnutrition in those with neuromuscular and skeletal disorders. Firstly, mobility may be too limited to obtain food without help.

Secondly, cooking and preparing food may be difficult and additionally there may be problems in using food utensils. The neuromuscular condition may also cause weakness of the masticatory muscles, and those involved in swallowing. Eating also leads to a temporary cessation of inspiration which may cause breathlessness. Aspiration of food or drink into the tracheobronchial tree or the fear of this may also limit nutritional intake. As a result there is often muscle wasting in addition to that due to disuse atrophy and the underlying neuromuscular disorder.

The details of the nutritional content that is required for patients with respiratory problems is outside the scope of this chapter, but in general there should be not only sufficient calorie intake but also adequate protein to maintain muscle mass or to reverse any wasting.

The value of supplements such as creatine which increases the energy available within muscle cells, is uncertain. Anabolic steroids, which enhance muscle mass, may also be useful in severely underweight subjects in whom nutritional supplementation is ineffective.

Oxygen

Oxygen is frequently prescribed for breathlessness in neuromuscular and skeletal disorders. In general it is contraindicated for use at rest because of the risk that it will worsen hypercapnia by abolishing any residual hypoxic drive. Oxygen should only be prescribed after careful estimation of blood gases during the day and also sleep studies, including transcutaneous PCO_2 recordings at night.

Oxygen may, however, be of value in relieving breathlessness on exertion, during which oxygen desaturation is common. Exertion itself increases the respiratory drive and reduces the risk of hypercapnia during oxygen treatment.

Walking tests, with or without oxygen, should be used to determine the optimal flow rate, and a small lightweight portable oxygen cylinder may be of help. Liquid oxygen is preferable, but may have limited availability. Oxygen can also be used briefly after exertion in order to speed recovery and reduce the time for which breathlessness is present.

Ventilatory support

Ventilatory support provides a back-up for patients with neuromuscular and skeletal disorders who have developed respiratory failure, and it may also improve respiratory function. It resets the respiratory drive, partly through relieving sleep deprivation and partly through reducing the cerebrospinal fluid bicarbonate concentration and thereby increasing the ventilatory response to hypercapnia. It probably improves respiratory muscle function and so increases the vital capacity and raises the threshold at which breathlessness is likely to develop. Respiratory muscle rest may also diminish respiratory muscle fatigue, but there is doubt about the clinical significance of this.

Non-invasive ventilation is usually required. This may be delivered by a nasal mask (Figure 13.2), or a full face mask. Pressure preset ventilators are usually preferred to volume preset equipment. Bi-level pressure support in which the expiratory pressure prevents distal airway collapse is usually used. The details of the ventilator settings probably

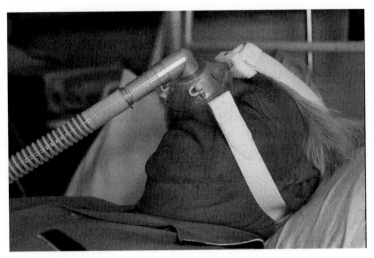

Fig. 13.2 Nasal ventilation.

have an important impact on the extent to which the respiratory muscles are unloaded, sleep architecture and the adequacy of alveolar ventilation (47).

An alternative, which is now much less frequently used, is a negative pressure system, such as a cuirass or jacket (Figure 13.3). With these systems the ribcage and abdomen are covered by an airtight and rigid enclosure from which air is evacuated by a negative pressure ventilator. This expands the ribcage and abdomen and air is drawn in through the mouth and nose. No appliance is required around the airway.

Both these non-invasive techniques can adequately ventilate most patients with respiratory failure due to neuromuscular and skeletal disorders. They are usually only required at night while the patient is asleep, but occasionally an extra 1–2h during the day is of benefit. In Duchenne muscular dystrophy this unloads respiratory muscles and relieves breathlessness more effectively than night time treatment alone (48).

Non-invasive ventilation can also be used while exercising. Inspiratory pressures of around 20cmH$_2$0 are required to increase exercise performance in scoliosis (49, 50) and following tuberculosis (51).

As respiratory muscle weakness worsens, the duration of the ventilation gradually increases. This is seen particularly with Duchenne muscular dystrophy and motor neuron disease, where in the later stages the ventilator may be used almost continuously to minimize breathlessness (52). Tracheostomy ventilation may be preferred to a non-invasive system if respiratory support is required for more than around 16 h/day, or if there is a weak cough or the airway needs to be protected (53).

The non-invasive systems can considerably improve the quality of life and reduce breathlessness at rest (54) in scoliosis (55, 56), motor neuron disease (57, 58) and Duchenne muscular dystrophy (59). As many of these patients find it difficult to communicate it is important to be aware that the quality of life with respiratory failure treated by non-invasive ventilation to relieve symptoms such as breathlessness is usually

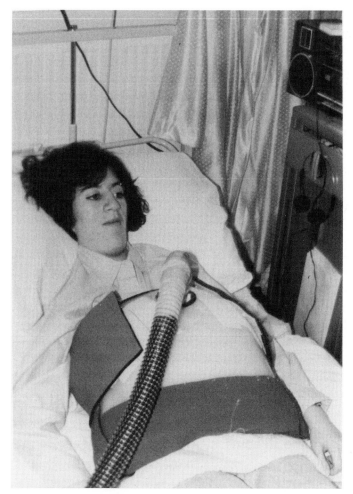

Fig. 13.3 Cuirass shell with connecting tubing which leads to the negative pressure ventilator. Reproduced with permission from Shneerson JM. *Handbook of Sleep Medicine*. Oxford: Blackwell Science, 2000.

underestimated by the carer, relative to the patient's own assessment (60, 61). Relief of breathlessness at night enables a better quality of sleep to be obtained with less subsequent tiredness during the day (58). There is also some evidence that sleep quality in patients who have had poliomyelitis is better with tracheostomy ventilation than with non invasive ventilation (62)

Sedative drugs

Opioids and other centrally sedating drugs may be of value in the preterminal phase and when patients are approaching death, to relieve intense breathlessness, but should not be initiated at an earlier stage in the natural history. Diazepam has been recommended to relieve breathlessness due to vocal cord adduction in motor neuron disease and may work either by relaxing the adductor muscles of the larynx or by reducing anxiety about the airway obstruction (see Chapter 7, this volume, for discussion of sedatives).

Obstructive sleep apnoea

Most of the symptoms of OPA resolve once effective treatment of the upper airway obstruction during sleep is established, whether this is by weight loss, surgical approach, such as tonsillectomy, a mandibular advancement device or a nasal CPAP system. This implies that most of the symptoms of OSA are due directly to the apnoeas themselves and the arousals and other physiological responses that they cause. Control of sleep apnoeas partially reverses the metabolic associations of OSA, and the residual abnormalities reflect the underlying cause of the OSA, such as obesity, rather than the effects of the apnoeas themselves (63).

There are however two groups of problems which may persist despite adequate treatment of OSA. Firstly, OSA may cause a stroke (64), or myocardial infarction which may leave a permanent or transient disability which requires conventional management. Secondly, there are some features which represent either permanent functional neurological or endocrine damage, or an aspect of OSA which is not amenable to treatment of the apnoeas themselves. Before initiating any treatment for these residual symptoms it is important to be sure that the OSA is adequately controlled. Apparent failure of CPAP treatment, for instance, may be due to any of the causes listed in Box 13.2. Each of these should be addressed before supportive treatment of residual symptoms is attempted.

The most important residual symptoms of OSA that may require supportive treatment are as follows.

Excessive daytime sleepiness and cognitive defects

The exact frequency of residual excessive daytime sleepiness from OSA after effective treatment with CPAP is uncertain, but is probably around 5–10% (65, 66). Excessive daytime sleepiness may be due to a pre-existing neurological abnormality, brain damage due to the apnoeas, probably as a result of the repeated oxygen desaturations and resaturations or to arousals or awakenings due to the CPAP system itself.

Modafinil, a non amphetamine wakefulness promoting drug, is often effective in relieving sleepiness in a dose of 200–400mg daily (67). The addition of modafinil has been

---

Box 13.2 Possible causes of failure to respond to CPAP treatment

Undiagnosed central sleep apnoeas
Undiagnosed non-respiratory sleep disorder
Inadequate CPAP level
Poor compliance
Sleep deprivation

shown not to reduce the compliance with CPAP. Although it improves daytime alertness, it does not prevent the other physiological changes of OSA and in particular would not be anticipated to reduce the risk of a subsequent myocardial infarction or stroke.

The cognitive defects associated with OSA, such as memory loss, may improve with modafinil if the deficit is primarily due to lack of alertness, but it is uncertain whether or not modafinil or any other treatment has any specific effect on the cause of the cognitive defects.

Mood disorders

Anxiety and depression are common associations with obstructive sleep apnoeas (68, 69), particularly in females (70). Magnetic resonance imaging scans have shown different abnormalities in those with anxiety (71) and depression (72) to subjects with OSA without these psychological problems.

CPAP has been shown to improve depression (73, 74), but may not relieve it completely. This may be because of abnormalities of neurotransmitters induced by the apnoeas themselves (68), and antidepressants may be required in addition to CPAP. Most antidepressants also reduce the duration of REM sleep which may be advantageous if the OSA is particularly frequent in this sleep state.

Erectile dysfunction

This is often associated with obstructive sleep apnoeas (75–77) and is partly due to reduction in testosterone secretion during REM sleep as a result of a fall in LH secretion (78). It would therefore be expected to be particularly a problem if the apnoeas occur predominantly in REM sleep.

CPAP is often effective (79, 80), but despite the theoretical problems with phosphodiesterase inhibitors, such as sildenafil which may alter pharyngeal muscle tone and cause an increase in nasal resistance (81). The combination of sildenafil and CPAP appears to be more effective than CPAP alone (82).

Key points

- Breathlessness in neuromuscular and skeletal disorders may be due to global respiratory muscle weakness or selective weakness (e.g. the diaphragm) and it is important to carefully assess the pattern of respiratory muscle weakness in order to plan appropriate treatment.

- Respiratory muscle weakness causes respiratory failure during sleep before this is apparent in wakefulness.

- Physiotherapy techniques such as relaxation, improvement of coordination, and education in specific types of respiratory breathing patterns may be of value.

- Cough assistance and prevention of tracheobronchial aspiration is often important, particularly in the presence of bulbar muscle weakness.

- Oxygen may induce carbon dioxide retention and non-invasive ventilatory techniques are usually preferable in respiratory failure.

- ◆ Central sedatives should be reserved for the advanced stages of disease.
- ◆ Residual symptoms after treatment of OSA respond to the addition of conventional pharmacological treatments.

References

1. Kohler M, Clarenbach CF, Boni L, Brack T, Russi EW, Bloch KE. Quality of life, physical disability, and respiratory impairment in Duchenne muscular dystrophy. *Am J Resp Crit Care Med* 2005; **172**:1032–6.

2. Cejudo P, Lopez-Marquez I, Lopez-Campos JL, *et al.* Factors associated with quality of life in patients with chronic respiratory failure due to kyphoscoliosis. *Disabilty Rehabil* 2009; **31**:928–34.

3. Miglioretti M, Mazzini L, Oggioni GD, Testa L, Monaco F. Illness perceptions, mood and health-related quality of life in patients with amyotrophic lateral sclerosis. *J Psychosmatic Res* 2008; **65**: 603–9.

4. Stromberg SF, Weiss DB. Depression and quality of life issues in patients with amyotrophic lateral sclerosis. *Current Treatment Options Neurol* 2006; **8**:410–14.

5. Bostrom K, Ahlstrom G. Quality of life in patients with muscular dystrophy and their next of kin. *Int J Rehabil Res* 2005; **28**:103–9.

6. Lanini B, Misuri G, Gigliotti F, Iandelli I, Pizzi A, Romagnoli I, Scano G. Perception of dyspnea in patients with neuromuscular disease. *Chest* 2001; **120**:402–8.

7. Laroche CM, Moxham J, Green M. Respiratory muscle weakness and fatigue. *Q J Med, NS* 1989; **71**(265):373–97.

8. Gibson GJ. Diaphragmatic paresis: pathophysiology, clinical features, and investigations. *Thorax* 1989; **44**:960–70.

9. McNicholas WT. Impact of sleep in respiratory failure. *Eur Respir J* 1997; **10**:920–33.

10. Midgren B, Petersson K, Hansson L, *et al.* Nocturnal hypoxaemia in severe scoliosis. *Br J Dis Chest* 1988; **82**:226–36.

11. Shneerson, J.M. Rehabilitation in neuromuscular disorders and thoracic wall deformities. *Monaldi Arch Chest Dis* 1998; **53**:415–18.

12. Ugalde V, Breslin EH, Walsh SA, Bonekat HW, Abresch RT, Carter GT. Pursed lips breathing improves ventilation in myotonic muscular dystrophy. *Arch Phys Med Rehabil* 2000; **81**:472–8.

13. Nardin R, O'Donnell C, Loring SH, *et al.* Diaphragm training in amyotrophic lateral sclerosis. *J Clin Neuromusc Dis* 2008; **10**:56–60.

14. Nitz J, Burke B. A study of the facilitation of respiration in myotonic dystrophy. *Physio Res Int* 2002; **7**:228–38.

15. Dail, C.W. Glossopharyngeal breathing by paralyzed patients. A preliminary report. *Calif Med* 1951; **75**:217–18.

16. Montero JC, Feldman DJ, Montero D. Effects of glossopharyngeal breathing on respiratory function after cervical cord transection. *Arch Phys Med Rehabil* 1967; **48**: 650–3.

17. Moloney E, Doyle S, Kinahan J, Burke CM. A case of frog breathing. *Irish Med J* 2002; **95**:81–2.

18. Bach JR, Bianchi C, Vidigal-Lopes M, Turi S, Felisari G. Lung inflation by glossopharyngeal breathing and 'air stacking' in Duchenne muscular dystrophy. *Am J Phys Med Rehabil* 2007; **86**:295–300.

19. Cup EH, Pieterse AJ, Ten Broek-Pastoor JM, *et al.* Exercise therapy and other types of physical therapy for patients with neuromuscular diseases: a systematic review. *Arch Phys Med Rehabil* 2007; **88**:1452–64.

20. Salhi B, Troosters T, Behaegel M, Joos G, Derom E. Effects of pulmonary rehabilitation in patients with restrictive lung diseases. *Chest* 2010; **137**:273–79.

21. Gross D, Ladd HW, Riley EJ, Macklem PT, Grassino, A. The effect of training on strength and endurance of the diaphragm in quadriplegia. *Am J Med* 1980; **68**:27–35.

22. Biering-Sorensen F, Knudsell JL, Schmidt A, Bundgaard A, Christensen I. Effect of respiratory training with a mouth-nose mask in tetraplegics. *Paraplegia* 1991; **9**:113–19.

23. Yeldan I, Gurses HN, Yuksel H. Comparison study of chest physiotherapy home training programmes on respiratory functions in patients with muscular dystrophy. *Clin Rehabil* 2008; **22**:741–8.

24. DiMarco AF, Kelling JS, DiMarco MS, *et al.* The effects of inspiratory resistive training on respiratory muscle function in patients with muscular dystrophy. *Muscle Nerve* 1985; **8**:284–90.

25. Martin AJ, Stern L, Yeates J, *et al.* Respiratory muscle training in Duchenne dystrophy. *Dev Med Child Neruol* 1986; **28**:314–8.

26. Smith PEM, Coakley JM, Edwards RHT. Respiratory muscle training in Duchenne muscular dystrophy. *Muscle Nerve* 1988; **11**:784–5.

27. Rodillo E, Noble-Jamieson CM, Aber V, *et al.* Respiratory muscle training in Duchenne muscular dystrophy. *Arch Dis Child* 1989; **64**:736–8.

28. Stern LM, Martin AJ, Jones N, *et al.* Training inspiratory resistance in Duchenne dystrophy using adapted computer games. *Dev Med Child Neurol* 1989; **31**:494–500.

29. Schiffman PL, Belsh JM. Effect of inspiratory resistance and theophylline on respiratory muscle strength in patients with amyotrophic lateral sclerosis. *Am Rev Respir Dis* 1989; **139**:1418–23.

30. Fregonezi GA, Resqueti Vr, Guell R, Pradas J, Casan P. Effects of 8-week, interval-based inspiratory muscle training and breathing retraining in patients with generalized myasthenia gravis. *Chest* 2005; **128**:1524–30.

31. Shneerson, J.M. Are there new solutions to old problems with weaning? *Br J Anaesth* 1997; **78**:238–40.

32. Siebens AA, Kirby NA, Poulos DA. Cough following transection of spinal cord at C-6. *Arch Phys Med Rehabil* 1964; **45**:1–7.

33. Barach AL, Beck GJ, Smith RH. Mechanical production of expiratory flow rates surpassing the capacity of human coughing. *Am J Med Sci* 1953; **226**:241–8.

34. Chatwin M, Ross E, Hart N, Nickol AH, Polkey MI, Simonds AK. Cough augmentation with mechanical insufflations/exsufflation in patients with neuromuscular weakness. *Eur Res J* 2003; **21**:502–8

35. Dohna-Schwake C, Ragette R, Teschler H, Voit T, Mellies U. IPPB-assisted coughing in neuromuscular disorders. *Ped Pulmonology* 2006; **41**:551–7.

36. Haas CF, Loik PS, Gay SE. Airway clearance applications in the elderly and in patients with neurologic or neuromuscular compromise. *Resp Care* 2007; **52**:1362–81.

37. Sancho J, Servera E, Vergara P, Marin J. Mechanical insufflation-exsufflation vs. tracheal suctioning via tracheostomy tubes for patients with amyotrophic lateral sclerosis: a pilot study. *Am J Phys Med Rehabil* 2003; **82**:750–3.

38. Mustfa N, Aiello M, Lyall RA, *et al.* Cough augmentation in amyotrophic lateral sclerosis. *Neurology* 2003; **61**:1285–7.

39. Liszner K, Feinberg M. Cough assist strategy for pulmonary toileting in ventilator-dependent spinal cord injured patients. *Rehabil Nurs* 2006; **31**:218–21.

40. Marchant WA, Fox R. Postoperative use of cough-assist device in avoiding prolonged intubation. *Br J Anaesth* 2002; **89**:644–7.

41. Linder SH. Functional electrical stimulation to enhance cough in quadriplegia. *Chest* 1993; **103**:166–9.

42. Trebbia G, Lacombe M, Fermanian C, Falaize L, Lejaille M, Louis A, Devaux C, Raphael JC, Lofaso F. Cough determinants in patients with neuromuscular disease. *Resp Phys Neurobiol* 2005; **146**: 291–300.

43. Toussaint M, Boitano LJ, Gathot V, Steens M, Soudon P. Limits of effective cough-augmentation techniques in patients with neuromuscular disease. *Resp Care* 2009; **54**:359–66.

44. Ishikawa Y, Bach JR, Komaroff E, Miura T, Jackson-Parekh R. Cough augmentation in Duchenne muscular dystrophy. *Am J Phys Med Rehabil* 2008; **87**:726–30.

45. Tate D, Kirsch N, Maynald F, *et al.* Coping with the late effects: differences between depressed and nondepressed polio survivors. *Am J Phys Med Rehabil* 1994; **73**:27–35.

46. Shneerson J. Quality of life in neuromuscular and skeletal disorders. *Eur Respir Rev* 1997; **7**:71–3.

47. Fanfulla F, Delmastro M, Berardinelli A, Lupo ND, Nava S. Effects of different ventilator settings on sleep and inspiratory effort in patients with neuromuscular disease. *Am J Resp Crit Care Med* 2005; **172**:619–24.

48. Toussaint M, Soudon P, Kinnear W. Effect of non-invasive ventilation on respiratory muscle loading and endurance in patients with Duchenne muscular dystrophy. *Thorax* 2008; **63**:430–4.

49. Highcock MP, Smith IE, Shneerson JM. The effect of noninvasive intermittent positive-pressure ventilation during exercise in severe scoliosis. *Chest* 2002; **121**:1555–60.

50. Menadue C, Alison JA, Piper AJ, Wong KK, Hollier C, Ellis ER. High and low level pressure support during walking in people with severe kyphoscoliosis. *Eur Respir J* 2010; **36**(2):370–8.

51. Tsuboi T, Ohi M, Chin K, Hirata H, Otsuka N, Kita H, Kuno K. Ventilatory support during exercise in patients with pulmonary tuberculosis sequelae. *Chest* 1997; **112**:1000–7.

52. Toussaint M, Chatwin M, Soudon P. Mechanical ventilation in Duchenne patients with chronic respiratory insufficiency: clinical implications of 20 years published experience. *Chronic Resp Dis* 2007; **4**:167–77.

53. Bach JR. A comparison of long-term ventilatory support alternatives from the perspective of the patient and care giver. *Chest* 1993; **104**:1702–6.

54. Brooks D, King A, Tonack M, Simson H, Gould M, Goldstein R. User perspectives on issues that influence the quality of daily life of ventilator-assisted individuals with neuromuscular disorders. *Canadian Resp J* 2004; **11**:547–54.

55. Pehrsson K, Olofson J, Larsson S, Sullivan M. Quality of life of patients treated by home mechanical ventilation due to restrictive ventilatory disorders. *Respir Med* 1994; **88**:21–6.

56. Nauffal D, Domenech R, Martinez Garcia MA, Compte L, Macian V, Perpina M. Noninvasive positive pressure home ventilation in restrictive disorders: outcome and impact on health-related quality of life. *Resp Med* 2002; **96**:777–83.

57. Piepers S, van den Berg JP, Kalmijn S, van der Pol WL, Wokke JH, Lindeman E, van den Berg LH. Effect of non-invasive ventilation on survival, quality of life, respiratory function and cognition: a review of the literature. *Amyotrophic Lateral Sclerosise* 2006; **7**:195–200.

58. Bourke SC, Bullock RE, Williams TL, Shaw PJ, Gibson GJ. Noninvasive ventilation in ALS: indications and effect on quality of life. *Neurology* 2003; **61**:171–7.

59. Narayanaswami P, Bertorini TE, Pourmand R, Horner LH. Long-term tracheostomy ventilation in neuromuscular diseases: patient acceptance and quality of life. *Neurorehabil* 2000; **14**:135–9.

60. Bach JR, Campagnolo DI, Hoeman S. Life satisfaction of individuals with Duchenne muscular dystrophy using long-term mechanical ventilatory support. *Am J Phys Med Rehabil* 1991; **70**:129–35.

61. Bach, J.R. Ventilator use by muscular dystrophy association patients. *Arch Phys Med Rehabil* 1992; **73**:179–83.

62. Klang B, Markstrom A, Sundell K, Barle H, Gillis-Haegerstrand C. Hypoventilation does not explain the impaired quality of sleep in postpolio patients ventilated noninvasively vs. invasively. *Scand J Caring Sci* 2008; **22**:236–49.

63. Levy P, Bonsignore MR, Eckel J. Sleep, sleep-disordered breathing and metabolic consequences. *Eur Respir J* 2009; **34**:243–60.

64. Dyken ME, Im KB. Obstructive sleep apnea and stroke. *Chest* 2009; **136**:1668–77.

65. Pepin JL, Viot-Blanc V, Escourrou P, *et al.* Prevalence of residual excessive sleepiness in CPAP-treated sleep apnoea patients: the French multicentre study. *Eur Respir J* 2009; **33**:1062–7.

66. Koutsourelakis I, Perraki E, Economou NT, *et al.* Predictors of residual sleepiness in adequately treated obstructive sleep apnoea patients. *Eur Respir J* 2009; **34**:687–93.

67. Abad VC, Guilleminault C. Pharmacological management of sleep apnoea. Sleep expert opinion. *Pharmacol Therapy* 2006; **7**:11–23.

68. Bilyukov RG, Georgiev OB, Petrova DS, Mondeshki TL, Milanova VK. Obstructive sleep apnea syndrome and depressive symptoms. *Folia Medica (Plovdiv)* 2009; **51**:18–24.

69. Harris M, Glozier N, Ratnavadivel R, Grunstein RR. Obstructive sleep apnea and depression. *Sleep Med Rev* 2009; **13**:437–44.

70. McCall WV, Harding D, O'Donovavn C. Correlates of depressive symptoms in patients with obstructive sleep apnea. *J Clin Sleep Med* 2006; **2**:424–6.

71. Kumar R, Macey PM, Cross RL, Woo MA, Yan-Go FL, Harper RM. Neural alterations associated with anxiety symptoms in obstructive sleep apnea syndrome. *Depression Anxiety* 2009; **26**:480–91.

72. Cross RL, Kumar R, Macey PM, *et al.* Neural alterations and depressive symptoms in obstructive sleep apnea patients. *Sleep* 2008; **31**:1103–9.

73. Schwartz DJ, Karatinos G. For individual with obstructive sleep apnea, institution of CPAP therapy is associated with an amelioration of symptoms of depression which is sustained long term. *J Clin Sleep Med* 2007; **3**:631–5.

74. Schwartz DJ, Kohler WC, Karatinos G. Symptoms of depression in individuals with obstructive sleep apnea may be amenable to treatment with continuous positive airway pressure. *Chest* 2005; **128**:1304–9.

75. Zias N, Bezwada V, Gilman S, Chroneou A. Obstructive sleep apnea and erectile dysfunction: still a neglected risk factor? *Sleep & Breathing* 2009; **13**:3–10.

76. Shin HW, Rha YC, Han DH, *et al.* Erectile dysfunction and disease-specific quality of life in patients with obstructive sleep apnea. *Int J Impotence Res* 2008; **20**:549–53.

77. Hoekema A, Stel AL, Stegenga B, *et al.* Sexual function and obstructive sleep apnea-hypopnea: a randomized clinical trail evaluating the effects of oral-appliance and continuous positive airway pressure therapy. *J Sexual Med* 2007; **4**:1153–62.

78. Andersen ML, Tufik S. The effects of testosterone on sleep and sleep-disordered breathing in men: its bidirectional interaction with erectile function. *Sleep Med Rev* 2008; **12**:365–79.

79. Karkoulias K, Perimenis P, Charokopos N, *et al.* Does CPAP therapy improve erectile dysfunction in patients with obstructive sleep apnea syndrome? *Clin Terapeutica* 2007; **158**:515–8.

80. Goncalves MA, Guilleminault C, Ramos E, Palha A, Paiva T. Erectile dysfunction, obstructive sleep apnea syndrome and nasal CPAP treatment. *Sleep Med* 2005; **6**:3s33–9.

81. Perimenis P, Giannitsas K. Safety of sildenafil in the treatment of erectile dysfunction in patients with obstructive sleep apnoea. *Expert Opinion Drug Safety* 2007; **6**:423–30.

82. Perimenis P, Konstantinopoulos A, Karkoulias K, Markou S, Perimeni P, Spyropoulos K. Sildenafil combined with continuous positive airway pressure for treatment of erectile dysfunction in men with obstructive sleep apnea. *Int Urol Nephrol* 2007; **39**:547–52.

Chapter 14

Hyperventilation syndrome

Julie Moore and Sally Singh

Introduction

In the last few decades there has been a growing interest in hyperventilation syndrome (HVS) mainly due to the improvement in assessment tools and the effectiveness of treating the condition (1, 2). The physiological understanding of the syndrome is currently under debate and HVS as a title has itself come under question (3–5). This chapter aims to unravel the problems with the definition and title of HVS, highlight the numerous and varied causes, explain how to identify the syndrome, establish what assessment tools are available, and provide a practical guide for assisting breathing re-education.

The terminology and history of hyperventilation syndrome

The first description of the condition was back in the 19th century when it was first described as a heart problem. Da Costa, the founder of the condition, used titles such as 'irritable heart' and 'soldier's heart' due to the predominance of fighting soldiers experiencing chest pains during the American Civil War (6). Other titles such as 'neurocirculatory asthenia' and 'autonomic imbalance' have also been used but were still not sufficient in providing a title which encompassed all the components of the syndrome (6, 7). In 1917, the UK described it as 'effort syndrome' and it was not long after this that the heart was excluded as the primary cause of the condition. Dr Paul Wood, a cardiologist, set up an 'Effort Syndrome Clinic' during World War II. An estimated 100,000 soldiers were diagnosed with the condition and taken out of battle. As a result of numerous studies performed by Dr Wood and his team it was found that through injecting lignocaine into the muscles of the chest wall, the chest pain was eradicated. This led to the conclusion that this was a respiratory problem rather than a cardiology problem (7).

For a period of time following the war, there was very little interest in the condition until the 1960s when patients who were complaining of breathlessness undertook spirometry testing. The introduction of these tests highlighted a group of patients that had no underlying respiratory disease to account for their symptoms and the term 'disproportionate breathlessness' was introduced. It soon became clear that some of these patients were overtly hyperventilating and the symptoms of hypocarbia appeared to provide a good explanation for the symptoms exhibited. Some patients, however, had carbon dioxide levels within the normal range even though they appeared to be hyperventilating (3). One explanation for this is that symptoms arise not so much from hypocarbia but from rapid changes in arterial carbon dioxide as a result of erratic breathing patterns (5). Furthermore, some patients when asked to hyperventilate voluntarily do not always experience symptoms of HVS (4). These conflicting theories cast a shadow of doubt over the physiological explanation and thus 'HVS' as the title of the condition.

More recently, a wide range of other terms have been used to describe the cluster of somatic symptoms, including 'dysfunctional breathing' and 'breathing pattern disorder'. These titles, however, have not yet superseded the term HVS as they still provide no further indication of the exact cause of the condition, merely just a description of the methods used to recognize it (4). It is agreed, however, that an inefficient breathing pattern is common to all ways in which the condition presents itself. This chapter will therefore focus on looking at what we currently have available to define, explain, identify, and treat the condition and leave the title for future discussions.

Definition of hyperventilation

The term hyperventilation, in itself, is straightforward to define. The most widely accepted definition is 'breathing in excess of metabolic requirements'. There are two types of hyperventilation: acute and chronic.

Acute hyperventilation

Acute hyperventilation manifests itself as a sudden increase in respiratory rate accompanied by an immediate sensation of breathlessness. Ventilation therefore exceeds metabolic requirements, resulting in hypocapnia and respiratory alkalosis. Respiratory alkalosis causes an array of terrifying symptoms such as paraesthesia, chest pain, cold fingers and toes, aching muscles and joints, exhaustion, fatigue, fainting, poor concentration, confusion, and emotional instability—the onset of which causes alarm, the patient panics and tries to take deeper breaths to relieve the symptoms, which just leads to worsening of the symptoms. The symptoms can mimic serious illnesses such as heart attacks, asthma attacks, or even a stroke. The patient may present to the Accident and Emergency department and require a multitude of tests, which all return as negative. This often leaves the doctor with no explanation to give to the patient who may then feel as if they are imagining their symptoms, which leads to further worry and anxiety. For some, this can then perpetuate the problem further, meaning the patient continues to overbreathe. As a result, chronic hyperventilation may develop.

Chronic hyperventilation

Chronic hyperventilation is much more subtle than acute hyperventilation. The symptoms may be the same but the degree of 'over' breathing exhibited is less. The anxiety about the bizarre and random symptoms prevents the poor breathing pattern from returning to its normal efficient pattern. The patient experiences a strong sensation of 'air hunger' which never quite gets satisfied. Acute episodes may only account for as little as 1% of the total number of patients diagnosed with HVS, leaving the remainder with the chronic form of hyperventilation (8). Panic tends to be more common in those with acute hyperventilation and high anxiety levels (5). Although there is a strong link between anxiety and breathlessness, anxiety is not always seen as the primary cause of HVS, indeed patients that are highly anxious do not always present with HVS and vice versa (3). Chronic hyperventilation can be asymptomatic and go unnoticed; minute volume can be doubled or even tripled before any signs of breathlessness or symptoms are felt. The best and most economic way to breathe is not always adopted and a poor breathing pattern often becomes habitual. This unhelpful habit can then provide a platform for chronic hyperventilation that for some leads to symptoms.

Prevalence

Patients of either gender can present with the condition at any age. During the war it was predominantly a male condition but more recently there appears to be a higher incidence of middle-aged females (5). Females generally have a higher rate of respiration which is exaggerated due to increases in progesterone, a respiratory stimulant that rises during the postovulation/premenstrual phase (luteal phase) of the menstrual cycle and throughout pregnancy (5). Various studies have found that between 6–10% of patients who attended a general practitioner's surgery demonstrated an abnormal breathing pattern and up to 30% of asthmatic patients have symptoms of HVS (8–10). It is thought that the figure could be as high as this amongst other chronic illnesses but no studies have shown this as yet (3).

Causes of hyperventilation

There are a wide range of physiological, psychological, and biomechanical reasons why breathing rate may be altered. There is no one singular cause of HVS; it is most likely due to a number of factors contributing to a poor breathing pattern.

Figure 14.1 highlights a few of the many factors that may alter the breathing pattern. The plethora of factors that may aggravate the breathing pattern will differ for each individual; thus contributing to the complexity of establishing an accurate diagnosis.

Anxiety, depression, and stress are amongst the most common causes of hyperventilation. Although there is some doubt as to whether they are the initiating primary cause or a secondary factor as a result of HVS (3). Hyperventilation is induced by pain but again there is not necessarily a strong correlation between the two as pain is rarely seen during voluntary over breathing (3).

Lifestyle can play an important role in the cause of HVS. Respiratory stimulants such as caffeine and nicotine are contributing factors that must be reduced to help correct the breathing pattern. Speech alters breathing and excessive speech can extenuate hyperventilation problems due to the habitual mouth breathing that coincides with fast speech.

Symptoms of hyperventilation

The symptoms of HVS are diverse and non-diagnostic in their own right. If the patient is classically hyperventilating, the effect of hypocapnia is widespread and includes vasoconstriction

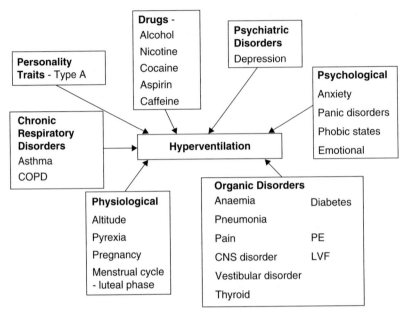

Fig. 14.1 Factors that can increase respiration and potentially cause hyperventilation.

of smooth muscle reducing blood flow to vital organs, reduced oxygen availability, increased lactic acid, and increased neuronal excitement. Patients usually show a unique set of symptoms which exacerbate intermittently and vary in intensity, frequency, and duration, adding to the complexity of diagnosis. The following is a break down of the potential physiological changes with the symptoms in italics:

- With hyperventilation there is a reduction in carbon dioxide which causes a rise in blood pH and this instigates the compensatory mechanism of increased bicarbonate excretion by the kidneys. If the compensation is prolonged, respiration is stimulated in order to avoid metabolic acidosis causing a further increase in *breathlessness*. The body fights to maintain homeostasis often to the detriment of the patients well being.

- Reduced levels of calcium ions in the plasma precipitates hyperirritability of the motor and sensory axons causing increased neuronal excitability. *Tingling* sensations in the tips of fingers and around the mouth are classic signs. *Hypertonicity, cramps,* and *carpo-pedal spasm* of the muscles due to nerve membrane destabilisation can be experienced but are not as common.

- Hypocapnia decreases blood flow to the brain which causes symptoms such as *headaches, memory lapses,* feelings of being '*detached from reality*' and *lack of concentration.*

- Vasoconstriction of the peripheral blood flow causes patients to complain of *cold extremities.* Reduced blood flow to skeletal muscle reduces capacity for aerobic metabolism, leading to increased lactic acid production and *fatigue.* Smooth muscle can also be affected including the gut and the bowel which presents, and is often diagnosed as *irritable bowel syndrome.*

- Muscle tissue can also become hypoxic due to the inability of haemoglobin (Hb) to release oxygen into the tissue. When blood pH rises as a result of low carbon dioxide levels, Hb has an increased affinity to pick up oxygen but not release it. Hypoxic muscle tissue leads to aggravation of trigger points which can lead to a variety of *musculoskeletal complaints.*

- Alkalosis alone is not the full picture; other mechanisms appear to cause some of the symptoms. For example, breathlessness can be present as bronchoconstriction, induced or aggravated by excessive mouth breathing. Non-adrenergic, non-cholinergic stimulatory fibres (C-fibres) found in the lung tissue are activated by cold air inhalation causing inflammation and bronchospasm. This *mimics asthma* and may result in misdiagnosis.

- *Palpitations* and *chest pains* are familiar symptoms. Chest pain is most likely due to musculoskeletal causes rather than coronary artery constriction. The chest pain felt in hyperventilation is typically described as dull and diffuse and is reproducible by palpating the intercostal muscles that are fatigued or in spasm due to excessive upper chest breathing. Hyperexcitability of the cardiac muscle fibres and electrical conduction systems may cause arrhythmias.

- *Bloatedness* and excess gas production are common manifestations due to excessive swallowing of air through unnecessary mouth breathing. When the diaphragm is not working optimally, the massaging effect on the stomach is lost which can also increase digestive problems.

- Sympathetic nervous system dominance is frequently experienced and causes an aroused state that the patient can find distressing. Adrenalin levels three times the normal range have been measured in some individuals with hyperventilation syndrome (8). Symptoms arising from an overactive sympathetic nervous system include *sweaty palms, hot flushes,* and an *inability to relax* and *poor sleep.*

Efficient breathing

To be able to diagnose HVS, it is essential to be able to identify an efficient breathing pattern.

The diaphragm is the most important muscle for breathing. During inhalation the central tendon of the diaphragm is pulled down, increasing the vertical space within the thorax. The diaphragm moves from a dome shape to a flattened position and is resisted by the abdominal viscera. This fixes the central tendon allowing the outer fibres of the diaphragm to displace laterally. As the lower ribs flare out, the sternum is lifted anteriorly and superiorly. The contraction of the diaphragm and intercostal muscles enables the ribcage to move in three dimensions, vertically, laterally and antero-superiorly. The volume of air drawn in due to the negative pressure inside the lungs is dependent on these three movements.

The intercostal muscles contribute to the mechanics of breathing through stabilizing and assisting the ribcage to move. If a larger volume of air is required, accessory muscles, such as the scalenes or sternomastoid muscles, are activated to further increase the thoracic volume. Use of these accessory muscles has high energy demands and in normal breathing is only required during activities that require high amounts of oxygen. Efficient breathing can use as little as 2% of total oxygen consumption. Excessive use of accessory muscles can increase this figure to up to 30%.

Efficient breathing *at rest* encompasses 80–90% diaphragm activity and 10–20% intercostal muscle activity. The diaphragm movement can be felt by placing a hand on the abdomen, which rises as the lungs expand vertically. The lower ribs move out like bucket handles which causes the lungs to expand laterally, this can be felt by placing the hands on the lower ribs at the waist region.

During exhalation, all the muscles should passively recoil to their original position. Exhalation should only become active if the respiratory rate rises in response to increased metabolic demand. At the end of exhalation a relaxed pause in respiration is crucial for the alteration in pressures between the abdominal and thoracic cavities.

Another essential component of an efficient breathing pattern is effective use of the nose. Nose breathing provides a multitude of benefits, such as warming, cleaning and humidifying inhaled air. It regulates the volume of air drawn into the lungs. The nose also has a protective function with a variety of mechanisms that defend against bacterial and viral infections. These include phagocytic engulfment of organisms and the production of nitric oxide, in large quantities, which is a powerful disinfectant. Thus bypassing the nose is detrimental in several ways and may increase the likelihood of a chest infection.

Inefficient breathing patterns

Upper chest breathing

Upper chest breathing is commonly adopted and is often a sign of HVS. The diaphragm cannot function optimally when the upper chest respiratory muscles are active. This changes the chest wall motion to predominantly anterior-superior movement, with very minimal vertical displacement. This breathing pattern creates a ventilation/perfusion mismatch as blood circulates mostly around the lower lobes whilst ventilation mainly supplies the upper lobes. Consequently, the respiratory rate or depth must be increased to meet the oxygen demands of the body. This further perpetuates the inefficient breathing pattern.

Upper chest breathing has several negative effects. Increased fuel is required to supply the highly demanding accessory muscles which are predominantly fast-fatiguing skeletal muscle. Their origin is the upper spine, base of the skull, and the clavicles; the constant movement causes a pulling action which can illicit a variety of musculoskeletal problems, such as neck, shoulder, and chest pain. Over time, this new, less efficient pattern of breathing becomes habitual and is adopted regardless of the original cause of the upper chest breathing pattern.

Practical tip: by placing one hand on the upper chest and one hand on the abdomen, just above the navel, you can identify which area is moving, this gives you a good indication of whether the diaphragm or the accessory muscles are more dominant.

Mouth breathing

Mouth breathing is easily adopted as the nose provides 50% more resistance to airflow. A lack of nasal airflow leads to constricted nasal smooth muscle which amplifies the difficulty of nose breathing, further perpetuating the problem.

Inhaling and exhaling through the mouth decreases the time for gas exchange to take place, because air enters and leaves the lungs more rapidly. Breathing regulation becomes more difficult because feedback to the brain triggered from nose breathing is reduced. Large volumes of air pass in and out of the lungs meaning hyperventilation is more likely. The mouth is unable to clean or warm the air as it enters and water loss is accelerated. Air travelling quickly through the mouth and into the upper airway can cause excessive airway drying and cooling that results in bronchospasm and inflammation. This can increase breathlessness and aggravate any underlying organic disease such as asthma.

Minute ventilation

Normal minute ventilation is around 5–6L per minute at rest. This figure can be doubled or even tripled (up to 20L per minute) before a sensation of breathlessness becomes apparent to the individual. Hyperventilation can therefore occur without any undue sense of breathlessness. The average respiratory rate at rest is between 8 and 12 breaths per minute (bpm). A respiratory rate up to around 18bpm can go unrecognized and may not be noticed by the patient until they become more active. The increased metabolic demand raises the respiratory rate further, potentially up to 20–30bpm. The mouth then opens in response to the increased respiratory rate, causing increased work of breathing disproportionate to the activity.

An average tidal volume is approximately 500–600mL, with little abdominal excursion.

A slight increase in this tidal volume can easily go unnoticed and is a complete waste of energy and may even cause symptoms of hypocarbia. For example, if a person's tidal volume increased by 250mL per breath, by the end of one day 3000L of air would have been moved in and out of the lungs unnecessarily.

Excessive sighing and yawning is another way in which the body increases tidal volume and so are frequently observed in patients with established HVS. A typical patient with HVS may complain of yawning frequently despite not feeling tired. Others may not even notice their excessive sighing. Filling the upper chest with over a litre of air every few minutes is fatiguing for the chest wall muscles and can be one of the causes of chest pain.

Diagnosis of hyperventilation syndrome

The diagnosis of HVS can easily be overlooked as the patient usually presents with a spectrum of physical symptoms which mimic other organic diseases. Gathering evidence from a variety of sources is essential. Initially, the most important aspect is to eliminate any organic disease, especially of the cardiorespiratory system. It is important to establish if there is any cardiac cause of breathlessness and eliminate pulmonary hypertension, pulmonary emboli, hyperthyroidism, or metabolic acidosis. Lung function tests, chest x-ray, and oxygen saturation at rest and during exercise are all important diagnostic tools to help eliminate respiratory disease as the primary cause of breathlessness. Multiple tests can be a cause for concern for the patient, thus continual reassurance to reduce any excess anxiety is important while a diagnosis is being established.

Once the elimination process is complete, the next step is confirmation of the syndrome.

Recording symptoms

Patients should be encouraged to explain *every* symptom even if they do not feel it is appropriate. A body chart can be helpful so the assessor can visually document the array of symptoms. The Nijmegen questionnaire (Table 14.1) is simple to complete and can be used to aid diagnosis and measure effectiveness of treatment (1). It has not been validated in patients with underlying lung disease and so care must be taken if it is used in this patient group.

Table 14.1 The Nijmegen Questionnaire: a total score of 23 or higher indicates hyperventilation

	Never (0) Rarely (1)	Sometimes (2)	Often (3)	Very often (4)
Chest pain				
Feeling tense				
Blurred vision				
Dizzy spells				
Feeling confused				
Faster/deeper breathing				
Short of breath				
Tight feelings in chest				
Bloated feeling in stomach				
Tingling in fingers				
Unable to breathe deeply				
Stiff fingers/arms				
Tight feelings around mouth				
Cold hands/feet				
Heart racing (palpitations)				
Feelings of anxiety				
Total score:				

While taking the subjective history, attention should be paid to the patient's breathing pattern. Establish if there are any abnormalities with their resting breathing pattern while they are unaware of being assessed. Look out for excessive upper chest movement, mouth breathing, increased respiratory rate, and any large or erratic movements of the chest. Be watchful of their breathing pattern while talking and take note of any excessive sighing or yawning.

The breath-hold test

A reduced breath-hold is used as an indication of a tendency to hyperventilate and essentially gives a measurement of the drive to breathe. This test has not been validated but is becoming increasingly popular as an outcome measure and aid to diagnosis. The breath-hold is usually done at the end of inspiration. One of the problems with the test is that the volume of air inspired before the breath-hold will affect the length of time that the breath can be held for (3). Reliability of the test is also reduced because time of day and motivation can influence the result. Despite the limitations, it has been described that those patients (without any underlying respiratory disease) whom cannot hold their breath for longer than 30s may have an increased drive to breathe and have increased potential to hyperventilate (3).

Measuring carbon dioxide

Measuring carbon dioxide has always been the gold standard for diagnosing hyperventilation but there are a variety of problems with this test. The primary problem with the test is the uncertainty of the lower limits of the normal range of carbon dioxide. Patients may have more problems with variable changes in carbon dioxide levels making the single measurement of carbon dioxide not appropriate (5). Performing the test through an arterial puncture can itself increase a patient's breathing pattern which may lead to a patient having a lower carbon dioxide level despite not having chronic hyperventilation, giving a false-positive result. The use of capnographs have overcome some of these problems and are becoming increasingly popular as they are non-invasive, measuring end-tidal carbon dioxide through a small catheter placed in the nostril over a longer period of time (3). The validity of the test is also questioned as it has been shown that patients can still experience their symptoms during voluntary hyperventilation even when carbon dioxide levels are maintained (4).

Provocation test

The provocation test has also been used to aid diagnosis. Patients are asked to take 20 or more deep breaths. Healthy subjects should only feel paraesthesia but if a patient's symptoms are reproduced then this can aid diagnosis of HVS. This test may be more helpful when the patient does not believe that their symptoms are related to their inefficient breathing pattern. Showing the patient that their symptoms can be reproduced through increasing the breathing pattern can help to convince them of the diagnosis.

Hospital Anxiety and Depression scale

Patients who exhibit high levels of anxiety or depression need to be assessed and managed appropriately. The Hospital Anxiety and Depression scale (HAD) is one way of identifying those patients who may require psychological input (11). This tool is recommended as part of the assessment and could also be used as an outcome measure.

Hyperventilation syndrome and other organic diseases

There appears to be a link between HVS and chronic disease (3, 5). Being diagnosed with a chronic illness can cause great concern and the anxiety related to the diagnosis could be sufficient to trigger HVS. With chronic respiratory disease, the likelihood of developing HVS may be higher as breathlessness is already a significant problem, making it more likely to worsen.

Asthma

Asthma and HVS appear to be closely related. There appears to be a high prevalence of HVS amongst patients diagnosed with asthma, although conversely a large proportion of HVS patients are in actual fact asthmatic (4, 12). Excessive airway drying and cooling appears to be the exacerbating factor. Hyperventilation could aggravate this process further causing the airways to constrict or become more inflamed leading to symptoms typical of asthma. Chronic inhalation of cold, dry air into hypersensitive airways could be detrimental for asthmatics. Thomas et al. (9) found that a large proportion of asthmatics demonstrated a dysfunctional breathing pattern. These authors reviewed Nijmegen scores on 217 asthmatic patients and found that 63 (29%) had a score greater than 23, which indicates potential hyperventilation. Notably, a large proportion of those with a positive score were female. These results must be interpreted with caution, however, as the Nijmegen questionnaire has not been validated in asthma. These patients may possibly score higher than healthy subjects simply due to their chronic lung disease symptoms.

It has even been suggested that hyperventilation is the direct cause of asthma (13). Konstantin Buteyko developed a theory based on the link between hyperventilation and a variety of conditions such as asthma, sleep apnoea, and general ill health. He created a breathing training programme that aimed to normalize breathing patterns, reversing symptoms, and reducing the need for medication: 'The Buteyko view is that asthma is not a disease, but rather that it is a collection of symptoms—bronchospasm, mucus production and inflammation of the lining of the airways' (14).

The theory of Buteyko is based on the consequences of low carbon dioxide levels in the blood and its link with chronic disease. Buteyko suggested that hypocapnia develops as a result of overbreathing which in turn causes bronchospasm of the smooth muscle lining the small airways. Inefficient breathing dries out the lungs causing increased inflammation and mucus production.

Buteyko's theory is limited by the fact that not all patients with asthma or HVS exhibit low carbon dioxide levels. Even when the breathing pattern is corrected, airway inflammation does not improve (12, 15). Until more recently, the Buteyko theory has not been accepted very readily in the Western medical world as it encouraged patients to reduce their asthma medication without any scientific evidence that it is safe or effective to do so. Bowler et al. (15) performed a blind, randomized control (RCT) trial to assess the effectiveness of the Buteyko breathing techniques in asthma patients (15). The results showed that those practising the Buteyko breathing technique had improved quality of life scores and a reduced use of their beta-2 agonist medication compared to a control group that was given education and relaxation techniques only. Minute volume was significantly less in the Butyeko breathing group compared to the control group and also correlated with reduced use of beta-2 agonist medications. The RCT showed no evidence that reducing breathing resulted in increased carbon dioxide levels—central to the theory of Buteyko.

Thomas et al. (12) also conducted an RCT demonstrating that breathing exercises for asthmatics showed no difference in quality of life at 1 month between the group that received the breathing retraining compared with the group that did not. At 6 months, however there was a significant difference between the two groups, favouring breathing retraining (12). The authors also found that there was no change in airway inflammation, airway physiology, or hyper-responsiveness in either group at any stage in the study. This led them to conclude that reducing anti-inflammatory medication is not appropriate for asthmatic patients after a breathing rehabilitation programme.

Chronic obstructive pulmonary disease

The mechanism of breathlessness with chronic obstructive pulmonary disease (COPD) is multifactorial and it is often difficult to establish the exact cause. Often COPD patients present with breathlessness disproportionate to the severity of their lung disease according to lung function tests. This does not, necessarily mean they are hyperventilating. Airway obstruction caused by chronic inflammation is certainly an important factor contributing to breathlessness in COPD but peripheral muscle deconditioning, particularly of the ambulatory muscles, is also now known to play an important role (16). Deconditioning from inactivity reduces the aerobic capacity of the muscle tissue, resulting in increased lactic acid production and further breathlessness on exertion. Exercise programmes in the form of pulmonary rehabilitation have shown highly significant improvements in reducing breathlessness (17).

Breathlessness in COPD is also caused by altered breathing mechanics due to hyperinflation. The loss of elasticity renders the lungs unable to passively recoil after inspiration, causing air trapping and distension of the alveoli. As a consequence, the diaphragm is pushed downwards into a flattened position, altering its length–tension relationship. With the diaphragm at a mechanical disadvantage, the patient will adopt an upper chest breathing pattern to compensate. Guidelines have highlighted that attempting to change the breathing pattern of a patient with severe hyperinflation can increase rather than reduce energy expenditure for breathing (2). However, COPD patients with less severe hyperinflation can still present with an upper chest breathing pattern. The reason for this has not yet been answered. Further research is required to establish if COPD patients with a milder form of diaphragm dysfunction who demonstrate a poor breathing pattern could respond to breathing retraining.

Bronchiectasis

Patients with bronchiectasis often present with an inefficient breathing pattern. Upper chest breathing leads to poorly ventilated basal areas and worsening sputum retention; hence a poor breathing pattern may in fact be a contributory factor to the recurrent chest infections commonly experienced by these patients. Breathing re-education should therefore be used in conjunction with effective chest clearance regimes to optimize the management of patients with bronchiectasis (2).

With chronic lung disease patients who demonstrate an inefficient breathing pattern, it can be difficult to establish whether breathing retraining is appropriate or indeed possible. The irreversible physiological and mechanical changes within the lungs may mean that upper chest breathing has developed because it is in fact the most efficient breathing pattern for a patient with established severe chronic lung disease.

Other chronic diseases

Diabetic patients could be at risk of developing HVS. Fluctuating sugar levels can cause an increase in respiratory rate, meaning that a poorly controlled diabetic patient can be at a high risk of becoming a habitual over-breather. Gastrointestinal reflux disease (GORD) has also been associated with HVS and asthma. The exact mechanism of the relationship is unknown (18). One explanation for the link could be that a breathing pattern that involves partial expiration or hyperventilation can have a significant influence on oesophageal motor control and inappropriate relaxation of the lower oesophageal sphincter which can exacerbate GORD (8). Further evidence is required to establish if correcting breathing patterns in patients with GORD can assist with management.

The management of hyperventilation syndrome

Most of the literature for the management of HVS has focused on breathing retraining, relaxation, medication, as well as a full explanation of the syndrome (2, 3, 5, 8, 12, 19). The latter is very important as giving a patient an explanation for their symptoms can immediately relieve some of the anxiety that perpetuates the condition. The explanation and breathing retraining written for this chapter is a regimen that is widely used by physiotherapists who have specialized in the management of HVS and is used in the studies by Holloway and West (19) and Thomas et. al (12). Both studies found significant improvements in asthma-related quality of life scores in those that received the explanation of dysfunctional breathing and the breathing retraining regimen compared to those that received education only (12, 19).

It is imperative at assessment to establish if the patient has any specific psychological needs which would require onward referral to psychological services. Often drug management such as beta blockers may be required for patients with high levels of anxiety (3).

Stress management and lifestyle advice is often imperative to provide a holistic approach and to help prevent recurrence of the symptoms.

Explanation

A thorough explanation of why the patient is experiencing such a wide range of symptoms is imperative for successfully reducing anxiety associated with the condition. Patients must be made aware of their inefficient breathing pattern and helped to understand how this alone can cause their varied and often bizarre symptoms. Providing written literature about hyperventilation is essential.

Breathing retraining

Nose breathing

The first step to correcting a breathing pattern is to re-instigate nose breathing. This can be difficult if the patient has had previous nasal problems and may need to be referred to an ear, nose, and throat specialist before any breathing retraining can be started effectively. Nose breathing for patients who hyperventilate is challenging because they are used to large volumes of air moving freely in and out through the mouth. Initially, nose breathing can be very uncomfortable and the patient often feels intense air hunger which can trigger further overbreathing to compensate. It is important to only make minor changes to the breathing pattern initially so that the body learns to adjust gradually, rather than fight against it and overcompensate. Give the patient small, achievable goals, such as breathing through the nose for 1 minute and then mouth breath for 1 minute, repeating five times per day, increasing the time spent nose breathing gradually.

Diaphragm breathing

It is important when performing any breathing re-education that the patient is comfortable. Semi-supine is usually the best position for most patients to start, with the exception of patients with other underlying lung or heart diseases who may need to be in upright sitting. Placing a pillow under the knees to release the hip flexors and loosening any tight clothing around the waist to enable the diaphragm to move freely. Achieving effective diaphragm activity can be very difficult at first. Patients often try to use their abdominal muscles, forcing their stomachs to rise and fall to mimic diaphragm activity. Care must be taken to eliminate this by placing one hand on the abdomen and feeling for any muscle activity. Patients may complain of sore stomach muscles if they are using them inappropriately.

Quiet breathing

At first, it may be appropriate to ask the patient to take larger volume breaths in order to identify and experience basal expansion, and to initiate diaphragm activity, but this should not be encouraged for more than a few breaths. Breathing should be quiet or even silent, to reduce air moving in and out of the lungs and excessive movement of the ribcage.

Rate of breathing

Once diaphragmatic, quiet, nose breathing is established, then the rate of breathing needs to be reduced to between 8–12 breaths per minute. Relaxation techniques can be very beneficial for reducing the respiratory rate by relaxing tense muscles and stimulating the parasympathetic nervous system.

Breathing in sitting and standing

Once an efficient breathing pattern is mastered at rest in semi-supine lying, breathing retraining can be progressed to more functional positions such as sitting and then standing. Sitting is often harder to achieve than standing due to the increased abdominal resistance and may need extra practice. Encouragement of basal expansion can help overcome the abdominal resistance in both sitting and standing.

Breathing and exercise

Once efficient breathing in standing has been established progression of breathing retraining during walking and more vigorous exercise can then be introduced. Further encouragement of basal expansion to maintain good diaphragm activity is crucial. The upper chest should become more active as the exercise becomes more challenging. Mouth breathing will become essential once the respiratory rate rises above 30 breaths per minute. It is important the patient breathes at a rate that feels as naturally as possible.

Patients with hyperventilation will often suffer from deconditioning, not that dissimilar to a patient with a chronic respiratory disease. A deconditioning cycle is often adopted as breathlessness is experienced on minimal exertion, causing a rapid spiral of inactivity to avoid the unpleasant sensation of breathlessness. Although to date no research has investigated the effect of pulmonary rehabilitation specifically in hyperventilation, other respiratory illnesses such as asthma and COPD, have shown significant improvements in both exercise tolerance and quality of life following pulmonary rehabilitation (17). Future research is required to establish if an exercise and self-management programme such as pulmonary rehabilitation is equally effective in HVS.

Talking and breathing

It is important to address any problems with the coordination of talking and breathing as speech can interfere with breathing patterns and vice versa. Patients who hyperventilate tend to take upper chest gasps through the mouth in between long sentences. Slowing speech down can help to improve HVS symptoms by enabling more time for a nose–diaphragm breath to take place between sentences. Lack of diaphragm activity during speech can also lead to reduced voice volume, especially towards the end of a sentence. Good diaphragmatic breathing is essential for an effective clear voice.

Lifestyle changes

An individualized approach to breathing retraining is paramount to address the specific needs of each patient. A reduction in stimulant intake, such as alcohol and caffeine, can be particularly important if identified as a potential aggravator. Promoting effective sleep is essential to reduce stress, anxiety, and tiredness, since disordered sleep patterns can exacerbate breathing dysfunction. A balanced diet is imperative as erratic blood sugar levels can increase the likelihood of overbreathing. An appropriate amount of protein should be ingested at each meal with a reduction of high sugary foods.

Musculoskeletal rehabilitation

Musculoskeletal techniques can also be effective for improving breathing patterns. Leon Chaitow has shown an improvement in breathing pattern through muscle energy techniques which inhibit the accessory muscles and promote good rib cage mobility (8). The diaphragm is a key muscle for core stability which should contribute to supporting the spine. During hyperventilation, the diaphragm can be severely inhibited which reduces the stability role it plays for the spine (8). Ensuring patients are able to appropriately breathe whilst maintaining a good posture is essential in the prevention of musculoskeletal problems.

Factors that can prevent successful breathing retraining

Evidence suggests that breathing retraining, involving reducing respiratory rate and/or tidal volume, relaxation training and exercise can significantly improve symptoms in patients with HVS and asthma (2). Generally it takes 2–3 months to show improvements in breathing patterns, but may take as long as 6 months to get clinically significant improvements (12, 19). If a patient does not improve however there maybe other factors inhibiting progression of breathing retraining that needs to be addressed. The following are some examples:

◆ Fluctuating and low blood sugar levels—respiratory rate can rise when blood glucose is within the lower half of the normal range (4.4mmol/L).

◆ Restriction of the diaphragm:
  • Food intolerance that causes bloatedness can restrict the diaphragm and prevent efficient breathing.
  • Patients who are keen exercisers and have performed excessive amounts of upper abdominal exercises may need specialist musculoskeletal therapy to help release the tight structures that are limiting diaphragm movement.

◆ Allergies—patients with poorly-controlled allergies who constantly sniff, sneeze, or cough can experience difficulty with breathing re-education due to excessive upper respiratory inspirations or expirations. Onward referral for optimal management of allergies would be required before breathing retraining can be effective.

◆ Progesterone—is a strong respiratory stimulant that makes it difficult for women to maintain a reduced breathing pattern during the premenstrual period. Progesterone is high during pregnancy, combine this with a raised diaphragm and breathlessness is a common symptom.

Conclusion

In summary, despite the problems with the title of the condition and the limited knowledge of the underlying physiology, once recognized and diagnosed, the symptoms can be rectified relatively easily without medication or lengthy procedures. Recognizing the condition can easily be missed due to subtlety of chronic hyperventilation; however, symptoms common to HVS provide the clue to identifying it. Once accurately diagnosed, time must be taken to explain the syndrome to the patient to ensure effective treatment. A knowledgeable physiotherapist with experience of breathing retraining is ideally suited to manage this patient group. Asthma appears to have the close links with HVS, and evidence suggests that breathing retraining can be effective in reducing asthmatic and hyperventilation symptoms. Some patients, however, may need additional help from a psychologist to help manage anxiety states that cannot be controlled though breathing retraining. A holistic approach to the management of this complex syndrome that is not fully understood is essential for successful treatment.

References

1. Van Dixhoorn J, Duivenvoorden HJ. Efficacy of Nijmegen Questionnaire in recognition of hyperventilation syndrome. *J Psychosom Res* 1985; **29**(2):199–206
2. Bott J, Blumenthal S, Buxton M, *et al.* Guideline for physiotherapy management of the adult, medical, spontaneously breathing patient. *Thorax* 2009; **64**(Suppl 1):i1–51.
3. Gardner W. The pathophysiology of hyperventilation. *Chest* 1996; **109**:516–34.
4. Morgan M. Dysfunctional breathing in asthma: is common, identifiable and correctable? *Thorax* 2002; **57**:31–5.
5. Lum L. Hyperventilation syndromes in medicine and psychiatry. *J Roy Soc Med* 1987; **80**:229–31.
6. Da Costa JM. On irritable heart: a clinical study of a form of functional cardiac disorder and its consequences. *Am J Med Science* 1871; **61**:17–53.
7. Wood P. Da Costa's syndrome. *BMJ* 1941; **1**:767.
8. Chaitow L. Breathing patterns, motor control and low back pain. *J Osteopath Med* 2004; **7**(1): 34–41.
9. Thomas M, McKinley R K, Freeman E. Foy C. Prevalence of dysfunctional breathing in patients treated for asthma in primary care: cross sectional survey. *BMJ* 2001; **322**:1098–100.
10. Kern B. *Hyperventilation Syndrome* [Internet], 2010. http://emedicine.medscape.com/article/807277-overview
11. Zigmond AS, Snaith RP. The hospital anxiety and depression scale. *Acta Psychiatr Scand* 1983; **67**(6):361–70.
12. Thomas M, McKinley RK, Mellor S, *et al.* Breathing exercises for asthma: a randomised controlled trial. *Thorax* 2004; **64**:55–61.
13. Stalmatski A. Freedom from asthma: Buteyko's revolutionary treatment. *Hale Clinic Health Library*, p. 175. London: Kylecathie Ltd, 1997.
14. http://www.buteykoairways.com/asthma.htm
15. Bowler SD, Green A, Mitchell CA. Buteyko breathing techniques in asthma: a blinded randomised controlled trial. *Med J Aust* 1998; **169**:575–8.
16. Pulmonary rehabilitation: joint ACCP/AACVPR evidence-based guidelines. ACCP/AACVPR Pulmonary Rehabilitation Guidelines Panel. American College of Chest Physicians. American Association of Cardiovascular and Pulmonary Rehabilitation. *Chest* 1997; **112**(5):1363–96.

17. Lacasse Y, Brosseau L, Milne S, *et al.* Pulmonary rehabilitation for chronic obstructive pulmonary disease. *Cochrane Database Syst Rev* 2002; **3**:CD003793.

18. Kasasbeh A, Kasasbeh E, Krishnaswamy G. Potential mechanisms connecting asthma, esophageal reflux, and obesity/sleep apnea complex—a hypothetical review. *Sleep Med Rev* 2007; **11**(1):47–58.

19. Holloway E, West R. Integrated breathing and relaxation training (the Papworth method) for adults with asthma in primary care: a randomized controlled trial. *Thorax* 2007; **62**:1039–42.

Part 5

Cough and expectoration

Chapter 15

Physiology and pathophysiology of cough

Ian D. Pavord

Introduction

Cough is an important defence mechanism that clears the airways of secretions and prevents entry of foreign bodies and irritants to the lower respiratory tract. It is a universal experience in health but also a non-specific presenting feature of most respiratory conditions and a number of non-respiratory conditions. Acute cough is one of the most common presenting symptoms to a general practitioner. Most cases result from viral and bacterial upper respiratory tract infection, are self-limiting, and do not require further evaluation but some patients have persistent cough that requires specialist opinion. Chronic cough is arbitrarily defined as a cough lasting more than 8 weeks. It is present in 3–10% of the general population and is responsible for between 10–20% of respiratory outpatient referrals. Chronic cough with significant sputum production is likely to be due to intrapulmonary disease such as chronic bronchitis or bronchiectasis. A chronic dry or minimally productive cough may be due to extrapulmonary factors but can also be unexplained; the cough is likely to be due to abnormal sensitization of the cough reflex secondary to the effects of local inflammation on sensory nerve endings. Chronic cough is often perceived as a trivial problem but can be a disabling symptom associated with impairment of quality of life, and distressing associated symptoms such as musculoskeletal chest pains, syncope, incontinence, disturbed sleep, and social embarrassment (1, 2). Treatment options are unsatisfactory (3) and a high proportion of patients with chronic cough have continued problems needing supportive care.

Cough can become particularly burdensome in the terminal phases of lung cancer, metastatic disease in the lung, and interstitial lung disease. Understanding the physiology, pathophysiology, and pharmacology of the cough reflex is thus also an important priority for clinicians with an interest in palliative care.

The cough reflex

As with all reflexes, the cough reflex involves an afferent and efferent pathway and a degree of central processing. The most sensitive sites for initiating cough are the larynx, the carina, and the points of bronchial branching. Cough receptors are also present in extrapulmonary structures including the oesophagus, diaphragm, and stomach. A broad group of 'rapidly adapting "irritant" receptors' (RARs) found in the larynx and tracheo-bronchial tree, can be stimulated by a wide range of stimuli. These all provoke cough and include cigarette smoke, ammonia, ether vapour, acid and alkaline solutions, hypotonic and hypertonic saline, and mechanical stimulation by direct contact, mucus, or dust. Another closely-related fibre is the slowly-adapting stretch receptor (SAR) which terminates inspiration and initiates expiration when the lungs are at an adequate level of inflation. SARs may also influence cough. Finally, C-fibre receptors are found in the laryngeal, bronchial, and alveolar walls. They are relatively insensitive to mechanical stimulation and lung inflation, but are exquisitely sensitive to chemicals such as bradykinin, capsaicin, and acid pH. Stimuli that are known to cause cough in human subjects such as capsaicin, bradykinin, and citric acid activate C-fibre afferents, particularly those located in the bronchi.

Cough receptors may possess mechanically-gated ion channels such as sodium channels, while acid stimuli can interact with voltage-gated sodium channels belonging to the acid-sensing ion channel family. A cationic ion channel, transient receptor potential vanilloid-1 (TRPV-1), found on RARs and C-fibres is the receptor for capsaicin and is activated by heat, acid, bradykinin, arachidonic acid derivatives, and adenosine triphosphate. TRPV-1 has been localized to epithelial nerves in human airways and this expression is increased in patients with chronic cough (4). TRPV-1 inhibitors inhibit the tussive response caused by allergen challenge in a sensitized guinea-pig model, raising the possibility that they may be active as antitussives (5). Bradykinin and prostaglandin (PG) E_2 and $F_{2\alpha}$ increase the tussive response to capsaicin, sensitizing effects that are mediated through specific voltage-gated sodium channels (6, 7).

Afferent fibres from cough receptors in the airways converge, via the vagus nerves, to sites of brainstem relaying in the nucleus tractus solitarius, where there are connections to respiratory-related neurons in the central respiratory generator, which coordinates the efferent cough response. These respiratory neurons are often referred to as the 'cough centre'. C-fibre activation interacts centrally with RARs or other afferents to promote coughing. Sensitization of the cough reflex could also be present at the level of the brain stem neurons. Finally, cough can be controlled by the higher cortical centres since we can voluntarily inhibit or produce a cough. The inhibitory effect of placebo treatment and sleep on cough may be related to the modulation of cortical control. Functional magnetic resonance measurements have shown that the urge-to-cough sensation is associated with activation of the insular cortex, the anterior cingulated cortex, the primary sensory cortex, and the cerebellum, supporting cortical influences in cough (8).

Patients with chronic cough have a cough response to inhaled stimuli such as citric acid or capsaicin, reflecting increased sensitivity of cough receptors (peripheral sensitization) or by changes in the central processing at the level of the ganglia or brainstem (central sensitization). The former could occur as the result of airway inflammation and the presence of an abnormally high concentration of tussive mediators such as prostaglandin E_2, histamine and substance P (9). Sensitization could also occur as a result of changes in sensory pathways with release of neurotransmitters or neuromodulators, increased excitability of the postsynaptic neuron, a change in the structure of the nerve or as a result of changes in central neural pathways. Under normal conditions, a mechanical deformation of the cough receptor leads to a protective cough reflex, but, under conditions of irritation or inflammation, the cough receptor may become responsive to stimuli that it does not usually respond to.

Clinical aspects of chronic cough

Cough in health and disease

Recent developments in cough detection systems and semi-automated computerized cough detection systems have made it possible to determine cough frequency in health and disease. Healthy adults cough once or twice an hour during day-time and hardly ever at night (Figure 15.1). Cough frequency is highest between 8 and 10 am and in mid-afternoon (10, 11). Healthy women cough twice as much as healthy men (11); they also have a heightened cough response to inhaled tussive stimuli such as capsaicin (12). Age, menopause status, and body mass index are not associated with any obvious difference in either measure. Cough frequency is 10–15 times higher in patients presenting with chronic cough (Figure 15.1) but the diurnal pattern of coughing is unchanged. The highest cough frequency occurs in patients with unexplained chronic cough.

The causes of cough can be conveniently divided into acute and chronic (Table 15.1). An acute cough is arbitrarily defined as a cough less than 3 weeks. Infectious and allergic conditions are by far the commonest aetiologies. Most acute coughs resolve by 3 weeks; they will not be discussed further.

Many conditions implicated in causing chronic cough such as chronic obstructive pulmonary disease (COPD), lung cancer, foreign bodies, pulmonary tuberculosis, sarcoidosis, idiopathic pulmonary fibrosis, and heart failure will be obvious after clinical assessment, spirometry, and a chest radiograph. The management of chronic cough in these situations is broadly the same as the management of the underlying conditions although there will be some patients whose cough is a disproportionate problem who require further evaluation and treatment along the lines suggested below. The majority of patients referred for investigation of chronic cough are non-smokers and have normal findings on physical examination and chest radiography. Most present with a non-productive or minimally productive cough and 60–75% are female. There is a tendency for cough to first present around the time of the menopause (3).

Evaluation of the patient

An initial assessment of a patient with chronic cough is directed at finding a specific cause, assessing severity and initiating trials of treatment. A careful history and physical examination is paramount to the evaluation of a patient with chronic cough (Table 15.2). Details of the factors surrounding the onset of cough and associated symptoms, and a careful assessment of the upper airways and the respiratory system are particularly important. Basic initial investigations should include an up-to-date chest radiograph, spirometry,

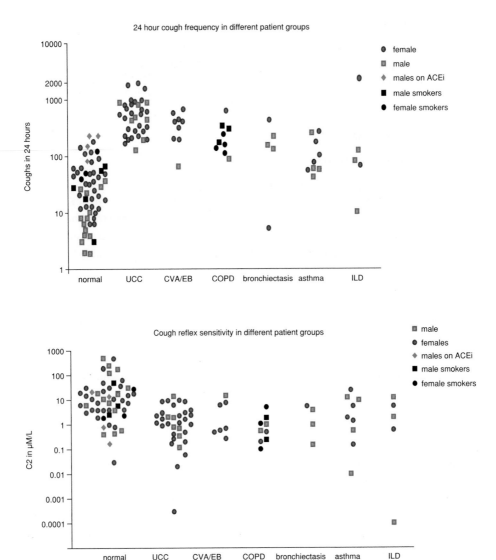

Fig. 15.1 Cough frequency and cough reflex sensitivity in health and disease. CVA, cough variant asthma; COPD, chronic obstructive pulmonary disease; EB, eosinophilic bronchitis; ILD, interstitial lung disease; UCC, unexplained chronic cough.

and bronchodilator reversibility if appropriate. An abrupt onset of coughing while eating or chewing should raise the possibility of an inhaled foreign body and the onset of cough shortly after introduction of angiotensin-converting enzyme (ACE) inhibitor therapy suggests ACE inhibitor-associated cough. The presence of significant quantities of sputum, haemoptysis, systemic symptoms, prominent breathlessness, wheeze, or abnormal physical signs increases the probability of intrinsic lung disease and should trigger appropriate investigations which may include a high-resolution computed tomography (CT) scan of the chest and a bronchoscopy even if there are no suggestive findings with more

Table 15.1a Common causes of acute cough

Acute cough
Upper respiratory tract infections
Acute sinusitis
Allergic rhinitis
Asthma

Table 15.1b Common conditions implicated in causing chronic cough

Diagnosis	Approximate incidence (%)
Rhinitis	25–30
Asthma/eosinophilic bronchitis	20–25
Gastro-oesophageal reflux	5–20
Post-viral cough	5–10
Chronic bronchitis	5–10
Bronchiectasis	5–10
ACE inhibitor induced cough	5–10
Unexplained	5–40

ACE, angiotensin converting enzyme

simple investigations. The onset of cough with symptoms suggesting an upper or lower respiratory tract infection raises the possibility of a post-infectious cough; prominent whoops, a very troublesome nocturnal cough and cough associated with vomiting are all associated with pertussis, a condition that is increasingly recognized in school-age children and adults. Otherwise there is little evidence that information on the timing, nature, complications, and potential aggravating factors is predictive of the underlying cause of the cough.

The history and physical examination is often unremarkable, in which case the evaluation of a patient focuses on the recognition of corticosteroid responsive conditions (i.e. asthma and eosinophilic bronchitis) and extra-pulmonary factors that may be aggravating the cough such as rhinitis and gastro-oesophageal reflux. One approach to the assessment of patients with chronic cough is outlined in Figure 15.2. There is emphasis on early recognition of corticosteroid responsive cough, which can be detected easily in most cases with appropriate investigations and/or treatment trials. In contrast, the management of patients with non-eosinophilic cough can be complex, time-consuming, and expensive; it is often associated with a disappointing response to specific therapy. It must be emphasized that it is far from clear whether extra-pulmonary factors implicated in causing cough are aggravating a pre-existing tendency to cough or are the underlying cause of the cough (3). Several factors suggest the former, including the tendency for non-asthmatic chronic cough to affect middle-aged women and the frequent clinical observation that

Table 15.2 An initial evaluation of a patient with chronic cough

History	Cough: onset, duration, character, triggers
	Sputum (volume, character)
	Smoking, occupation
	Upper respiratory tract infection
	Drug history (ACE inhibitors)
	Asthma: breathlessness, wheeze, nocturnal symptoms, atopy
	Gastro-oesophageal reflux: reflux associated symptoms
	Rhinitis: post nasal drip, sinusitis, throat clearing, nasal congestion
	Adverse quality of life: musculoskeletal chest pains, incontinence, syncope, social embarrassment, anxiety, disturbed sleep
Examination	Clubbing
	External nasal: polyps
	Oropharyngeal: signs of post nasal drip, tonsillar enlargement
	Chest: signs of airflow obstruction, crackles
Investigations	Chest radiograph
	Spirometry ± bronchodilator reversibility
	Serial peak expiratory flow
	Full blood count and eosinophil differential cell count
Optional investigations	Methacholine challenge test, induced sputum, allergen skin tests
	Sinus x-ray/CT sinus
	24 hour oesophageal pH and manometry
	CT chest/bronchoscopy in selected patients
Treatments	Directed at cause(s)

ACE: angiotensin converting enzyme; CT: computed tomography.

interventions against potential causes of chronic cough often help, but rarely cure the cough. It is perhaps best to have no preconceptions about the underlying causal factors in non-asthmatic cough and to view extra-pulmonary factors such as rhinitis and gastro-oesophageal reflux as potential aggravating factors rather than causes of the problem. This model has the advantage of providing a basis for the incomplete response to the treatment of these conditions seen in many patients; it should also stimulate research into the cause and treatment of the underlying heightened cough reflex sensitivity.

A further difficulty in evaluating patients with non-asthmatic chronic cough is that there is a poor correlation between the presence of symptoms or abnormalities on investigation of the potential aggravating factor and the success of treatment directed against that factor. Thus the diagnosis is largely secured by demonstrating improvement in the cough after a suitable trial of treatment, an approach that may be flawed because of the marked placebo effect seen with most therapies directed against chronic cough. Multiple potential aggravating factors are commonly present, which further complicates matters.

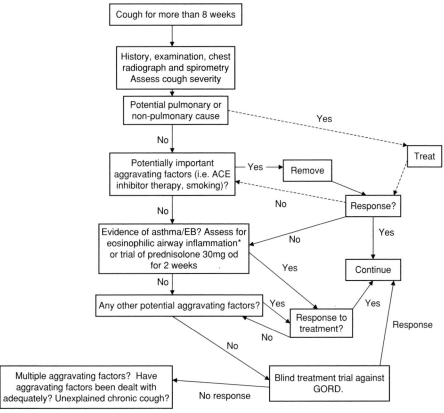

Fig. 15.2 Diagnostic algorithm for patients with chronic cough. *i.e. induced sputum eosinophils >3% and/or exhaled nitric oxide >50 ppb. ACE, angiotensin-converting enzyme; EB, eosinophilic bronchitis; GORD, gastro-oesophageal reflux disease.

Treatment trials are more easily interpreted when combined with attempts to assess cough severity objectively before and after treatment. Relapse of cough after withdrawal of treatment directed against a potential aggravating factor also increases confidence of a real causal relationship. Suitable methods to assess cough objectively include simple cough visual analogue scores, cough specific health related-quality of life scores such as the Leicester Cough Questionnaire (2) and evaluation of cough reflex sensitivity. A greater than 15-mm change in cough visual analogue score, more than 2-point change in Leicester Cough Questionnaire quality of life score, and a/or two doubling dose change in the concentration of capsaicin that causes two coughs could be regarded as evidence of a significant response to treatment. The remainder of this section focuses on the evaluation of the commoner conditions implicated in causing chronic cough.

Cough variant asthma/eosinophilic bronchitis

Some of the important differences between cough due to asthma/eosinophilic bronchitis and non-asthmatic chronic cough are summarized in Table 15.3. Asthma is a condition

Table 15.3 Differences between cough due to eosinophilic airways disease and cough due to other factors

	Eosinophilic airway diseases	Non-eosinophilic chronic cough
Age	Any	40–60
Gender	Equal	Female predominant
Response to corticosteroids	Good	Poor
Pathology	Eosinophilic	Non-eosinophilic
Exhaled [nitric oxide]	Raised	Low
Variable airflow obstruction	Present in asthma	Absent
Airway hyper-responsiveness	Present in asthma	Absent

characterized by airway hyper-responsiveness, and variable airflow obstruction. Most patients with asthma present with variable symptoms of cough, dyspnoea, and wheeze. A subgroup can present with an isolated chronic cough, a condition widely known as cough variant asthma. Eosinophilic bronchitis is characterized by a sputum eosinophilia, heightened cough reflex sensitivity, but no evidence of variable airflow obstruction or airway hyper-responsiveness. Both conditions are associated with eosinophilic airway inflammation but there is a difference in the site of mast cell localization in the airway with infiltration of the epithelium occurring in eosinophilic bronchitis and infiltration of the airway smooth muscle occurring in asthma (13). These differences may be responsible for the different functional associations of eosinophilic airway inflammation in asthma and eosinophilic bronchitis.

Asthma and eosinophilic bronchitis are distinguished by the demonstration of variable airflow obstruction and/or airway hyper-responsiveness. The absence of these features in eosinophilic bronchitis is a consistent finding within patients (14). However, from a clinical standpoint the distinction is not important. What is important is that the great majority of patients with cough due to asthma or eosinophilic bronchitis respond well to corticosteroid therapy. Tests suggesting the presence of eosinophilic airway inflammation such as a raised induced sputum eosinophil count, an increased peripheral blood eosinophil count, and increased exhaled nitric oxide concentration are associated with the success of corticosteroid therapy; they are arguably the most helpful way of making the distinction between cough due to asthma/eosinophilic bronchitis and non-asthmatic chronic cough (15). In the absence of these tests, current guidelines recommend a carefully controlled 2-week trial of oral prednisolone (16). Management of identified cases of asthma/eosinophilic bronchitis should then be along the lines suggested by current guidelines (Table 15.4).

Angiotensin-converting enzyme inhibitor associated cough

Approximately 8% of patients taking ACE inhibitors develop a persistent cough. The risk is higher in females and is similar with all types of angiotensin converting enzyme inhibitors. Excess cough is not seen with angiotensin-converting receptor antagonists.

Table 15.4 Specific therapy for chronic cough

Cause	Treatment
Rhinitis	Nasal corticosteroids
	Selected patients: topical ipratropium, topical decongestants, oral antihistamines, surgery
Asthma	Inhaled corticosteroids, as required inhaled bronchodilators, leukotriene antagonists
Eosinophilic bronchitis	Inhaled corticosteroids, oral corticosteroids in selected cases
GOR associated cough	Self-help measures: weight loss, smoking cessation, reduce alcohol intake, elevate head of bed, avoid eating within 2 hours of bedtime
	Acid suppression: proton pump inhibitors
	Prokinetic agents: metaclopramide in selected patients
	Surgery: laproscopic fundoplication in selected patients
Chronic bronchitis	Smoking cessation
ACE cough	Drug withdrawal. Substitution of alternative if appropriate
Post viral cough	Observation
Bronchiectasis	Chest physiotherapy and postural drainage, antibiotics
Unexplained chronic cough	Antitussives (dextromethorphan, codeine), nebulized lidocaine

ACE: angiotensin converting enzyme; GOR: gastro-oesophageal reflux.

Increased airway concentrations of airway tussive mediators such as bradykinin and prostaglandins are thought to be responsible for heightened cough reflex sensitivity and cough in patients with ACE inhibitor cough (7). The cough usually resolves within 2 months of treatment withdrawal. Persistence may suggest asthma, the onset of which has been linked to the use of ACE inhibitors (17).

Rhinitis/upper airway cough

Rhinitis, often associated with sinusitis and post-nasal drip is one of the most common conditions implicated as an aggravating factor in chronic cough. Allergy and infection are common causes of rhinitis and are thought to result in cough by mechanical stimulation from a post-nasal drip and extension of local inflammation to the pharyngeal and laryngeal area where the cough receptors are most concentrated. Patients usually report nasal congestion, nasal discharge, and facial pain, and may be aware of a post-nasal drip and the need to frequently clear their throat. Careful examination of upper airways may reveal a nasal quality to the voice, nasal polyps, sinus tenderness, inflammation of the posterior pharyngeal wall with evidence of draining secretions. Investigations for rhinitis include nasal endoscopy and x-ray or CT scan of the sinuses, which may reveal mucosal thickening and fluid levels. An ear, nose, and throat specialist opinion is helpful when there is diagnostic uncertainty or in the presence of severe disease. The mainstay of management is nasal topical corticosteroids with antihistamines if there is prominent sneezing or itching and nasal ipratropium bromide for watery nasal discharge (Table 15.4).

Gastro-oesophageal reflux

Symptoms suggesting gastro-oesophageal reflux and abnormalities of oesophageal function are common in patients with chronic cough of all age groups and the frequent clinical observation that effective treatment of gastro-oesophageal reflux is associated with improvement of cough supports a causal association. However, there is a paucity of data from good quality clinical trials supporting such an association (18). Conceivably microaspiration of oesophageal contents to the tracheobronchial tree and stimulation of neural oesophageal-tracheobronchial reflexes might occur.

Gastro-oesophageal reflux-related cough is thought to be associated with the relaxation of the lower oesophageal sphincter and often occurs during eating, talking, and on waking. Although most patients recognize heartburn, dysphagia, sore throat, globus, and dysphonia, up to a third of patients with gastro-oesophageal reflux associated cough have no such symptoms. Investigations for gastro-oesophageal reflux such as 24-hour oesophageal pH studies have limited value in the investigation of cough since they are poor predictors of response to therapy and are usually limited to patients with persistent cough despite adequate therapy or when considering more invasive therapy. Recent studies have suggested that oesophageal dysmotility and non-acid gastro-oesophageal reflux may be aggravating factors for cough but there are few data to support the routine evaluation of these conditions in the investigation of cough. In the presence of so much uncertainty it is difficult to make definitive statements about management. A reasonable approach is outlined in Table 15.4.

Chronic productive cough

A minority of patients present with a chronic productive cough, somewhat arbitrarily defined as a cough productive of more than 5mL of sputum per day. Few studies have evaluated this sub-group separately but there is a perception that they are more likely to have a definable and treatable cause for their symptoms. Bronchiectasis is commonly identified on imaging (19) and appropriate physiotherapy input with antibiotics might lead to important benefits. Chronic bronchitis is a common cause of cough in smokers and may occur in non-smokers with dusty occupations. By definition, patients have a productive morning cough for more than 3 months/year. Community studies have shown that active smoking is associated with a 2–3-fold (20) and passive smoking a 1.3–1.6-fold (21) increase in the prevalence of cough and other respiratory symptoms including sputum production. There is good evidence of a dose–response relationship and the prevalence of cough is reduced to near normal in ex-smokers. This strongly suggests that the effect of smoking on cough is reversible. Smoking cessation is essential in all patients with a troublesome chronic cough.

Diffuse panbronchiolitis is a well-recognized cause of corticosteroid resistant adult onset chronic productive cough in Japan and other parts of South East Asia (22). It is an important diagnosis to consider as treatment with low dose macrolide antibiotics is associated with a sticking improvement which appears to be independent of the antimicrobial effects of these drugs. Patients with diffuse panbronchiolitis typically have sinusitis and prominent small airway changes such as centrilobular nodules and tree-in-bud shadows on imaging. Whether less clinically overt cases occur in a general productive cough population is unclear.

Other causes of chronic cough

Community surveys suggest that most coughs related to upper respiratory tract infections resolve within 3 weeks. However, the cough can take several months to resolve in a small proportion of subjects. The infection in most cases remains unidentified but respiratory viruses, *Mycoplasma pneumoniae*, *Chlamydia pneumoniae*, and *Bordetella pertussis* have been implicated in adults. Other conditions recently reported to be associated with isolated chronic cough include asymptomatic enlarged tonsils (23), obstructive sleep apnoea (24), Horner's syndrome (25), and familial peripheral neuropathy (26). The mechanism of the associations remains to be determined. Further study is required as a better understanding may increase our understanding of chronic cough and may open up new treatment possibilities.

Unexplained chronic cough

Cough remains unexplained after extensive investigations and treatment trials in up to 40% of patients (27). These patients are predominantly middle-aged females; they have objective evidence of airway abnormalities including increased cough reflex sensitivity and airway inflammation. Organ-specific autoimmune diseases, a peripheral blood lymphopenia, and a mild bronchoalveolar lavage lymphocytosis are common suggesting that the airway abnormalities might have an auto-immune basis (28, 29). Patients with unexplained chronic cough suffer considerable physical and psychological morbidity which, in some domains, can be equivalent to that experienced by patients with severe COPD (1). Some patients with unexplained chronic cough are labelled with a diagnosis of psychogenic cough although there is little evidence to support this view and it is perhaps more likely that any abnormal illness behaviour is secondary to the adverse impact of cough on psychosocial aspects of quality of life. Drug therapy for idiopathic chronic cough is disappointing and is largely limited to non-specific antitussive therapy such as dextromethorphan, codeine, and drugs with weak evidence of benefit such as baclofen and nebulized local anaesthetics (lidocaine, mepivicaine). There is therefore a large unmet need for better antitussive treatment in these patients.

Treatment of chronic cough

Treatment directed at the specific cause of chronic cough is summarized in Table 15.4. Using the anatomical diagnostic protocol, success rates of up to 95% in the management of chronic cough have been reported although there is wide variability in the reported literature. The success rate goes down to 60–80% in specialist cough clinics, possibly due to the complexity of cases referred. Reassessment of the patient after treatment and excluding additional aggravating factors or causes form an integral part of managing a patient with chronic cough. A common dilemma faced by physicians managing patients with chronic cough is that the diagnosis of cough often depends on successful trials of treatment, which if unsuccessful leads to the difficult question as to whether the underlying condition has not responded or is not responsible for the cough. In some situations the use of objective tests to make a diagnosis and careful validation of the effect of therapy and withdrawal of this therapy for the underlying condition should minimize this problem.

General supportive care

A recent study has shown improvement in chronic cough in a randomized placebo controlled trial of a speech therapy intervention (30); similar benefits have been shown in an uncontrolled study of outpatient physiotherapy (31). The key components of these interventions are unclear. An important part of the advice is voluntary cough suppression suggesting that excess coughing may be partly due to the continuation of a vicious cycle where coughing leads to airway trauma and activation of the cough reflex. More research in this important area is needed.

Patients presenting with common cough fear serious disease and a relentless deterioration in their already troublesome symptoms. An important part of general supportive care is to address these concerns head on. The majority of patients with chronic cough can be reassured that they do not have serious pathology, and although relatively little is known about the long-term prognosis, what is known is reassuring.

Antitussive therapies

It is becoming clear that in a significant number of patients the cause of the heightened cough reflex will remain at least partly unexplained and that treatments directed against potential aggravating factors will not achieve perfect results. In many such patients there is a need for antitussive therapies. Codeine and dextromethorphan are the most commonly prescribed opioid-derived antitussives. However, clinical trial data are not consistent (32, 33) and there remains uncertainty about the role of these agents in the management of chronic cough. The use of morphine and diamorphine has been restricted to the severe painful and distressing cough occurring in advanced lung cancer. There is evidence of efficacy of a slow-release formulation of morphine in chronic cough (34) but whether this agent can be justified in this setting is unclear. Lignocaine delivered by aerosol or nebulizer has been used to treat chronic cough (35) although good evidence of the efficacy and safety of this approach is lacking.

Potentially new antitussive therapies are summarized in Table 15.5. Much of the existing work evaluating the pharmacological manipulation of the cough reflex is limited as it has been carried out in animal models that are poorly predictive of effects in man. Moreover, those agents that have been investigated in man have been tested against models of questionable relevance to the at-need population including simple capsaicin challenge protocols in normal volunteers and subjectively assessed cough in patients

Table 15.5 Potential new antitussive agents

Target	Agent	Comment
Peripheral opioid receptors	BW443C (μ-opioid receptor agonist, SB-221122 (δ-opioid receptor agonist	BW443C effective in animal models; no efficacy against capsaicin-induced cough in man (36). SB-221122 inhibits citric acid induced cough in guinea pigs (37). No human data
NOP$_1$ receptor	Nociceptin	Effective against mechanical and capsaicin-induced cough in animal models (38). No human data
Transient receptor potential vanilloid receptor-1 (TRPV-1)	Capsazepine, iodo-resiniferatoxin	Activated by capsaicin and protons. Expression is increased in airway nerves of patients with chronic cough (4). Capsazepine blocks capsaicin and citric acid-induced cough in animal models (39); iodo-resiniferatoxin is more potent (40). No human data
Bradykinin B$_2$ receptor	Icatibant and HOE-140 (both B$_2$ receptor antagonsts)	Icantibant inhibits citric acid-induced cough (41) and HOE-140 inhibits ACE inhibitor associated increase in the cough reflex in animal models (7). No data in man
Tachykinin receptor	CP-99994 (NK$_1$ antagonist), SR-48968 (NK$_2$ antagonist), SB-235375 (NK$_3$ antagonist)	CP-99994 ineffective against hypertonic saline-induced cough in asthma (42). SR-48968 and SB-235375 inhibit citric acid induced cough in animal models (43, 44)
Cannabinoids	JWH-133 (CB$_2$ agonist)	Inhibits citric acid induced cough in animal models (45). No human data
Ion channel modulators	NS-1619 (Opens large-conductance Ca^{2+}-activated channel), pinacidil (K$^+$ channel opener, Furosemide (Na/Cl cotransport inhibitor)	NS-1619 inhibits citric acid induced cough (46) and pinacidil capsaicin induced cough (47) in animal models. Inhaled furosemide inhibits cough induced by low chloride solutions but not by capsaicin in man (48). The mode of action is unknown.
GABA$_B$ receptor	Baclofen (GABA$_B$ agonist)	Baclofen inhibits capsaicin induced cough via a central effect in animal models (49); also active in man (50)

with COPD. There is an urgent need for clinical trials of new drugs using objective measures of cough severity and frequency as well as cough specific quality of life and symptom scores in patients with chronic cough.

Cough in malignancy and palliative care

A new or changed cough is the commonest mode of presentation of lung cancer, reported by 70% of patients. Cough is also reported by 25% of patients with advanced cancers outside the lung; in many cases due to the presence of pulmonary or mediastinal metastases but also as a result of pulmonary toxicity secondary to chemotherapy and radiotherapy.

Bleomycin is particularly likely to cause pulmonary toxicity and does so in a dose-dependent and, to some extent, predictable manner. Chronic cough can occur as a result of permanent lung damage due to chemotherapy and radiotherapy given well in the past. Cryptogenic organizing pneumonia (COP), which has been associated with radiotherapy, is a particularly important condition to pick up as there is a high potential for confusion with metastatic disease but it responds well to corticosteroid treatment. A common scenario is for patients with COP to present with a common cough and flitting chest x-ray changes some time after radiotherapy. Patients with breast cancer also commonly cough as a result of minor lung scarring secondary to past radiotherapy. In the terminal phases of cancer care, cough may reflect sputum retention and respiratory tract infection as a result of opiate therapy, dehydration, and inhibition of cough by pain.

Cough is also important in non-malignant terminal conditions such as AIDS, neurodegenerative diseases, heart failure, and interstitial lung disease. Persistent dry cough in patients with interstitial lung disease is a particular clinical challenge as the severity of cough often bears little relation to the severity of other symptoms or the underlying lung disease. Moreover, treatment directed at the lung disease is often ineffective against the cough. Sometimes cough is due to identifiable and treatable comorbid conditions such as airway inflammation, rhinitis, or gastro-oesophageal reflux but this is the exception rather than the rule and most patients with cough associated with interstitial lung disease have an important unmet need for better treatments.

Opioid therapy is the mainstay of palliation of cough in the setting of cancer or other terminal illnesses. In cases where retained secretions are an important cause of the cough, physiotherapy, antibiotics, humidified oxygen, and mucolytic agents may help. Some patients develop a death rattle in the advanced terminal stages of their disease as a result of thick mucus retained in the upper and larger intrathoracic airways. This can be distressing to patients, relatives, and their carers; it can be helped by local suction and by injections of a sedative antimuscarinic agent such as hyoscine.

Cough in children

There are some important differences in chronic cough in children and adults. Conditions such as lung cancer and pulmonary fibrosis are extremely rare in children whereas cystic fibrosis, congenital abnormalities, and inhaled foreign body are more common, particularly in children who have always coughed or in whom the cough has a clearly defined beginning. Cough due to RSV and pertussis infection is more common and both infections are more likely to lead to a severe and chronic cough in children.

The opportunities to investigate children can be more limited than adults so clinical features and physical signs are important. Paediatricians commonly draw a distinction between cough in an otherwise well child, which may be normal and physiological or due to asthma, eosinophilic bronchitis, aggravating factors such as rhinitis or gastro-oesophageal reflux disease, or unexplained; and cough due to a specific serious disease. Pointers towards the latter include other respiratory symptoms, persistent physical signs in the chest or abnormalities on chest x-ray or spirometry, a chronic productive cough, and failure to thrive. Non-specific, unexplained dry cough in a well child with no abnormal physical signs or investigation findings is common as is repeated cough linked to viral upper-respiratory tract infection. Both are thought to have an excellent prognosis and it is important that clinicians guard against over-investigating and over-treating patients.

Conclusion

All pulmonary and many non-pulmonary conditions can present with cough. Most will be evident after a simple clinical assessment that includes a history, physical examination, a chest radiograph, and a spirogram. Cough that remains unexplained after such an assessment is a common reason for referral to secondary care. Potential causes include asthma, eosinophilic bronchitis, rhinitis and gastro-oesophageal reflux. Satisfactory outcomes can be achieved in some patients with a management strategy that includes targeted investigations and carefully controlled treatment trials. However, complete cure is often not possible, particularly in patients with cough thought to be due to extra-pulmonary factors, and a significant number of predominantly middle-aged women have unexplained chronic cough. Whether this reflects failure to identify important causes or inadequate treatment of established factors is unclear. The considerable morbidity due to unexplained chronic cough needs to be better recognized and there is an urgent need for better treatments.

References

1. French CL, Irwin RS, Curley FJ, Krikorian CJ. Impact of chronic cough on quality of life. *Arch Intern Med* 1998; **158**(15):1657–61.
2. Birring SS, Prudon B, Carr AJ, Singh SJ, Morgan MD, Pavord ID. Development of a symptom specific health status measure for patients with chronic cough: Leicester Cough Questionnaire (LCQ). *Thorax* 2003; **58**(4):339–43.
3. Pavord ID, Chung KF. Management of chronic cough. *Lancet* 2008; **371**(9621):1375–84.
4. Groneberg DA, Niimi A, Dinh QT, *et al*. Increased expression of transient receptor potential vanilloid-1 in airway nerves of chronic cough. *Am J Respir Crit Care Med* 2004; **170**(12):1276–80.
5. McLeod RL, Fernandez X, Correll CC, *et al*. TRPV1 antagonists attenuate antigen-provoked cough in ovalbumin sensitized guinea pigs. *Cough* 2006; **2**:10.
6. Choudry NB, Fuller RW, Pride NB. Sensitivity of the human cough reflex: effect of inflammatory mediators prostaglandin E2, bradykinin, and histamine. *Am Rev Respir Dis* 1989; **140**(1):137–41.
7. Fox AJ, Lalloo UG, Belvisi MG, Bernareggi M, Chung KF, Barnes PJ. Bradykinin-evoked sensitization of airway sensory nerves: a mechanism for ACE-inhibitor cough. *Nat Med* 1996; **2**(7):814–17.
8. Mazzone SB, McLennan L, McGovern AE, Egan GF, Farrell MJ. Representation of capsaicin-evoked urge-to-cough in the human brain using functional magnetic resonance imaging. *Am J Respir Crit Care Med* 2007; **176**(4):327–32.
9. Birring SS, Parker D, Brightling CE, Bradding P, Wardlaw AJ, Pavord ID. Induced sputum inflammatory mediator concentrations in chronic cough. *Am J Respir Crit Care Med* 2004; **169**(1):15–19.
10. Birring SS, Fleming T, Matos S, Raj AA, Evans DH, Pavord ID. The Leicester Cough Monitor: preliminary validation of an automated cough detection system in chronic cough. *Eur Respir J* 2008; **31**(5):1013–18.

11. Yousaf N, Matos S, Birring SS, Pavord ID. Factors affecting cough frequency in a mixed population. *Thorax* 2009; **64**:A151.

12. Prudon B, Birring SS, Vara DD, Hall AP, Thompson JP, Pavord ID. Cough and glottic-stop reflex sensitivity in health and disease. *Chest* 2005; **127**(2):550–7.

13. Brightling CE, Bradding P, Symon FA, Holgate ST, Wardlaw AJ, Pavord ID. Mast-cell infiltration of airway smooth muscle in asthma. *N Engl J Med* 2002; **346**(22):1699–705.

14. Berry MA, Hargadon B, McKenna S, *et al.* Observational study of the natural history of eosinophilic bronchitis. *Clin Exp Allergy* 2005; **35**(5):598–601.

15. Chatkin JM, Ansarin K, Silkoff PE, McClean P, Gutierrez C, Zamel N, *et al.* Exhaled nitric oxide as a noninvasive assessment of chronic cough. *Am J Respir Crit Care Med* 1999; **159**(6):1810–13.

16. Morice AH, McGarvey L, Pavord I. Recommendations for the management of cough in adults. *Thorax* 2006; **61**(Suppl 1):i1–24.

17. Lunde H, Hedner T, Samuelsson O, *et al.* Dyspnoea, asthma, and bronchospasm in relation to treatment with angiotensin converting enzyme inhibitors. *BMJ* 1994; **308**(6920):18–21.

18. Chang AB, Lasserson TJ, Kiljander TO, Connor FL, Gaffney JT, Garske LA. Systematic review and meta-analysis of randomised controlled trials of gastro-oesophageal reflux interventions for chronic cough associated with gastro-oesophageal reflux. *BMJ* 2006; **332**(7532):11–17.

19. Kastelik JA, Aziz I, Ojoo JC, Thompson RH, Redington AE, Morice AH. Investigation and management of chronic cough using a probability-based algorithm. *Eur Respir J* 2005; **25**(2): 235–43.

20. Jansen DF, Schouten JP, Vonk JM, *et al.* Smoking and airway hyperresponsiveness especially in the presence of blood eosinophilia increase the risk to develop respiratory symptoms: a 25-year follow-up study in the general adult population. *Am J Respir Crit Care Med* 1999; **160**(1):259–64.

21. Janson C, Chinn S, Jarvis D, Zock JP, Toren K, Burney P. Effect of passive smoking on respiratory symptoms, bronchial responsiveness, lung function, and total serum IgE in the European Community Respiratory Health Survey: a cross-sectional study. *Lancet* 2001; **358**(9299):2103–9.

22. Koyama H, Geddes DM. Erythromycin and diffuse panbronchiolitis. *Thorax* 1997; **52**(10):915–18.

23. Birring SS, Passant C, Patel RB, Prudon B, Murty GE, Pavord ID. Chronic tonsillar enlargement and cough: preliminary evidence of a novel and treatable cause of chronic cough. *Eur Respir J* 2004; **23**(2):199–201.

24. Chan KK, Ing AJ, Laks L, Cossa G, Rogers P, Birring SS. Chronic cough in patients with sleep-disordered breathing. *Eur Respir J* 2010; **35**(2):368–72.

25. Kimber J, Mitchell D, Mathias CJ. Chronic cough in the Holmes-Adie syndrome: association in five cases with autonomic dysfunction. *J Neurol Neurosurg Psychiatry* 1998; **65**(4):583–6.

26. Kok C, Kennerson ML, Spring PJ, Ing AJ, Pollard JD, Nicholson GA. A locus for hereditary sensory neuropathy with cough and gastroesophageal reflux on chromosome 3p22–p24. *Am J Hum Genet* 2003; **73**(3):632–7.

27. McGarvey LP. Idiopathic chronic cough: a real disease or a failure of diagnosis? *Cough* 2005 23(1):9.

28. Birring SS, Brightling CE, Symon FA, Barlow SG, Wardlaw AJ, Pavord ID. Idiopathic chronic cough: association with organ specific autoimmune disease and bronchoalveolar lymphocytosis. *Thorax* 2003; **58**(12):1066–70.

29. Birring SS, Murphy AC, Scullion JE, Brightling CE, Browning M, Pavord ID. Idiopathic chronic cough and organ-specific autoimmune diseases: a case-control study. *Respir Med* 2004; **98**(3): 242–6.

30. Vertigan AE, Theodoros DG, Gibson PG, Winkworth AL. Efficacy of speech pathology management for chronic cough: a randomised placebo controlled trial of treatment efficacy. *Thorax* 2006; **61**(12):1065–9.

31. Watkin G, Willig BW, Mutalithas K, Pavord IDBSS. Improvement in health status following outpatient chest physiotherapy for patients with refractory chronic cough. *Thorax* 2006; **61**:iii92.

32. Smith J, Owen E, Earis J, Woodcock A. Effect of codeine on objective measurement of cough in chronic obstructive pulmonary disease. *J Allergy Clin Immunol* 2006; **117**(4):831–15.

33. Matthys H, Bleicher B, Bleicher U. Dextromethorphan and codeine: objective assessment of antitussive activity in patients with chronic cough. *J Int Med Res* 1983; **11**(2):92–100.

34. Morice AH, Menon MS, Mulrennan SA, *et al.* Opiate therapy in chronic cough. *Am J Respir Crit Care Med* 2007; **175**(4):312–15.

35. Howard P, Cayton RM, Brennan SR, Anderson PB. Lignocaine aerosol and persistent cough. *Br J Dis Chest* 1977; **71**(1):19–24.

36. Choudry NB, Gray SJ, Posner J, Fuller RW. The effect of 443C81, a mu opioid receptor agonist, on the response to inhaled capsaicin in healthy volunteers. *Br J Clin Pharmacol* 1991; **32**(5):633–6.

37. Kotzer CJ, Hay DW, Dondio G, Giardina G, Petrillo P, Underwood DC. The antitussive activity of delta-opioid receptor stimulation in guinea pigs. *J Pharmacol Exp Ther* 2000; **292**(2):803–9.

38. McLeod RL, Parra LE, Mutter JC, *et al.* Nociceptin inhibits cough in the guinea-pig by activation of ORL(1) receptors. *Br J Pharmacol* 2001; **132**(6):1175–8.

39. Lalloo UG, Fox AJ, Belvisi MG, Chung KF, Barnes PJ. Capsazepine inhibits cough induced by capsaicin and citric acid but not by hypertonic saline in guinea pigs. *J Appl Physiol* 1995; **79**(4):1082–7.

40. Trevisani M, Milan A, Gatti R, *et al.* Antitussive activity of iodo-resiniferatoxin in guinea pigs. *Thorax* 2004; **59**(9):769–72.

41. Featherstone RL, Parry JE, Evans DM, *et al.* Mechanism of irritant-induced cough: studies with a kinin antagonist and a kallikrein inhibitor. *Lung* 1996; **174**(4):269–75.

42. Fahy JV, Wong HH, Geppetti P, *et al.* Effect of an NK1 receptor antagonist (CP-99,994) on hypertonic saline-induced bronchoconstriction and cough in male asthmatic subjects. *Am J Respir Crit Care Med* 1995; **152**(3):879–84.

43. Girard V, Naline E, Vilain P, Emonds-Alt X, Advenier C. Effect of the two tachykinin antagonists, SR 48968 and SR 140333, on cough induced by citric acid in the unanaesthetized guinea pig. *Eur Respir J* 1995; **8**(7):1110–14.

44. Hay DW, Giardina GA, Griswold DE, *et al.* Nonpeptide tachykinin receptor antagonists. III. SB 235375, a low central nervous system-penetrant, potent and selective neurokinin-3 receptor antagonist, inhibits citric acid-induced cough and airways hyper-reactivity in guinea pigs. *J Pharmacol Exp Ther* 2002; **300**(1):314–23.

45. Patel HJ, Birrell MA, Crispino N, *et al.* Inhibition of guinea-pig and human sensory nerve activity and the cough reflex in guinea-pigs by cannabinoid (CB2) receptor activation. *Br J Pharmacol* 2003; **140**(2):261–8.

46. Fox AJ, Barnes PJ, Venkatesan P, Belvisi MG. Activation of large conductance potassium channels inhibits the afferent and efferent function of airway sensory nerves in the guinea pig. *J Clin Invest* 1997; **99**(3):513–19.

47. Morita K, Kamei J. Involvement of ATP-sensitive K(+) channels in the anti-tussive effect of moguisteine. *Eur J Pharmacol* 2000; **395**(2):161–4.

48. Ventresca PG, Nichol GM, Barnes PJ, Chung KF. Inhaled furosemide inhibits cough induced by low chloride content solutions but not by capsaicin. *Am Rev Respir Dis* 1990; **142**(1):143–6.

49. Bolser DC, DeGennaro FC, O'Reilly S, *et al.* Peripheral and central sites of action of GABA-B agonists to inhibit the cough reflex in the cat and guinea pig. *Br J Pharmacol* 1994; **113**(4):1344–8.

50. Dicpinigaitis PV, Dobkin JB. Antitussive effect of the GABA-agonist baclofen. *Chest* 1997; **111**(4):996–9.

Chapter 16

Expectoration: pathophysiology, measurement, and therapy

Alyn H. Morice

The therapy of expectoration

Expectoration—the removal of secretions from the chest—is a symptom which may be triggered by a wide range of respiratory conditions. Because of this diversity, an extensive armamentarium of therapeutic options may be used which are specifically directed at individual causal agents. In general this strategy has a high success rate. Alternatively (and usually less efficaciously), therapy can be given to improve the act of expectoration itself or to suppress the desire to expectorate. Finally, expectoration can be aided by manoeuvres designed to increase the ease and convenience of expectoration.

Because treatment of the *cause* of expectoration is our most successful strategy, efforts should be directed to establishing a diagnosis. There are two major subdivisions of disease leading to expectoration. Firstly, inflammatory conditions such as asthma or bronchiectasis are frequently associated with copious expectoration. Removal of the inflammatory stimulus by either specific therapy aimed at a particular organism or generalized anti-inflammatory therapy (such as the use of inhaled or parenteral corticosteroids for asthma), leads to reduction of symptoms. Secondly, neoplastic diseases, most notably alveolar cell carcinoma, produce expectoration through uncontrolled production of mucus. Specific therapy to control expectoration in individual conditions will not be considered further in this chapter other than to list the main therapeutic areas in Table 16.1.

Pathophysiology

The desire to expectorate arises from sensory nerves within the upper airways stimulating the cough reflex. In the normal lung, airways secretions contain a mixture of submucosal gland products together with secretions of the airways surface cells such as goblet cells. The resultant mixture contains mucous glycoproteins and electrolytes. The airways' surface liquid forms two layers, a sol phase which has contact with the cilia and a gel phase which rests on top and traps inhaled particles. The tips of the epithelial cell cilia drive the mucous blanket towards the upper airways and on their return stroke, the cilia dip from the gel phase into the sol phase (1). As the mucus blanket travels centrally water and electrolytes are reabsorbed and the volume of secretions is reduced. It has been suggested that approximately 10mL of secretions are expectorated daily in normal subjects, but quantification has proven difficult (2).

Table 16.1 Specific disease-related therapy for expectoration

Underlying diagnosis	Specific therapy for expectoration
Bronchiectasis	Antibiotics
	Intermittent
	Continuous (dependent on bacteria (sensitivities) or non-specific (e.g. high-dose amoxicillin or amoxicillin with probenecid))
Cystic fibrosis	RhDNase
Asthma, eosinophilic bronchitis, and chronic obstructive pulmonary disease	Corticosteroids inhaled or oral bronchodilators
Alveolar cell carcinoma	Macrolides, resection, lung transplantation

Expectoration may be due to excessive mucus production or poor clearance. In most diseases the excess secretions are produced by a combination of these factors. Thus in cystic fibrosis, excessive sodium absorption reduces the salt and consequently water content of the airways surface liquid. This increases mucus viscoelasticity and decreases ciliary motility. In addition, colonization of the airways by bacteria causes inflammation and abnormal secreted mucins which further impair mucociliary clearance. Release of pro-inflammatory cytokines such as tumour necrosis factor alpha, interleukin (IL)-1 beta, IL-8, and IL-6 (3) enhance macrophage activity giving rise to a cycle of lung damage and repair. Thus, a combination of poor clearance and increased mucus production summate to produce excessive mucus requiring expectoration.

The clinical approach to expectorant therapy

Measurement

In many studies of cough and expectoration the endpoints chosen to demonstrate efficacy are difficult to translate into clinical practice. Tracheobronchial clearance as measured by gamma camera studies has been recommended as the gold standard for assessing mucoactive agents (4) but studies using this methodology do not accurately assess small airways and are unable to examine the effect of agents on mucus production as opposed to clearance. Measurement of sputum volume is similarly difficult to interpret. A decrease in expectorated volume *may* indicate clinical improvement but many patients claim that their inability to expectorate thickened secretions is a major cause of morbidity due to excessive ineffective cough. Measures of lung function may provide useful information and it is hypothesized that the improvements in FEV_1 (forced expiratory volume in 1s) seen in diseases characterized by limited reversibility of airflow obstruction such as chronic obstructive pulmonary disease (COPD) and cystic fibrosis are due to reduced mucus secretion. The two most useful methods of clinical assessment in chronic airflow obstruction, whilst they are not focused specifically at expectoration, are probably quality of life and exacerbation rate. Simple questionnaires are used to evaluate quality of life in expectoration (5, 6). In the ISOLDE study (7) of inhaled steroids in severe COPD, the St Georges Questionnaire demonstrated clinically useful improvements in quality of life which were associated with a reduction in exacerbation rate. Unfortunately very few studies in expectoration provide us with such large numbers of patients and much of the evidence concerning therapy is of poor quality.

Mucolytic agents

The lysis of pathologically thickened mucus in order to aid expectoration has been attempted by two strategies each directed at combating the underlying pathological processes causing this increased sputum viscosity. Firstly the abnormal mucins released during airways inflammation can be targeted by preventing cysteine bridging between their glycoprotein molecules, by using sulphydryl moieties. *In vitro*, agents such as acetylcysteine, reduce sputum viscosity (8). However, the *therapeutic* effects of such drugs are debated. Two studies show no demonstrable effect of oral N-acetylcysteine and S-carboxymethylcysteine on mucociliary clearance (9, 10). In contrast studies using clinical endpoints have demonstrated beneficial effects of mucolytic therapy (11, 12). Oral acetylcysteine reduces the exacerbation rate in chronic bronchitis, reduces days of illness and has been claimed to improve well-being (13). The two largest studies have shown little effect (14, 15) and a recent Cochrane review concluded there was a slight but clinically significant reduction in exacerbation (16).

The alternate strategy for mucolysis is to disrupt the tangled mesh of DNA derived from dead bacteria and leucocytes. *In vitro*, enzymatic degradation of DNA is a highly effective means of reducing sputum viscosity. Its use has been associated with modest improvements in spirometry and a reduced rate of exacerbations in cystic fibrosis (17). This specific condition is described in detail elsewhere in this volume. In exacerbations of COPD, DNase has not been a success. A multinational study of DNase following admission to hospital with a COPD exacerbation was abandoned because of increased mortality in the active treatment arm. Surprisingly, the results of this study have never been published in full (18).

Mucolytic therapy can be used in an alternative fashion. Patients presenting with mucus plugging leading to distal segmented or lobar collapse have been treated with acetylcysteine or rhDNase instilled through the bronchoscope. Whilst it is logical, this therapy has not been subjected to randomized controlled study and it could be difficult to differentiate any mucolytic effects from the effects of the procedure itself, including suction.

Secretagogues

The hypothesis that expectoration will be eased by increasing the volume and liquidity of secretions is attractive. However, evidence for clinical benefit from the group of substances classed in pharmacopoeias as secretagogues is tenuous. They are mainly compounds which in previous times have been used as emetics. Guaifenesin, bromhexine, iodide, ipecacuanha, and ammonium chloride have all been used and have remained in the national formularies of many countries particularly as part of a combination of over the counter cough remedies. Of these agents guaifenesin (19) has been shown to increase mucus secretion in animals, but clinical evidence, mainly in chronic bronchitis, is either of poor quality or negative (20–22).

Mucokinetic agents

The ideal palliative therapy for intractable expectoration would increase the rate of ciliary mucus transport to enable the patient to clear secretions before bronchial obstruction, infection and inflammation supervenes. Two methods of achieving this therapeutic goal can be envisaged. Either the properties of the mucus itself can be altered to enable more rapid transport or the mucociliary escalator can be stimulated to enhance tracheobronchial clearance.

Water and saline

Inhalations of water, steam and saline have been used for centuries to promote expectoration. Most modern interest has centred on the use of hypertonic saline. Even in normal subjects inhalation of 4–7% saline causes expectoration and such 'induced' sputum may be used for diagnostic and research purposes. In cystic fibrosis we have used hypertonic saline to induce sputum in patients who are unable or unwilling to provide bacteriological samples. The main problem with routine clinical use is the propensity for bronchoconstriction in patients with reactive airways. Pretreatment with bronchodilators will prevent this side effect. Therapy with hypertonic saline in cystic fibrosis has been shown to improve FEV_1 when compared with isotonic saline (23). It is interesting to speculate whether this therapeutic effect has any specific link to the proposed pathophysiological defect in cystic fibrosis, namely an alteration in chloride handling in the airways surface liquid (24).

The use of isotonic saline and water as expectorants is previously widespread, either in the form of nebulized solutions or as steam inhalations. In contrast to hypertonic saline the evidence for efficacy of these treatments is poor although a single study has reported benefit when combined with physiotherapy (25).

Beta agonists and other bronchodilators

The use of nebulized beta agonists to aid expectoration has some rational basis. Beta agonists have been shown to stimulate ciliary beat frequency *in vitro* and some studies *in vivo* have shown effects on mucociliary transport (26). However, in patients with chest disease as opposed to normal subjects the effects of beta agonists are of doubtful clinical significance (27). Ipratropium bromide has no effect on mucociliary clearance (28).

Despite the poor scientific base for the use of bronchodilators as expectorants they are widely prescribed. Patients with respiratory failure from obstructive pulmonary disease frequently comment that the nebulizers aid expectoration. It is my own practice to offer patients a trial of nebulized saline or bronchodilator and to continue therapy with the preferred substance. If saline is chosen it is cheaper, and does not have side effects such as tremor and hypoxemia secondary to alterations in V/Q matching after $beta_2$ agonists.

Anticholinergics

The anticholinergic drugs act by blocking muscarinic receptors both on airway smooth muscle and preganglionically on airway nerves. Because there is intrinsic cholinergic tone, particularly in chronic pulmonary disease, these agents are effective bronchodilators, but their activity in expectoration is variable. Tertiary ammonium compounds such as atropine and hyoscine are claimed to reduce bronchial gland secretion although no change in sputum viscosity is seen (29). A number of studies have demonstrated a decrease in mucociliary transport with tertiary ammonium compounds when given systemically to normal subjects (30–32). In contrast a considerable body of evidence suggests either no effect or an increase in mucociliary clearance with quaternary ammonium compounds in patients (33–35). No effect on sputum rheology is seen in chronic bronchitis (28).

Whatever the explanation for the contrasting effects on mucociliary clearance seen with the two classes of antimuscarinic the differential effects can be exploited clinically. If bronchodilation alone is required then quaternary compounds should be used. If suppression of mucus secretion is an additional objective then systemic tertiary ammonium compounds are the treatment of choice provided the patient can tolerate the inevitable systemic side effects.

Physiotherapy for expectoration

Autogenic drainage

Unlike conventional physiotherapy, autogenic drainage is specifically designed to aid expectoration in a fashion eminently suitable for supportive and palliative care. The technique was devised by the Belgian physiotherapist Jean Chevallier and uses inspiration at increasing lung volumes to collect and then expectorate mucus (36).

It consists of three phases—unstick, collect, and evacuate. Patients begin diaphragmatic breathing at low lung volume. Inspiration is slow and initially terminates with a pause at the end of tidal respiration. Forced expiration is then performed with an open glottis down to expiratory reserve volume. As secretions begin to move the patient is encouraged to breathe at medium and then high lung volumes. When the patient has completed breathing at near total lung capacity and the secretions are felt to have progressed as far as possible they are asked to expectorate. Coughing is suppressed during the performance of autogenic drainage and the technique is described as physically undemanding and is therefore highly applicable to debilitated patients. Patient cooperation is required and it may be difficult to teach in children. Ideally a physiotherapist skilled in the technique and trained in its application should be used to initiate treatment.

Studies of autogenic drainage have compared it with conventional physiotherapy such as active cycle of breathing (ACBT). In the largest randomized study in cystic fibrosis, Miller (37) found that autogenic drainage cleared mucus faster than ACBT and that both methods improved ventilation and pulmonary function.

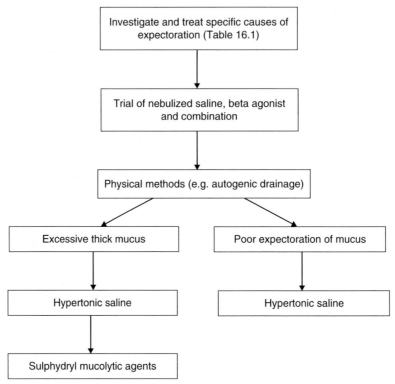

Fig. 16.1 Expectoration care pathway.

Conclusions

The most effective therapy for expectoration is aimed at the underlying pathophysiological process. If specific therapy is impossible or unhelpful then measures to aid expectoration directly by a combination of pharmacological and physical means can produce clinical benefit. Because the literature supporting the use of individual agents is, in general, of poor quality and often with conflicting conclusions, individual therapeutic trials should be undertaken to maximize patient benefit. A suggested expectoration care pathway is provided in Figure 16.1.

References

1. Lucas AM, Douglas MJ. Principals underlying ciliary activity in the respiratory tract. *Arch Otolaryngol* 1934; **20**:518–41.
2. Rogers DF. Airway goblet cells – responsive and adaptable front-line defenders. *Eur Respir J* 1994; **7**(9):1690–706.
3. Bonfield TL, Panuska JR, Konstan MW, *et al.* Inflammatory cytokines in cystic-fibrosis lungs. *Am J Respir Crit Care Med* 1995; **152**(6):2111–18.
4. Wills PJ, Cole PJ. Mucolytic and mucokinetic therapy. *Pulmonary Pharmacology & Therapeutics* 1996; **9**:197–204.

5. Curtis JR, Deyo RA, Hudson LD. Health-related quality-of-life among patients with chronic obstructive pulmonary-disease. *Thorax* 1994; **49**(2):162–70.

6. Hansen NCG, Skriver A, Brorsenriis L, *et al*. Orally-administered n-acetylcysteine may improve general well- being in patients with mild chronic-bronchitis. *Resp Med* 1994; **88**(7):531–5.

7. Burge PS. EUROSCOP, ISOLDE and the Copenhagen City Lung Study. *Thorax* 1999; **54**(4):287–8.

8. Scheffner AL, Medler EM, Jacobs LW, Sarett HP. The *in vitro* reduction in viscosity of human tracheobronchial secretions by acetylcysteine. *Am Rev Respir Dis* 1964; **90**:721–9.

9. Millar AB, Pavia D, Agnew JE, Lopezvidriero MT, Lauque D, Clarke SW. Oral n-acetylcysteine has no demonstrable effect on mucus clearances in chronic-bronchitis. *Thorax* 1984; **39**(3):238.

10. Thomson ML, Pavia D, Jones CJ, McQuiston TAC. No demonstrable effect of S-carboxymethylcysteine on clearance of secretions from the human lung. *Thorax* 1975; **30**:669–73.

11. Boman G, Backer U, Larsson S, Melander B, Wahlander L. Oral acetylcysteine reduces exacerbation rate in chronic- bronchitis - report of a trial organized by the Swedish society for pulmonary-diseases. *Eur J Respir Dis* 1983; **64**(6):405–15.

12. Rasmussen JB, Glennow C. Reduction in days of illness after long-term treatment with N-acetylcysteine controlled-release tablets in patients with chronic bronchitis. *Eur Respir J* 1988; **1**:351–5.

13. Grassi C. Long-term oral acetylcysteine in chronic bronchitis. A double-blind controlled study. *Eur J Respir Dis* 1980; **61**:93–108.

14. Decramer M, Rutten-van Molken M, Dekhuijzen PN, *et al*. Effects of N-acetylcysteine on outcomes in chronic obstructive pulmonary disease (Bronchitis Randomized on NAC Cost-Utility Study, BRONCUS): a randomised placebo-controlled trial. *Lancet* 2005; **365**(9470):1552–60.

15. Zheng JP, Kang J, Huang SG, *et al*. Effect of carbocisteine on acute exacerbation of chronic obstructive pulmonary disease (PEACE Study): a randomised placebo-controlled study. *Lancet* 2008; **371**(9629):2013–18.

16. Poole P, Black PN. Mucolytic agents for chronic bronchitis or chronic obstructive pulmonary disease. *Cochrane Database Syst Rev* 2010; **2**:CD001287.

17. Fuchs HJ, Borowitz DS, Christiansen DH, *et al*. Effect of aerosolized recombinant human DNase on exacerbations of respiratory symptoms and on pulmonary function in patients with cystic fibrosis. The Pulmozyme Study Group (see comments). *N Engl J Med* 1994; **331**(10):637–42.

18. Anon. Pulmonzyme disappoints in COPD. *Script* 1995; **2043**:16.

19. Perry WF, Boyd EM. Method for studying expectorant action in animals by direct measurement of the respiratory tract fluids. *J Pharm Exp Ther* 1941; **73**:65–77.

20. Anon. Guaiphenesin and iodide. *Drug Ther Bull* 1985; **23**:62–64.

21. Anon. A controlled trail of the effects of bromhexine on the symptoms of out-patients with chronic bronchitis. *Br J Dis Chest* 1973; **67**:49–60.

22. Guyatt GH. A controlled trial of ambroxol in chronic bronchitis. *Chest* 1987; **92**:618–20.

23. Eng PA, Morton J, Douglass JA, Riedler J, Wilson J, Robertson CF. Short-term efficacy of ultrasonically nebulized hypertonic saline in cystic fibrosis. *Pediatr Pulmonol* 1996; **21**(2):77–83.

24. Rogers DF. Physiology of airway mucus secretion and pathophysiology of hypersecretion. *Respir Care* 2007; **52**(9):1134–46.

25. Conway JH, Fleming JS, Perring S, Holgate ST. Humidification as an adjunct to chest physiotherapy in aiding tracheobronchial clearance in patients with bronchiectasis. *Resp Med* 1992; **86**(2):109–14.

26. Wong LB, Miller IF, Yeates DB. Stimulation of ciliary beat frequency by autonomic agonists – in vivo. *J Appl Physiol* 1988; **65**(2):971–81.

27. Mortensen J, Hansen A, Falk M, Nielsen IK, Groth S. Reduced effect of inhaled beta 2-adrenergic agonists on lung mucociliary clearance in patients with cystic fibrosis. *Chest* 1993; **103**(3):805–11.

28. Taylor RG, Pavia D, Agnew JE, *et al.* Effect of four weeks' high dose ipratropium bromide treatment on lung mucociliary clearance. *Thorax* 1986; **41**(4):295–300.

29. Lopez-Vidriero MT, Costello J, Clark TJ, Das I, Keal EE, Reid L. Effect of atropine on sputum production. *Thorax* 1975; **30**(5):543–47.

30. Yeates DB, Aspin N, Levison H, Jones MT, Bryan AC. Mucociliary tracheal transport rates in man. *J Appl Physiol* 1975; **39**(3):487–95.

31. Foster WM, Bergofsky EH, Bohning DE, Lippmann M, Albert, RE. Effect of adrenergic agents and their mode of action on mucociliary clearance in man. *J Appl Physiol* 1976; **41**(2):146–52.

32. Pavia D, Thomson ML. Inhibition of mucociliary clearance from the human lung by hyoscine. *Lancet* 1971; **1**(7696):449–50.

33. Pavia D, Bateman JR, Sheahan NF, Clarke SW. Effect of ipratropium bromide on mucociliary clearance and pulmonary function in reversible airways obstruction. *Thorax* 1979; **34**(4):501–7.

34. Pavia D, Bateman JR, Sheahan NF, Clarke SW. Clearance of lung secretions in patients with chronic bronchitis: effect of terbutaline and ipratropium bromide aerosols. *Eur J Respir Dis* 1980; **61**(5):245–53.

35. Bell JA, Bluestein BM, Danta I, Wanner A. Effect of inhaled ipratropium bromide on tracheal mucociliary transport in bronchial asthma. *Mt Sinai J Med* 1984; **51**(2):215–17.

36. Schoni MH. Autogenic drainage – a modern approach to physiotherapy in cystic-fibrosis. *J R Soc Med* 1989; **82**:32–7.

37. Miller S, Hall DO, Clayton CB, Nelson R. Chest physiotherapy in cystic-fibrosis – a comparative-study of autogenic drainage and the active cycle of breathing techniques with postural drainage. *Thorax* 1995; **50**(2):165–9.

Part 6

Pain

Chapter 17

Pain assessment in respiratory disease

Elaine Cachia, Jason Boland, and Sam H. Ahmedzai

Introduction

Pain is a subjective experience, and influenced by the individual's personality and complex multifactorial networks involving emotions, memory, and cognition, and pathological and genetic factors. Also the response to pain is based on the particular situation and the appropriate response. Chest pain is a common symptom and numerous structures within the respiratory system can give rise to a painful sensation including chest wall and musculoskeletal, pleura, vascular, and lung parenchyma and airway; pain can also be referred to the chest from distant sites. Most patients will present to the doctor when their underlying disorder leads to a symptom, especially pain.

Pain arising in the chest can be either nociceptive and/or neuropathic in origin. Nociceptive pain can be divided into somatic or visceral pain mechanisms; somatic pain is usually well-defined and located (e.g. inflammatory pain) whilst visceral pain generates a dull ache which is often poorly-localized (e.g. stimuli to lung interstitium).

The different aetiologies of chest pain can range from the trivial to the potentially life-threatening and therefore it is of utmost importance to have a good anatomical knowledge of the structures within the thorax, the sensory innervations, and associated pathology likely to give rise to chest pain and how this arises (see Chapter 2).

It is important to ascertain any prior beliefs and misconceptions that the patient may have about pain and its treatment as these can affect compliance. Common fears about pain treatment include addiction, side effects, that they will get tolerant to their analgesic effects before they 'really need them', and that they are entering the terminal phase of their illness (1). Therefore, discussion with the patient and/or their family about the goals of care, hopes, wishes, and expectations must take place as this will allow the clinician to decide on whether investigations and interventions are relevant.

Evaluation of pain

Pain can be either a new manifestation of the respiratory disease and therefore the presenting symptom or it can be a continuing symptom of a known condition. Diagnostic evaluation begins with a review of all reported symptoms and a physical examination and this would lead to a list of differential diagnoses which can be further refined with appropriate investigations.

The speed of onset of pain is an indication as to whether the cause is more of a life-threatening situation, like acute chest pain following a myocardial infarction, rather than a dull ache that has been present for months. The severity of the pain does not usually influence the diagnosis but helps the clinician judge the speed of assessment and appropriate management.

Assessment

History

Pain should be evaluated with a systematic approach as this may help differentiate between respiratory, cardiac, musculoskeletal, oesophageal, and other causes. A detailed history of the pain should include: the location, intensity, frequency, and character; presence of radiation; any aggravating or relieving factors; how pain impairs activities of daily living; and the psychosocial factors (Table 17.1). Listen carefully to what the patients and their relatives have to say as this can point out the actual problem. Also consider any symptoms associated with the pain, especially in respiratory disease, like shortness of breath and haemoptysis. It is essential to understand the patients coping skills, together with any history of anxiety or depression. A detailed history sets in motion further testing and management.

Assessment tools

A variety of assessment tools exist that are based on the patient's perception and self-report of pain. Other assessment tools are observer-dependent and can be used, for example, in patients with dysphasia or dementia.

At the bedside a simple way of assessing pain is by using the verbal rating scale (2) (mild, moderate, severe) or a numeric rating scale (3) where the patient grades their pain on a 0–10 scale (0=no pain, 10=worst pain imaginable). It is important that after analgesia

Table 17.1 Assessment of pain–history

Description	*Timing*: onset, duration, pattern, and frequency
	Intensity or *severity*
	Location and *Radiation*: localization to specific landmarks—diffuse or systemic
	Distress: the degree to which a symptom bothers an individual
	Exacerbating factors: factors that precipitate or worsen a symptom
	Alleviating factors: factors that reduce or relieve a symptom
	Interference/impact: the degree to which the symptom influences activity or function
Previous history of pain	
Context	Social, cultural, emotional, spiritual factors
Interventions	What has been tried?
Medications taken	Dose, route, frequency, duration, efficacy, adverse effects

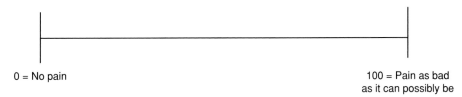

0 = No pain

100 = Pain as bad
as it can possibly be

Fig. 17.1 Visual analogue scale.

has been given, its effectiveness is assessed by re-evaluating the patient's pain and by using the same assessment tool.

Another tool that might be useful, especially in patients with communication difficulties, is the 'faces' pain scale (4). It is easy to use as the patient is asked to point to the words or faces on the scale to show how severe their pain is. In patients with cognitive impairment, there are specific tools to assess their pain. The pain assessment checklist for seniors with limited ability to communicate (PACSLAC) is a screening tool that could be used to assess pain by a healthcare professional. It has four subscales: facial expressions, activity/body movements, social/personality/mood, and physiological indicators/eating and sleeping changes/vocal behaviours. Behavioural observation scores should be considered alongside knowledge of existing painful conditions (5).

The visual analogue scale (VAS) (6) is another well-established measurement instrument, with which the patient indicates a position along a continuous 100-mm line between two endpoints to indicate how severe the pain is (Figure 17.1). This scale is more suited to research than use in everyday practice.

For neuropathic pain, several tools exist to identify pain of predominantly neuropathic origin, as distinct from nociceptive pain, without the need for clinical examination (7).

Overall, these assessments are subjective and therefore these scales are of most value when looking at change within individuals.

When a more comprehensive pain evaluation is needed, a multidimensional pain assessment is utilized. These are more commonly used in research settings. Two widely used assessment tools are the McGill Pain Questionnaire (8) and the Brief Pain Inventory (9). The McGill Pain questionnaire consists primarily of three classes of word descriptors: sensory, affective, and evaluative, these are used by patients to specify the subjective pain experience (Figure 17.2). It also contains an intensity scale and other items to determine the properties of pain experience. On the other hand, the Brief Pain Inventory (BPI) is a simple and easy to use tool which has been translated into many different languages (10). It provides information on the intensity of pain, how pain interferes with function, and also asks questions about pain relief, pain quality, and the patient's perception of the cause of pain.

Pain and quality of life

Pain is a multidimensional phenomenon with sensory-discriminative, affective-motivational, motor, and autonomic components (11). Therefore, these aspects are important to consider when looking at a patient's pain experience. Quality of life questionnaires refer to an

Sections:

(1) What does your pain feel like?

(2) How does your pain change with time?

(3) How strong is your pain?

Statement: People agree that the following 5 words (mild discomforting distressing horrible excruciating) represent pain of increasing intensity. To answer each question below write the number of the most appropriate word in the space beside the question.

Interpretation: The higher the pain scores the greater the pain.

Question	Response	Points
Which word describes your pain right now?	mild	1
	discomforting	2
	distressing	3
	horrible	4
	excruciating	5
Which word describes it at its worst?	mild	1
	discomforting	2
	distressing	3
	horrible	4
	excruciating	5
Which word describes it when it is least?	mild	1
	discomforting	2
	distressing	3
	horrible	4
	excruciating	5

Fig. 17.2 The McGill Pain Questionnaire.

individual's emotional, social, and physical well-being together with their functional ability (see Chapter 3, this volume). To improve accurate and reliable reporting of the health-related quality of life and pain, several assessments have been developed including the EORTC QLQ-C30: this is a 30-item self-reporting questionnaire developed to assess the quality of life of cancer patients (12) and the lung module EORTC QLQ-LC13 (13) which measures lung cancer associated symptoms and side-effects from treatment (Table 17.2).

Table 17.2 EORTC QLQ-LC13

Have you had tingling hands or feet?	1	2	3	4
Have you had hair loss?	1	2	3	4
Have you had pain in your chest?	1	2	3	4
Have you had pain in your arm or shoulder?	1	2	3	4
Have you had pain in other parts of your body?	1	2	3	4
If yes, where_____				
Did you take any medicine for pain?				
1 No 2 Yes				
If yes, how much did it help?	1	2	3	4

These are useful measures for evaluating progress in health goals and measuring the effectiveness of a clinical intervention as an important outcome is the change in the patient's own perceived state of health. On the other hand, the SF-36 health survey questionnaire is a multipurpose health survey used in general and specific populations and consists of eight scaled scores looking at vitality, physical functioning, bodily pain, general health perceptions, physical role, emotional and social functioning, and mental health (14).

A pain diary is another way of assessing pain and this involves recording, usually on a daily or several times a day basis, the level of pain as well as any medications taken and the effect. This is particularly helpful in establishing any pattern to the pain and the efficacy of medications.

Utility of assessment tools

Both in research and in clinics, patients are often asked to fill in questionnaires and diaries. However, it is important that the patients are able to understand and complete these assessments. Therefore the choice of the assessment tool to be given to the patient to complete has relevance as studies have shown that poor compliance, visual impairments, poor physical condition, and illiteracy are influencing factors in patients not completing these assessment tools (15). No matter which assessment tool is used, the ultimate goals are in making the right diagnosis, giving the appropriate treatment, and following-up the patient. It is thus important that the physician checks the questionnaire or diary as otherwise these will not impact on the pain control (16).

Physical examination

After taking a history, a thorough physical examination should follow as this can indicate a diagnosis. Initial observation includes looking at facial expression, body position, and asymmetry such as muscle atrophy or spasm and chest wall deformity. Inspection of the chest skin for erythema, lesions indicating current or previous herpes zoster infection, or post-surgical or biopsy scars should be performed. Palpation is an important aspect as it will detect masses, warmth, or localized tenderness. If an area of the thorax is tender on palpation, this might indicate a musculoskeletal cause, such as costochondritis or a fractured rib. Percussion and auscultation may detect signs of consolidation, pleurisy, or pneumothorax. The rest of the examination is guided by the presenting features and examination findings.

Investigations

A chest radiograph is the most frequently requested radiological examination and together with an electrocardiogram (ECG) are usually ordered when someone presents with new-onset chest pain. Laboratory tests may be helpful in investigating the cause of thoracic pain, e.g. raised serum alkaline phosphatase and calcium could indicate bone metastases. A computed tomography pulmonary angiogram (CTPA) would be appropriate if there is a suspicion of pulmonary embolism. If a patient presents with symptoms of thoracic back pain and neurological signs such as leg weakness and loss of sensation, an urgent magnetic resonance imaging (MRI) scan is required to exclude spinal cord compression. Abnormal findings on any of these tests might confirm diagnosis or might suggest the need to pursue further investigations, e.g. computed tomography (CT) or ultrasound of thorax.

Pain assessment in research

Neuroimaging in pain, both experimentally and clinically, has modernized the way we understand the central mechanisms of the pain processing. Changes in brain activity in response to painful stimuli have been studied using neuroimaging techniques like positron emission tomography (PET) and functional MRI (fMRI). These studies have mainly been carried out on healthy volunteers following induction of acute pain, e.g. by hot or cold stimulation. This research has led to the characterization of a network of brain areas that consistently activate in response to pain, forming a so-called 'pain matrix' (17). In a meta-analysis, haemodynamic studies of acute pain in normal subjects using PET and fMRI showed the six most commonly reported areas that are activated in pain: anterior cingulate gyrus (ACC), primary (S1) and secondary somatosensory cortex (S2), insular cortex (IC), thalamus, and prefrontal cortex (18). In a study on healthy subjects, Strigo and colleagues compared brain activations produced by contact heat on the chest and oesophageal distension. Cortical activations in the cutaneous and visceral pain included S1, S2, ACC, and IC, but the exact loci within the regions differed for the two types of pain (19).

Summary

Assessment of the patient's experience of pain in respiratory disease is crucial to providing effective pain management. A systematic approach for evaluating pain includes a thorough history followed by a pain assessment tool, physical examination, and any relevant investigations. It must be remembered to re-evaluate the pain frequently. It is important to: 1) illustrate the pain report and its impact of activities of daily living and quality of life and this could be aided with an assessment tool; 2) understand the pathophysiology of pain; 3) be sure of the extent of the disease and any reversible symptoms and any available treatment; 4) know what has already been done with regards to investigations and interventions for the pain and what helped; 5) be aware of comorbidities and psychosocial factors that could influence pain experience.

References

1. Weiss SC, Emanuel LL, Fairclough DL, Emanuel EJ. Understanding the experience of pain in terminally ill patients. *Lancet* 2001; **357**(9265):1311–15.

2. Jensen MP, Karoly P, Braver S. The measurement of clinical pain intensity: a comparison of six methods. *Pain* 1986; **27**(1):117–26.

3. Paice JA, Cohen FL. Validity of a verbally administered numeric rating scale to measure cancer pain intensity. *Cancer Nurs* 1997; **20**(2):88–93.

4. Herr KA, Mobily PR. Comparison of selected pain assessment tools for use with the elderly. *Appl Nurs Res* 1993; **6**(1):39–46.

5. Fuchs-Lacelle S, Hadjistavropoulos T. Development and preliminary validation of the pain assessment checklist for seniors with limited ability to communicate (PACSLAC). *Pain Manag Nurs* 2004; **5**(1):37–49.

6. Huskisson EC. Measurement of pain. *Lancet* 1974; **2**(7889):1127–31.

7. Bennett MI, Attal N, Backonja MM, Baron R, et al. Using screening tools to identify neuropathic pain. *Pain* 2007; **127**(3):199–203.

8. Melzack R. The McGill Pain Questionnaire: major properties and scoring methods. *Pain* 1975; **1**(3):277–99.

9. Daut RL, Cleeland CS, Flanery RC. Development of the Wisconsin Brief Pain Questionnaire to assess pain in cancer and other diseases. *Pain* 1983; **17**(2):197–210.

10. Cleeland CS, Ryan KM. Pain assessment: global use of the Brief Pain Inventory. *Ann Acad Med Singapore* 1994; **23**(2):129–38.

11. Treede RD, Kenshalo DR, Gracely RH, Jones AK. The cortical representation of pain. *Pain* 1999; **79**(2–3):105–11.

12. Aaronson NK, Ahmedzai S, Bergman B, *et al.* The European Organization for Research and Treatment of Cancer QLQ-C30: a quality-of-life instrument for use in international clinical trials in oncology. *J Natl Cancer Inst* 1993; **85**(5):365–76.

13. Bergman B, Aaronson N, Ahmedzai S, Kaasa S, Sullivan M. The EORTC QLQ-LC13: A modular supplement to the EORTC core quality of life questionnaire (QLQ-C30) for use in lung cancer clinical trials. *Eur J Cancer* 1994; **30A**(5):635–42.

14. Jenkinson C, Coulter A, Wright L. Short form 36 (SF36) health survey questionnaire: normative data for adults of working age. *BMJ* 1993; **306**(6890):1437–40.

15. Stahl E, Jansson SA, Jonsson AC, Svensson K, Lundback B, Andersson F. Health-related quality of life, utility, and productivity outcomes instruments: ease of completion by subjects with COPD. *Health Qual Life Outcomes* 2003; **1**:18.

16. Trowbridge R, Dugan W, Jay SJ, *et al.* Determining the effectiveness of a clinical-practice intervention in improving the control of pain in outpatients with cancer. *Acad Med* 1997; **72**(9):798–800.

17. Melzack R. From the gate to the neuromatrix. *Pain* 1999; Suppl **6**:S121–6.

18. Apkarian AV, Bushnell MC, Treede RD, Zubieta JK. Human brain mechanisms of pain perception and regulation in health and disease. *Eur J Pain* 2005; **9**(4):463–84.

19. Strigo IA, Duncan GH, Boivin M, Bushnell MC. Differentiation of visceral and cutaneous pain in the human brain. *J Neurophysiol* 2003; **89**(6):3294–303.

Chapter 18

Pain in respiratory disease: mechanisms and management

Jason Boland, Elaine Cachia, Russell K. Portenoy, and Sam H. Ahmedzai

Anatomical basis of pain in the thorax

Pain is a common symptom in patients with disease arising from, or affecting, the respiratory system. The capacity for pain sensation is found in many of the tissues of the thorax. The most important areas to consider are: the skeletal system, the pleura, the intercostal nerves, and the brachial plexus.

Pain arising from the thoracic skeletal system is frequently seen in diseases affecting the vertebrae, e.g. osteoporosis; sometimes seen after long-term corticosteroid treatment, and leading to wedge collapse; degenerative diseases; fracture, e.g. of the ribs with excessive coughing; malignancy. In the last case, pain can also be associated with malignant disease of the ribs as well as vertebrae. Bony pains in the thorax are often well localized by the patient, especially in the ribs or sternum.

The pleura are innervated on the parietal side, and diseases which cause pleural inflammation or irritation can cause diffuse lateralized pain, which may be related to the respiratory cycle (pleuritic pain). The intercostal nerves run beneath each of the ribs and are involved in pleural pain, or may be stimulated by diseases affecting the ribs themselves.

The brachial plexus is, strictly speaking, outside the thorax, but diseases affecting the apex of the lung can easily invade this anatomical area and give rise to severe pain which radiates down one or more nerve trunks to the shoulder or upper limb. This is commonly seen in patients with Pancoast tumour of lung, or locally advanced breast cancer (1).

Types of pain

It is traditional to divide pain into two main types—nociceptive and neuropathic. This classification is helpful at a rudimentary level, potentially suggesting next steps in diagnosis, if any are needed, and various strategies for pain control.

'Nociceptive' pain refers to pain that appears to be sustained predominantly by continuing tissue injury. In clinical practice the classification needs to be more sophisticated, as there are many subtypes of nociceptive pain. Some classifications separate out `inflammatory' pain; others subsume this under nociceptive pain. Among pains considered to be nociceptive, classifications distinguish somatic pain and visceral pain types. Somatic pain itself can be subdivided into cutaneous, soft tissue (myofascial), and bony. Within the thorax, visceral pain mainly arises from the mediastinal structures such as the oesophagus, heart, and aorta. The upper airways are very sensitive to foreign bodies and noxious gases, but true pain sensation is largely absent from the lungs.

Somatic nociceptive pain involves injury to somatic structures like bone, joints, or muscles. It often is described by patients as 'aching', 'stabbing', 'throbbing', or 'pressure-like' in quality. Visceral nociceptive pain involves injury to viscera and usually is characterized as 'gnawing' or 'crampy' when arising from the obstruction of a hollow viscus, and as 'aching' or 'stabbing' when arising from other visceral structures, such as organ capsules, myocardium, or pleura.

Pain is labelled as 'neuropathic' if the results of evaluation suggest that it is sustained by abnormal somatosensory processing in the peripheral or central nervous system. Neuropathic mechanisms are involved in approximately 40% of cancer pain syndromes and can be caused by the disease or by cancer treatment. Dysaesthesias, or uncomfortable sensations that are perceived as abnormal and described using terms such as 'burning', 'shock-like' or 'electrical,' are suggestive of neuropathic mechanisms. Upon physical examination, the presence of allodynia (i.e. pain induced by non-painful stimuli), hyperalgesia (i.e. increased perception of painful stimuli), or other sensory findings also suggest the presence of neuropathic pain. Patients may have other concomitant neurological findings, such as weakness or changes in reflexes, and some patients have autonomic dysfunction in the distribution of the pain.

Many pain syndromes have been described in relation to the thoracic structures, in both cancer and benign diseases (2). Table 18.1 summarizes the more important of these, which should be considered in the diagnostic work-up of a patient presenting with new or worsening thoracic pain. It is important always to bear in mind systemic or non-respiratory disease processes, e.g. herpes zoster virus (shingles) causing radicular or diffuse pain long before the eruption of vesicles. Sickle cell disease may present with vague pains affecting the upper limbs, shoulders, and chest.

Iatrogenic causes include localized pain from a biopsy or chest drain site; occasionally these may be due to a subcutaneous neuroma that may respond to infiltration with local anaesthetic. However, the major iatrogenic syndrome is post-thoracotomy pain, which is increasingly recognized as a significant cause of morbidity after diagnostic or curative surgery for cancer (3, 4). Like the post-mastectomy pain syndrome seen in breast cancer patients, this has a high priority for early detection and management because they both interfere with functioning and activities of daily living, and can prevent rehabilitation after curative resections. In the context of lung cancer, post-thoracotomy pain also suggests recurrent disease somewhere in the thorax, and repeated imaging will be needed until a conclusion about this possibility is clear.

Breakthrough pain is well-recognized syndrome, which refers to the periodic exacerbations of pain that arise in the context of a background pain. Originally described in the cancer population (5), patients with pain, e.g. from osteoporosis, can experience peaks of breakthrough pain. Breakthrough pain is often much more severe than the background pain, can arise in a different part of the body, and may be either predictable or unpredictable (6, 7). Predictable varieties include 'incident' pain, or pain on voluntary

Table 18.1 Painful conditions involving the thorax

Type of pain	Disease/syndrome	Causes
Non-malignant	Coronary syndromes—acute, chronic	Cardiac ischaemia
	Sickle cell crisis—acute chest syndrome	Ischaemia following vascular occlusion, fat embolism
	Herpes zoster	Infection affecting intercostal nerve roots
	Osteoporosis	Multiple rib, vertebral fractures
	Gastro-oesophageal reflux	Hyperacidity in oesophagus
	Pleurisy	Infection; trauma; pneumothorax; embolism
	Central chest pain	Pericarditis; cardiac ischaemia
Cancer-related	Rib destruction	Mesothelioma; metastatic cancer; myeloma
	Vertebral fracture	Metastatic cancer; myeloma
	Pleurisy	Mesothelioma
	Brachial plexopathy	Pancoast tumour; locally advanced breast cancer
Iatrogenic	Steroid-induced osteoporosis	Multiple rib, vertebral fractures
	Post-surgical pain	Thoracotomy; mastectomy; biopsy and chest drain sites
	Mediastinitis	High-dose radiation treatment

action, e.g. pain in a limb with a malignant deposit whenever it is used, e.g. weight-bearing in the leg, or lifting articles in the arm. (Another predictable type of pain exacerbation, which is usually not included in official taxonomy of breakthrough pain, is 'end of dose failure': this is the situation where a modified-release analgesic (usually an opioid) is given, say, twice a day but pain builds up a few hours before the second dose. In such situations the background dose may need to be increased, or the scheduling could be changed to three times daily.)

Unpredictable breakthrough pains are spontaneous, not related to activity or drug dosing, and are often described as sharp, shooting, or hot. They may be caused by abnormal peripheral neural activity, e.g. associated with nerve damage from tumour or chemotherapy; or they may be manifestations of the newly recognized condition of opioid-induced hyperalgesia (see below).

Biological basis of pain

In the past decade there have been major advances in our understanding of the molecular, cellular, and genomic mechanisms in the generation and persistence of pain. There are numerous specialist texts which the reader can consult for detailed descriptions of pain science (8–10). How analgesics work—and may cause harm too—have also been elucidated through preclinical and clinical studies (11–13). This section will review some of the new knowledge, which may not be familiar to clinicians dealing with respiratory disease patients.

Pain usually starts with the transduction of a signal—actually an action potential on a sensory neuron—most commonly at a nerve ending which is being stimulated in one of many ways (8, 9). Sensory nerves have numerous receptors or channels which can be activated or opened by inflammatory molecules (bradykinin, cytokines, chemokines) (14); acid from cellular breakdown; heat or cold (see Figure 18.1). Some of the receptors are multipotential, e.g. the TRPV1 receptor is sensitive to heat and H^+ ions. (This is also the

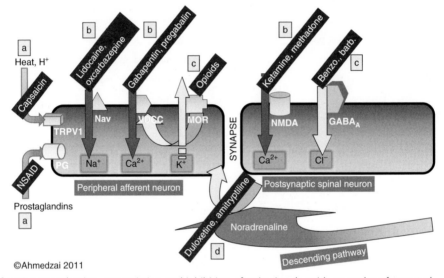

©Ahmedzai 2011

Fig. 18.1 Transduction, transmission and inhibition of pain signals, with examples of targeted blocking by drugs.

a. Peripheral pain signal transduction. Two examples are given: i) heat or acid stimulating the TRPV1 channel–targeted by capsaicin; ii) prostaglandins stimulating the PG receptor—targeted by NSAIDs.

b. Mechanisms facilitating pain signal transmission. Three examples are given: i) Nav channel allowing sodium entry into neuron—targeted by lidocaine, oxcarbazepine; ii) VDCC channel allowing calcium entry into neuron—targeted by gabapentin, pregabalin; iii) NMDA channel allowing calcium entry into cell—targeted by ketamine, methadone.

c. Mechanisms facilitating pain signal inhibition. Two examples are given: i) MOR receptor allows potassium to leave cell—targeted by opioids (note that MOR activation also block VDCC through intracellular downstream signalling); ii) $GABA_A$ receptor allows chloride to enter cell—targeted by benzodiazepines, barbiturate.

d. Mechanisms facilitating descending inhibition. Example is given of noradrenaline re-uptake—targeted by duloxetine, amitryptiline.

Key: TRPV1, transient receptor potential vanniloid 1; PG, prostaglandin; NSAID, non-steroidal anti-inflammatory drug; Nav, Sodium channel; VDCC, voltage dependent calcium channel; MOR, mu-opioid receptor; NMDA, N-methyl-D-aspartate channel; $GABA_A$, gamma-aminobutyric acid receptor type A; Benzo, benzodiazepine; Barb, barbiturate.

receptor in the mouth for capsaicin, which explains why chilli tastes hot—and also why we experience heat in an area of painful inflammation.)

The action potential propagates centrally to the first synapse in the dorsal horn of the spinal cord. Along the neuron, sodium and calcium channels are responsible for the maintenance of depolarizations and so are key to nerve transmission (10). In peripheral nerve damage, sodium channels are increased in the normal neurons, and these may be responsible for the increased firing which is seen in neuropathy and may be experienced as unpredictable spontaneous or breakthrough pain.

Opioid receptors are present on neuronal cell membranes throughout the nervous system, indeed throughout the body as the small endogenous opioid peptides are involved in numerous homeostatic and immunoregulatory functions. When activated by endogenous peptides or by pharmacological opioids, opioid receptors have two important membrane actions—they open K^+ channels and inactivate Ca^{2+} channels, both of which events reduce neural sensitivity and hence pain signal transmission. Opioid receptor activation has other complex intracellular downstream signalling effects, which paradoxically, can lead to pain up-regulation—this is thought to be one of the mechanisms of the newly recognized opioid-induced hyperalgesia.

At the dorsal horn of the spinal cord, afferent neurons synapse in a complex way with neurons that eventually cross over and rise to the brain in the ascending spinothalamic tracts. At these synapses, many critical events occur. Neurotransmitters are released in response to incoming pain signals and these traverse the synapse and stimulate postsynaptic receptors and channels. The commonest transmitter is glutamate and in short-term pain, it usually activates the AMPA receptor in a linear way. However, in chronic pain situations, glutamate also activates the NMDA channel, which allows calcium entry into the postsynaptic nerve—this key event leads to downstream second messenger signalling changes involving nitric oxide, that ultimately lead to increased sensitivity of the central nervous system (8, 10, 15). A consequence of this is the rapid development of structural, neuroplastic changes in the dorsal horn involving increased glial cell activation, which in turn cause increased postsynaptic sensitivity (9, 14). Neurons which originally only conduct touch now start to transmit pain signals, and neurons from adjacent areas are recruited so that the perception is that the painful area increases in size. Thus chronic pain—especially well demonstrated *in vivo* in animal neuropathic pain models—is a state of central sensitization which is characterized by disproportionately increased neural transmission to the brain and clinical manifestations like hyperalgesia and allodynia. Similar changes are now also seen with iatrogenic peripheral neuropathy, e.g. following cytotoxic chemotherapy and the new biological anticancer treatments (16).

In the brain, incoming neurons relay at the thalamus and radiate to several cortical and subcortical structures. Recent advances in human and animal neuroimaging have shown how the sensorimotor cortex, the anterior cingulate cortex, the amygdala, and the pre-frontal cortex are all activated in acute and chronic pain states—this has led to the description of the so-called 'pain matrix' (17–19). Connections to the limbic system are responsible for the mood or emotional response to pain, and these are also closely related to the arousal system. From the brain, descending pathways carry adrenergic and serotoninergic fibres which interact with the dorsal horn synapses. The former are inhibitory (i.e. reduce pain transmission), while the latter may be largely excitatory (i.e. increase pain transmission).

Rational approach to pharmacological pain management

The preceding brief summary of pain signalling opens the possibility of managing pain by specific targeting of the molecular and cellular processes that have been identified in the laboratory and early clinical studies. However, the actual management of pain is still lagging behind the scientific evidence and is largely based on 1980s and 1990s models, which were devised in order to achieve simple solutions to the complex problem of global cancer pain. The World Health Organization (WHO) three-step analgesic ladder was first published in 1986 as an empirical guide to the treatment of cancer pain, and is still used to this day, even though in the past decade many authorities have questioned its evidence base and clinical relevance in most developed countries (20, 21).

Whilst the three step analgesic ladder may be useful as a general educational tool, suggesting the gradual stepping up of pharmacological response to increasing levels of pain, many of its central tenets have been refined. Thus, the recommendation for using oral morphine has become superseded by experience showing that there are no special benefits from this drug; indeed intra-individual variation in the response to the different opioids is very large, and is the rationale for so-called opioid rotation as a strategy to find the best drug. Although most patients find oral drugs to be satisfactory, for many patients, the greater convenience and potentially improved gastrointestinal side effect profile of transdermal fentanyl suggests a trial of this formulation (22, 23). The recommendation for starting with 'weak opioids' like codeine may be helpful for some, but others have found that starting with low doses of 'strong opioids' is as good and may give faster pain relief (21). But perhaps the most outdated aspect of the WHO analgesic ladder approach is its reliance on opioids, with all other analgesic drugs being relegated to a secondary, even optional, position as 'adjuvants'. The term 'adjuvant analgesic' was originally coined to refer to a small number of drugs that were marketed for use other than for analgesia, but which can also be used for pain relief in select circumstances. These non-traditional drugs were meant to supplement opioid therapy, the mainstay of cancer pain analgesia, and thus give rise to the term 'adjuvant analgesia'. The number, diversity, and conventional use of these drugs have increased dramatically in the last few years to the extent that 'adjuvant analgesia' is really a misnomer. Several of these drugs are now indicated and promoted as first-line therapy for certain types of pain and in cancer and non-cancer populations. Moreover, it has been customary to name classes of so-called adjuvant drugs according to their original marketing indications, e.g. antidepressants, anticonvulsants: this makes no sense in pain management and especially now that many of these drugs are hardly used for those original purposes.

A new taxonomy of analgesic drugs has rejected this nomenclature and proposes that drugs that work on reducing pain should be classified according to their molecular actions (24). Table 18.2 summarizes the old and proposed new taxonomies. The main benefit of looking at analgesic drugs in this new way is that we may begin to target pain according to the

Table 18.2 Modern classification of analgesic drugs

Old WHO ladder-based description	Mechanistic description	Examples
Non-opioid	Antinociceptive non-opioid	NSAID, paracetamol (acetaminophen)
Opioid	Antinociceptive opioid	Morphine, fentanyl
Neuropathic agent	Antihyperalgesic—NMDA antagonist	Ketamine, methadone (mixed effect)
Co-analgesic; adjuvant; anticonvulsant	Peripheral transmission modulator—sodium channel blocker	Carbamazepine, oxcarbazepine, topiramate
Co-analgesic; adjuvant; anticonvulsant	Antihyperalgesic transmission modulator—calcium channel blocker	Gabapentin, pregabalin; lamotrigine
Local anaesthetic	Peripheral transmission modulator—sodium channel blocker	Lidocaine, bupivacaine
Tricyclic antidepressant; adjuvant	Modulator of descending inhibition	Amitriptyline, nortriptyline
Antidepressant; adjuvant	Modulator of descending inhibition	SNRI (e.g. duloxetine)
Adrenergic; adjuvant	Modulator of descending inhibition	Clonidine
Opioid with neuropathic effect	Mixed antinociceptive (opioid) with modulation of descending inhibition	Tramadol, tapentadol
Not previously described as analgesics	Bisphosphonate	Zolendronate, pamidronate
Not previously described as analgesics	Modulator of signal transduction	Capsaicin, menthol
Not previously described as analgesics	Anti-nociceptive analgesic—cannabinoid	Sativex™

NMDA, N-methyl-D-aspartate; NSAID: non-steroidal anti-inflammatory drug; SNRI, serotonin noradrenaline reuptake inhibitor; SSRI, selective serotonin reuptake inhibitor.

Notes:

1. Many of the older descriptions of the drugs were based on their original marketing licence, e.g. amitriptyline as an antidepressant, carbamazepine as an anticonvulsant. These terms no longer make sense as: a) the drugs as now used as much for pain control as their 'original' use and b) they do not describe the pharmacological action of the drugs.

2. According to the older WHO ladder based classification, many drugs whose actions were unclear were classed as 'adjuvants' or co-analgesics'. This is now considered illogical as we understand their actions and they are as important in pain management as so-called 'analgesics' such as opioids.

3. Some of the newer classes of drugs (bisphosphonates, capsaicin, cannabinoids) were either not known in the days when the WHO ladder was devised, or were not regarded as being relevant in pain control.

Adapted from (24).

presumed pathological mechanism and also, we can see logical ways of combining drugs to maximize actions on multiple targets, rather than the sequential approach of old. Thus, the new way of managing pain pharmacologically will be increasingly seen as mechanism-based and multi-modal. Figure 18.1 shows how presently used drugs can be used logically to stop pain at every stage: inception (peripheral and central signal transduction), neuronal transmission, synaptic modulation, central processing, and descending inhibition.

Clearly this new approach to pain management is more complicated and therefore requires a higher degree of sophistication by the clinician. The old WHO approach was characterized by its sheer simplicity and may still be useful in non-specialist settings and in developing countries with very limited access to modern drugs. But in developed countries and where specialists in supportive and palliative care or in pain management services are available, it makes sense to adopt the more complex approach. One way to embrace the complexity is to visualize not a two-dimensional ladder, but a three-dimensional pyramid, which increases the options for therapeutic manoeuvres (Figure 18.2) (25). Thus the patient should be considered from the outset, depending on the location and type of pain, for initiation with peripherally acting, anti-inflammatory, ion-channel modifying, gabapentinoid, noradrenaline re-uptake inhibiting, GABA-ergic, or other drugs.

Opioids clearly have a special place in pain management, but there is increasing evidence of the multifaceted adverse effects associated with this class of drug (26–28). Because opioid mechanisms are involved in almost every body system, it is not surprising that patients experience gastrointestinal, urinary, respiratory, cutaneous, endocrine, and immunological as well as cognitive side effects (11, 13, 29). There is some evidence that fentanyl has a better side effect profile for the gastrointestinal and cognitive effects (22, 23, 30), but in the clinic, the intra-individual variation in the response to different drugs is so large that no single agent can be said to be the mainstay of treatment. When using the transdermal system, the potential benefits also must be balanced by its reduced flexibility in unstable pain, increased cost and adhesion limitations.

For breakthrough pain—whether in cancer or non-malignant chronic pain—it may make sense to use more rapid-acting drugs and formulations. Thus, transmucosal preparations of fentanyl again have shown superiority and are more preferred by patients to oral morphine, particularly in terms of speed of action. The rapid-onset fentanyl formulations are far more expensive than readily-available oral formulations, however, and the most appropriate positioning of these drugs is not yet clear. Their use is most rational when breakthrough pain has a very rapid onset or after oral drugs have been shown to be insufficiently effective. Regardless of the specific drugs selected, it is feasible and rational

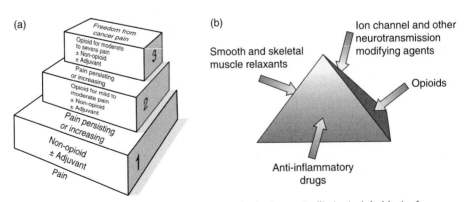

Fig. 18.2 (a) WHO analgesic ladder (http://www.who.int/cancer/palliative/painladder/en/). (b) Pyramid model (25).

now to prescribe two different opioids concurrently, i.e. one in a modified-release format for background pain (e.g. twice daily oxycodone or morphine) and another as a rapid-acting oral or nasal transmucosal fentanyl for breakthrough exacerbations.

Methadone is an old opioid drug which has become more widely used in recent years for chronic pain. This is partly because its potency and maximal efficacy may be relatively higher than expected, presumably because its d-isomer has intrinsic NMDA-blocking activity (31). There are other reasons why methadone may have advantages over other opioids, e.g. it increases receptor recycling, and it is also cheap. On the other hand, it is associated with the potential for serious toxicity unless used cautiously, both because of its unanticipated high potency in some patients and also its long and variable half-life, which may predispose to delayed accumulation and toxicity when the drug is first started or the dose increased. It also is associated with prolongation of the ECG QTc interval, which is associated with serious arrhythmia (torsade de Pointe) if above 500 ms.

Table 18.3 gives the clinician an overview of the main actions, formulations, routes, advantages, and disadvantages of the main opioids, at least which are available in the UK. Other parts of the world have local variations, e.g. hydromorphone, oxymorphone, and hydrocodone are used in North America; ketobemidone is used in Scandinavia. Methadone is very widely available but is best reserved for specialist use by supportive and palliative care, or pain management, physicians.

Bisphosphonates

Bisphosphonates have been shown to be useful in preventing skeletal-related events, including fracture and pain, and may improve the quality of life in cancer patients with bone pain (32). They act by directly inhibiting osteoclast activity, stimulating osteoblasts to produce osteoclast-inhibiting factor, and causing osteoclast apoptosis. There is substantial evidence that the commercially-available bisphosphonates can reduce bone pain. Intravenous pamidronate has been shown in large studies to reduce bone pain in breast cancer and was superior to oral clodronate in a 3-month trial. These studies demonstrated that analgesia following pamidronate infusion did not maximize until several doses at monthly intervals had been administered. Zoledronic acid, which may be infused over minutes compared to hours needed for pamidronate infusion, has been shown to reduce bone pain in some but not all studies of populations with metastatic bone pain. A direct comparison between zoledronic acid and pamidronate in breast cancer and multiple myeloma patients did not show any significant differences in control of bone pain.

Surgical techniques

The 'pyramid approach' which was introduced a decade ago to broaden the number of therapeutic options in symptom management can also show the place of surgery for some patients (see Figure 18.2b) (25). In respiratory disease patients with back pain due to vertebral collapse due to tumour or osteoporosis, the techniques of vertebroplasty and balloon kyphoplasty are available in many parts of the world (33). Vertebroplasty involves injecting bone cement directly into one or more collapsing vertebrae, leading to cessation

Table 18.3 Summary of commonly used opioids in pain management

Opioid	Receptors	Routes	Equivalent 24-hour dose (30mg daily oral morphine as reference point)	Advantages	Disadvantages	Renal failure	Hepatic failure	Other information
Morphine	MOR agonist	PO, IV, SC, Sp	30mg PO = 15mg SC, IV	Familiarity; cheap; available as normal release and modified-release tablets	Sedation; hallucinations; nausea; constipation; immuno-suppression	Avoid high risk of toxic metabolites in renal failure	Caution if prothrombin time prolonged	Nausea usually resolves—CNS side effects and constipation usually persist; metabolized by glucuronidation
Tramadol	MOR agonist; SNRI	PO, IM	150mg PO (maximum recommended dose is 400mg per 24 hours)	Less constipation than morphine; SNRI action may help with neuropathic pain maybe immune-enhancing	Risk of serotonin syndrome	Caution	Caution	Efficacy highly dependent on CYP2D6 phenotype; SNRI activity potentially blocked by 5HT3 antagonists
Codeine	MOR agonist (after conversion to morphine)	PO	300mg PO (NB this is higher than maximum daily dose of 240mg)	Familiarity; OTC	Constipation; sedation;	Unsafe—as for morphine	Caution—as for morphine	Pro-drug of morphine; CYP2D6 dependent; Often combined with paracetamol

Oxycodone	MOR, KOR agonist	PO, IV, SC	15mg PO = 7.5mg SC, IV	Reduced sedation, hallucinations cf. morphine	Oral liquid unpleasant taste—use capsules; For parenteral use, concentrate (50mg/mL) now available as substitute for diamorphine)	Caution—plasma concentrations may rise	Safe	Females may have greater response; CYP3A4 and CYP2D6 dependent
Fentanyl	MOR agonist	TM (buccal, sublingual, nasal), TD, IV, Sp	12mcg/hour TD patch over 72 hours	Reduced sedation, emesis, constipation cf. morphine; Convenience of 3-day patch	TM applications very short-acting (1–2 hours)—best reserved for incident (movement-related) pains and dressing changes, etc;	Safe in renal failure (Alternative for parenteral use is alfentanil)	Probably Safe	Use rapid acting TM formulations with caution in patients with addictive tendencies; Affected CYP3A4-acting drugs
Buprenorphine	MOR, ORL1 agonist; KOR, DOR antagonist	TM (sublingual), TD, IV	20mcg/h TD patch over 7 days	Reduced respiratory depression constipation; Convenience (5–20mcg dose TD patches can last 7 days; 35mcg. hour and higher-dose patches last 4 days)	Nausea with initiation of higher dose TD patch; TM tablet causes nausea	Safe	Safe	Ceiling dose for respiratory depression makes it safer for COPD patients; does not reverse other MOR opioids at normal therapeutic doses

(Continued)

Table 18.3 Summary of commonly used opioids in pain management (*Cont.*)

Opioid	Receptors	Routes	Equivalent 24-hour daily dose (30mg daily oral morphine as reference point)	Advantages	Disadvantages	Renal failure	Hepatic failure	Other information
Diamorphine	MOR agonist after conversion to morphine	IV, SC	10mg SC, IV	Familiarity (in the UK only); high water solubility	As for morphine	Unsafe—as for morphine	Caution -as for morphine	Pro-drug of morphine; Has no advantages apart from high water solubility (only used in UK—elsewhere hydromorphone or oxycodone)

Notes:

1. This table has been complied by one of the authors (SHA) as a guide for non-specialists in pain management on how to use the common opioids that are available in the UK. Other opioids, e.g. methadone and hydromorphone, are for specialist use only by palliative medicine and pain management services. Many of the routes described are out of the product licence for the drugs cited. The new fast-acting transmucosal fentanyl products are also usually restricted to specialist initiation only. For further details, consult a palliative medicine or pain management text or drug database, e.g. British National Formulary, available at: http://bnf.org/bnf/index.htm (accessed 17 September 2010).

2. Although there is a perception that there is no effective ceiling dose for morphine or other strong opioids, it is advised to seek specialist advice when total daily doses reach these levels—morphine 200mg PO, 100mg parenteral; oxycodone 100mg PO, 50mg parenteral; buprenorphine patch 70mcg/hour; fentanyl patch 50mcg/hour; diamorphine 50mg parenteral.

Key: MOR, mu-opioid receptor; KOR, kappa-opioid receptor; DOR delta-opioid receptor; ORL1, opioid-receptor-like receptor; SNRI, serotonin noradrenaline reuptake inhibitor; PO, oral; IV, intravenous; SC, subcutaneous; Sp, spinal (epidural or intrathecal); TD, transdermal; TM, transmucosal (sublingual, buccal or nasal).

of further collapse and rapid pain relief. Kyphoplasty uses a balloon placed in the vertebral body, which may help to regain lost height; cement is injected as with vertebroplasty (34). These techniques are clearly limited by virtue of the need for specialist equipment and training, and cost.

Where metastatic disease is affecting a long bone such as the humerus or femur, surgical correction by pinning or even hip replacement can quickly reduce pain and allow resumption of activities of daily living. The limitations are cost and the general fitness of the patient to undergo a major surgical procedure.

Interventional (anaesthetic) procedures

The dominance of the WHO analgesic approach has led, not intentionally, to a great reliance on pharmacological pain control and the potential for under-usage of interventional techniques. Clearly it is not advisable to go in too early with invasive procedures when analgesics have not been properly tried. However, it is not reasonable to persist with increasing doses of multiple drugs, with the inevitable adverse effects and 'tablet burden', when a brief intervention may give significant extra pain relief and perhaps also allow for reduction in drugs (35).

Table 18.4 shows the range of interventional approaches which may be helpful for respiratory disease patients with thoracic, back, or Pancoast tumour pains. The simplest intervention is a direct local nerve block with local anaesthetic (sodium channel blockers) (35). If this is successful, it could be followed up by a longer-lasting radiofrequency or other neurolytic procedure. These may be helpful for very localized pains

Table 18.4 Interventional approaches for managing thoracic pain

Site	Intervention	Application	Notes
Intercostal nerve	Local anaesthetic injection	Before intercostal drain insertion; pain management of rib fracture	Short-lasting (hours)
Intercostal nerve	Radiofrequency nerve destruction	Pain management of rib fracture; pain at site of biopsy or VATS procedure	Long-lasting (weeks–months)
Paravertebral nerve roots	Radiofrequency nerve destruction	Multiple levels for post-thoracotomy pain	May also be used for post-mastectomy pain
Cervical spinothalamic tract	Cervical cordotomy	Hemi-body pain relief, e.g. mesothelioma	See (41, 42)
Brachial plexus	Posterior brachial plexus continuous infusion	Upper thoracic and shoulder pain, e.g. Pancoast tumour	See (40)
Spinal cord	Intrathecal or epidural catheter with external or implanted pump delivering opioid and local anaesthetic	Thoracic pain refractory to above procedures	See (38, 39)

affecting a biopsy, VATS (video-assisted thoracoscopic surgery), or operation wound site, or rib pain in one or two thoracic dermatomes. In some cases it is helpful to administer systemic local anaesthetic agents, e.g. by intravenous infusion for severe pain or orally (36, 37). If there are several thoracic or other vertebral sites of pain, an epidural or intrathecal infusion with either an external or implanted pump for delivering local anaesthetic with an opioid may be preferable. The doses employed are a fraction of those delivered systemically and, as a result, neuraxial analgesia can be particularly helpful when systemic drug therapy is associated with an unacceptable degree of somnolence. Algorithms have been published which guide the clinician towards different types of spinal intervention, depending on the extent of disease and the prognosis of the patient (38). Spinal analgesic delivery has been shown to be safe and cost-effective even in patients with advanced cancer, if they are well selected and supported (39).

Many cancers cause extensive chest wall invasion with severe and refractory pain—notably mesothelioma. In this situation, a technique which has been increasingly used is percutaneous cervical cordotomy (40, 41). This can only be done in specialist centres and with x-ray or ideally computed tomography (CT) screening (42). There are no randomized trials of this technique but experience has shown that many patients achieve major and rapid reduction in hemi-body pain, which can last for several months.

Non-pharmacological therapies

There are numerous non-pharmacologic therapies for pain and other symptoms. These include various psychological approaches (e.g. guided imagery), transcutaneous electrical nerve stimulation and other modalities applied to the skin, a large number of specific nerve blocks, and treatments that are usually considered alternative or complementary (43)—these include acupuncture, massage, and other mind–body approaches.

The decision to try any of these adjunctive approaches must take into consideration the severity of disease, the patient's ability to work with the therapist, safety issues, availability, and cost. Some require specialist consultants and others could be considered within the purview of primary care providers. The role of specialist nurses working in supportive and palliative care is especially important in this context, as nurses are skilled at eliciting when patients have reached the limits of tolerability of drug therapies and when non-pharmacological approaches should be sought.

Pain at the end of life

In patients who are approaching the end of life with cancer, chronic diseases like chronic obstructive pulmonary disease (COPD) or major infections like HIV/AIDS and tuberculosis, pain may take on a special importance. In the last days or weeks of life, patients and families are generally keen to prioritize quality of life over yet more attempts to prolong living. If pain is present, it can seriously undermine the peace of mind that patients need to come to terms with the impending death and for families to say goodbyes. For some, spiritual distress may come to the fore—even in non-religious people, questions like 'Why me?' and difficulties in letting go may provoke severe existential crisis. Often this is misinterpreted by unskilled clinicians as increasing physical pain, and the natural response is to increase analgesic and sedative medication. However, it is vitally important to ascertain if indeed psychological, social, or spiritual issues are still unresolved and these are the cause of agitation, not pain. Referral to a counsellor, psychologist, or spiritual adviser (e.g. chaplain) may be of great value, if the patient is open to such a visit.

Unfortunately, physical pain does frequently become more problematic at the end of life. As patients become weaker, they may not be able to swallow oral medication, even liquids. Palliative care teams are familiar with the use of subcutaneous injections or infusions, using small portable battery-powered pumps. However, in many places such as busy surgical or medical wards, such patients may instead receive frequent deep intramuscular injections, which are unnecessary and often themselves painful. Intravenous medication is not usually required, unless the patient has widespread oedema, peripheral circulatory shut-down or has other reasons to avoid subcutaneous route.

Patients who are on a well-controlled transdermal patch delivery system (fentanyl or buprenorphine) and are approaching the end of life, should ideally remain on the same doses unless the pain rapidly escalates. Even then, it is advisable to maintain the patch but initiate new parenteral medication to cope with new or increasing pain. Spinal infusions can similarly be continued until death, which helps to minimize the need for additional medication.

In many settings now, the management of refractory symptoms at the end of life includes the option of palliative sedation. Palliative sedation is a therapeutic intervention defined as the intentional use of a therapy to reduce consciousness with the goal of eliminating suffering at the end of life. The use of this intervention requires understanding of its ethical foundation and the medical guidelines that have been developed to assist appropriate patient selection and treatment (44). Although it must be acknowledged that administration of any centrally sedating drug in critically ill patients could hasten death, and this is the basis for much of the controversy surrounding palliative sedation, clinicians who understand and adhere to the well accepted ethical principle of 'double effect' are following an approach that has now achieved broad acceptance. Adherence to the principle of double effect means that the intent of the intervention is beneficent—the relief of intolerable suffering—and the potential for a serious negative outcome—hastening of death—is recognized but not intended, and in this setting, proportionately less imperative than the good outcome. Palliative sedation should never be confused with physician-hastened death, e.g. assisted suicide or euthanasia (see Chapter 1, this volume).

Future developments in pain control

The recent revolution in understanding the mechanisms of pain generation and maintenance have not yet led to a similar radical change in pain management outcomes. With increasing shift away from the outdated WHO ladder approach and the growth of new taxonomies for classifying pain states and analgesic interventions, there is optimism for the coming decade. The future trend in pain management is towards mechanism-based, multimodal analgesia using pharmacological and non-pharmacological approaches. Combinations of drugs at lower doses are more likely to achieve success with reduced adverse effects, than the previous generation's use of high doses of opioids, at least in cancer patients. Because we are more aware of the long-term toxicities of opioids—and not forgetting the abuse potential for patients who may be living for several years with cancer—there will be greater reliance on non-opioid medications (45).

Current research which will bear fruit in the coming decade includes: the exploration of the role and limitations of cannabinoid analogues; antibodies for nerve growth factor (NGF) which is at the heart of pain initiation; antibodies and blockers of cytokines and chemokines; reduction of the glial response to chronic pain which increases hyperalgesia; and ways of modulating and increasing the descending inhibitory pathways (16, 46, 47). It is likely also that more 'personalized' pain management, based on a knowledge of the patient's phenotype for the expression of pain-related receptors and the uptake or metabolism of pain drugs, will lead to more targeted therapy with reduced side effects. Ultimately, the greatest advance in pain management will undoubtedly come with much higher emphasis given to pain education, training and awareness in all types of healthcare professionals who come into contact with patients with pain.

References

1. Arcasoy SM, Jett JR. Superior pulmonary sulcus tumors and pancoast's syndrome. *N Engl J Med* 1997; 337:1370–6.
2. Gordin V, Weaver MA, Hahn MB. Acute and chronic pain management in palliative care. *Best Pract Res Clin Obstet Gynaecol* 2001; **15**(2):203–34.
3. Maguire MF, Ravenscroft A, Beggs D, Duffy JP. A questionnaire study investigating the prevalence of the neuropathic component of chronic pain after thoracic surgery. *Eur J Cardiothorac Surg* 2006; **29**:800–5.
4. Wildgaard K, Ravn J, Kehlet H. Chronic post-thoracotomy pain: a critical review of pathogenic mechanisms and strategies for prevention. *Eur J Cardio-thoracic Surg* 2009; **36**:170–80.
5. Portenoy RK, Hagen NA. Breakthrough pain: definition, prevalence and characteristics. *Pain* 1990; **41**:273–81.
6. Davies AN, Dickman A, Reid C, Stevens AM, Zeppetella G. The management of cancer-related breakthrough pain: Recommendations of a task group of the Science Committee of the Association for Palliative Medicine of Great Britain and Ireland. *Eur J Pain* 2009; **13**:331–8.
7. Svendsen KB, Andersen S, Arnason S, *et al.* Breakthrough pain in malignant and non-malignant diseases: a review of prevalence, characteristics and mechanisms. *Eur J Pain* 2005; **9**:195–206.
8. Mantyh PW, Clohisy DR, Koltzenburg M, Hunt SP. Molecular mechanisms of cancer pain. *Nature Rev Cancer* 2002; **2**:201.
9. Marchand F, Perretti M, McMahon SB. Role of the immune system in chronic pain. *Nature Rev Neurosci* 2005; **6**:521.
10. Urch CE. Pathophysiology of cancer pain. In Walsh TD, Caraceni AT, Fainsinger R, *et al.* (eds). *Palliative Medicine*, pp. 1378–84. Philadelphia, PA: Saunders, 2009.
11. Davis MP, Pasternak GW. Opioid receptors and opioid pharmacodynamics. In Davis MP, Glare P, Hardy JR, Quigley C (eds) *Opioids in cancer pain*, 2nd edn, pp. 1–27. Oxford, Oxford University Press, 2009.
12. Tracey I. Getting the pain you expect: mechanisms of placebo, nocebo and reappraisal effects in humans. *Nature Med* 2010; **16**(11):1277.
13. Ahmedzai SH, Boland J. Opioids for chronic pain: molecular and genomic basis of actions and adverse effects. *Curr Opin Supp Palliat Care* 2007; **1**:117–25.

14. Sommer C, White F. Cytokines, chemokines, and pain. In Beaulieu P, Lussier D, Porreca F, Dickenson AH (eds) Pharmacology of pain, pp. 279–302. Seattle, WA: IASP Press, 2010.

15. Hucho T, Levine JD. Signaling pathways in sensitization: toward a nociceptor cell biology. *Neuron* 2007; **55**; 365.

16. Mantyh PW. Cancer pain and its impact on diagnosis, survival and quality of life. *Nature Rev Neurosci* 2006; **7**:797.

17. Tracey I, Mantyh PW. The cerebral signature for pain perception and its modulation. *Neuron* 2007; **55**;377.

18. Apkarian AV, Baliki MN, Geha PY. Towards a theory of chronic pain. *Prog Neurobiol* 2009; **87**:81–97.

19. Strigo IA, Duncan GH, Boivin M, Bushnell MC. Differentiation of visceral and cutaneous pain in the human brain. *J Neurophysiol* 2003; **89**:3294–303.

20. Ahmedzai SH, Boland J. The total challenge of cancer pain in supportive and palliative care. *Curr Opin Support Palliat Care* 2007; **1**(1):3–5.

21. Bennett MI. What evidence do we have that the WHO ladder is effective in cancer pain? In McQuay HJ, Kalso E, Moore RA (eds) *Systematic review in pain research*, pp. 303–13. Seattle, WA: IASP Press, 2008.

22. Ahmedzai S, Brooks D. Transdermal fentanyl versus sustained-release oral morphine in cancer pain: preference, efficacy, and quality of life. *J Pain Sympt Manage* 1997; **13** (5):254–61.

23. Tassinari D, Sartori S, Tamburini E, *et al.* Adverse effects of transdermal opiates treating moderate-severe cancer pain in comparison to long-acting morphine: a meta-analysis and systematic review of the literature. *J Palliat Med* 2008; **11**(3):492–501.

24. Lussier D, Beaulieu P. Toward a rational taxonomy of analgesic drugs. In Beaulieu P, Lussier D, Porreca F, Dickenson AH (eds) *Pharmacology of pain*, pp. 27–40. Seattle, IASP Press, 2010.

25. Ahmedzai SH, Clayson H. Supportive and palliative care in mesothelioma. In O'Byrne K, Rusch V (eds) *Malignant Pleural Mesothelioma*, pp. 403–33. Oxford, Oxford University Press, 2006.

26. Glare P, Walsh D, Sheehan D. The adverse effects of morphine: a prospective survey of common symptoms during repeated dosing for chronic cancer pain. *Am J Hosp Palliat Care* 2006; **23**:229.

27. Moore RA, McQuay HJ. Prevalence of opioid adverse events in chronic non-malignant pain: systematic review of randomised trials of oral opioids. *Arthritis Res Ther* 2005; **7**:R1046–R1051.

28. Villars P, Dodd, M, West C, *et al.* Differences in the prevalence and severity of side effects based on type of analgesic prescription in patients with chronic cancer pain. *J Pain Sympt Manage* 2007; **33**(1):67.

29. Ballantyne JC, Mao J. Opioid therapy for chronic pain. *N Engl J Med* 2003; **349**:1943–53.

30. Meert TF, Vermeirsch HA. A preclinical comparison between different opioids: antinociceptive versus adverse effects. *Pharmacol, Biochem Behav* 2005; **80**:309–26.

31. Shimoyama N, Shimoyama M, Elliott KJ, Inturrisi CE. d-Methadone is antinociceptive in the rat formalin test1. *JPET* 1997; **283**:648–52.

32. Hoskin PJ (2003) Bisphosphonates and radiation therapy for palliation of metastatic bone disease. *Cancer Treat Rev* 2003; **29**:321–7.

33. Wu, AS, Fourney DR. Supportive care aspects of vertebroplasty in patients with cancer. *Support Cancer Ther* 2005; **2**(2):98–104.

34. Siemionow K, Lieberman IH. Vertebral augmentation in osteoporosis and bone metastasis. *Current Opinion in Supportive and Palliative Care* 2007; **1**:323–7.

35. Hicks F, Simpson KH. *Nerve blocks in palliative care.* Oxford, Oxford University Press, 2004

36. Kvarnstrom A, Karlsten R, Quiding H, Emanuelsson BM, Gordh T. The effectiveness of intravenous ketamine and lidocaine on peripheral neuropathic pain. *Acta Anaesthesiol Scand* 2003; **47**:868–77.

37. Challapalli V, Tremont-Lukats IW, McNicol ED, Lau J, Carr DB. Systematic administration of local anesthetic agents to relieve neuropathic pain. *Cochrane Database Syst Rev* 2005; **19**(4):CD003345.

38. Burton AW, Rajagopal A, Shah HN, *et al.* Epidural and intrathecal analgesia is effective in treating refractory cancer pain. *Pain Med* 2004; **5**(3):239–47.

39. Smith TJ, Coyne PJ, Staats PS, *et al.* An implantable drug delivery system (IDDS) for refractory cancer pain provides sustained pain control, less drug-related toxicity, and possibly better survival compared with comprehensive medical management (CMM). *Ann Oncol* 2005; **16**:825–33.

40. Vranken JH, Zuurmond WW, de Lange JJ. Continuous brachial plexus block as treatment for the Pancoast syndrome. *Clin J Pain.* 2000; **16**(4):327–33.

41. Crul BJP, Blok LM, van Egmond J, van Dongen RTM. The present role of percutaneous cervical cordotomy for the treatment of cancer pain. *J Headache Pain* 2005; **6**:24–9.

42. Kanpolat Y, Ugur HC, Ayten M, Elhan AH. Computed tomography-guided percutaneous cordotomy for intractable pain in malignancy. *Neurosurgery* 2009; **64**(Suppl 3):187–94.

43. Raphael J, Ahmedzai SH, Hester J, *et al.* Cancer Pain: Part 1: Pathophysiology; oncological, pharmacological, and psychological treatments: a perspective from the British Pain Society endorsed by the UK Association of Palliative Medicine and the Royal College of General Practitioners. *Pain Med* 2010; **11**:742–64.

44. Hasselaar JG, Verhagen SC, Vissers KC. When cancer symptoms cannot be controlled: the role of palliative sedation. *Curr Opin Support Palliat Care* 2009; **3**(1):14–23.

45. Passik SD. Issues in long-term opioid therapy: unmet needs, risks, and solutions. *Mayo Clin Proc* 2009; **84**(7):593–601.

46. Rice ASC, Lever I, Zarnegar R. Cannabinoids and analgesia, with special reference to neuropathic pain. In McQuay HJ, Kalso E, Moore RA (eds) *Systematic review in pain research*, pp. 233–46. Seattle, WA: IASP Press, 2008.

47. Verri WA Jr, Cunha TM, Parada CA, Poole S, Cunha FQ, Ferreira SH. Hypernociceptive role of cytokines and chemokines: targets for analgesic drug development? *Pharmacol Therapeut* 2006; **112**:116–38.

Part 7

Specific diseases

Chapter 19

Supportive care in cystic fibrosis

Andrew Clayton

Introduction

Cystic fibrosis (CF) is the most common autosomal recessive disease in Caucasian populations affecting approximately 1 in 2500 live births. It's most striking clinical feature is progressive lung inflammation and infection. The lungs of CF infants are structurally normal at birth but the production of abnormally thick mucus leads to chronic infection. Overall *Pseudomonas aeruginosa* is the most common isolate, followed by *Staphylococcus aureus*, *Haemophilus influenzae*, and *Stenotrophomonas maltophilia*. Persistent infection and resulting intense neutrophil-driven inflammation lead to progressive bronchiectasis. Respiratory symptoms of persistent productive cough, shortness of breath, and haemoptysis are the commonest clinical features of the disease. Persistent and progressive lung disease is responsible for the majority of morbidity and mortality in most patients.

Other organ systems are almost invariably also affected—90% of patients have exocrine pancreatic insufficiency leading to gastrointestinal malabsorption. This problem is exacerbated by the hypermetabolic state associated with persistent endobronchial infection. Later on in disease progression pancreatic destruction affects Langerhans cells leading to diabetes mellitus. Approximately 20% of CF patients are diabetic (1) and the incidence of this complication rises with age. CF-related diabetes comprises features of type 1 and 2 disorder; a combination of reduced and delayed insulin secretion with insulin resistance is present in most patients. At least 30% of patients have abnormal liver function tests; the commonest histological finding is fatty infiltration, present in up to 70% of older patients. This progresses to biliary cirrhosis in fewer than 10% of these patients.

Infertility is almost universal in CF males due to atretic or absent seminal vesicles despite normal spermatogenesis and sexual potency.

The most significant advance in our understanding of cystic fibrosis occurred in 1989 with the identification of a 230-kb gene on the long arm of chromosome seven, mutations of which were shown to be the underlying cause of CF (2). Inheritance follows an autosomal recessive pattern; the heterozygous carrier state affects 1 in 22 individuals in the UK. Our knowledge of mutations in this gene is not comprehensive and new mutations are frequently described. There are currently over 1600. Worldwide the commonest mutation is ΔF 508, a 3-base pair substitution which leads to a single amino acid substitution at position 508 of the 1480-amino acid polypeptide for which the gene codes, the cystic fibrosis transmembrane conductance regulator (CFTR). Survival has increased rapidly over the last 50 years, in 2008 median survival was 38.8 years (3). Survival continues to improve; individuals born with CF today have a projected life expectancy well into their sixth decade.

Medical management in cystic fibrosis

This chapter is not intended as a comprehensive guide to the medical management of CF, a wide variety of textbooks exist covering this topic. Detailed guidelines are available from national organizations such as the UK CF trust (http://www.cftrust.org.uk/). Broadly speaking there are three central principles to optimizing outcomes in CF: aggressive use of antibiotics, airway clearance, and maintaining adequate nutrition. These strategies aim to prevent chronic infection for as long as possible (particularly colonization with *Pseudomonas aeruginosa*) and robustly treat acute exacerbations to minimize decline in lung function, improve quality of life, maintain independence and maximize life expectancy (4).

Supportive care in cystic fibrosis

Supportive measures are widely used in the care of patients with CF. CF is a complex multisystem disorder and it is now accepted that optimal CF care is delivered by a multi-disciplinary team (MDT). This multidisciplinary, holistic approach to patient care is central to modern CF medicine. In this respect CF teams are able to offer far more to their patients than is often the case for other respiratory subspecialities. This can lead to striking inequality between patients with similar needs. This is most obvious when comparing the care of CF patients with similar patients who have a diagnosis of non-CF bronchiectasis. In the following sections we will consider in more detail specific areas of supportive care in CF.

Specialist cystic fibrosis care

It is now widely accepted that optimal CF care is best delivered in specialist centres. Furthermore most CF patients and their families prefer to be looked after in this context (5). Specialist centres generally look after at least 50 patients. Typically the CF MDT is made up of the following members: CF clinicians; physiotherapists; dieticians; specialist nurses; social workers; and increasingly psychologists and specialist pharmacists. Patients receive input from all these professionals when seen in both outpatient and inpatient settings.

The cystic fibrosis medical team

This should be led by an experienced chest physician with extensive CF experience. Their job plan should be set up to ensure a majority of time is devoted to CF care. The lead clinician may be supported by one or more consultant colleague(s) depending on the number of patients accessing the service. Ideally the medical team will also be involved in CF specific research projects.

The specialist nurse

The specialist nurse is often the first point of access for patients when they encounter problems; they provide practical and emotional support for patients and their families. They have a key role in leading the ward nurses, educating them about specific aspects of CF care and providing support and expertise for practical issues such as the use of implantable intravenous (IV) access devices. They will often triage clinical, emotional, or practical problems to the MDT member best equipped to deal with it and increasingly are taking on additional responsibilities and skills such as prescribing, IV access or management roles.

The specialist physiotherapist

Facilitating the delivery of optimal airway clearance is the fundamental role of the CF physiotherapist. This is achieved not only through direct therapy sessions with patients but though education of patients and their families. Assessment of exercise tolerance and the use of structured exercise programmes to both augment airway clearance and enhance physical fitness are also vital roles. The role of the physiotherapist is becoming increasingly diverse with subspecialty interests such as posture management, incontinence, or non-invasive ventilation.

The specialist dietician

Maintenance of a normal body mass index (BMI) is very important in cystic fibrosis. A low BMI has consistently been shown to be a negative prognostic factor (6). The specialist dietician achieves this by close monitoring of patients dietary intake, the correct use of pancreatic enzyme supplementation, tight diabetic control, and fat-soluble vitamin supplements. Their help is essential in the management of gastrointestinal complications of CF, particularly distal intestinal obstructive syndrome (DIOS). Correcting low body weight in CF patients is often very challenging; patients with advanced lung disease will have very high basal calorie requirements, generally CF patients are thought to require 20–50% more calories than age- and gender-matched healthy individuals (7). Enteral feeding supplements are frequently required to deliver the calories needed for weight gain and have been shown to also stabilize lung function (8, 9). Other challenges are disordered eating behaviours and the pregnant CF patient (discussed later).

The social worker

The CF social worker has a very different role to that found on a typical medical ward. As CF patients are a young population their needs can be very different. There is considerable overlap with the work of the psychologist, assisting and supporting patients and their families. The social worker often visits patients at home; this frequently provides a telling insight into issues that can be unknown to the other members of the team, e.g. poor concordance, financial hardship, domestic abuse, or even child protection issues.

As patients now survive well into adult life they are increasingly completing higher education and joining the workforce as well as having families of their own. The social worker is an important advocate for those in the workplace—most employers will not be familiar with CF and the social worker can help to reinforce patients' needs. Many patients will be unable to work full time and may need frequent periods of prolonged absence to receive courses of IV antibiotics. For those unable to work due to declining health the social worker can help to decipher the increasingly complex benefit system and the need for adaptations in the home.

The psychologist

Attention to psychological well-being is essential in CF as with all chronic diseases. Untreated or unaddressed psychological issues are likely to lead to the failure of medical management and ultimately lead to worse outcomes for patients. The work of the psychologist is examined in more depth later.

Home care services

The burden of treatment for CF patients is substantial; even those in good health may need to spend several hours a day on their treatment. Physiotherapy, time-consuming medication such as nebulized drugs, and enteric feeding are common in all but the mildest cases. As health deteriorates, the intensity and number of treatments increases. Maintaining an active independent life in the face of these demands is not easy. Naturally most patients and families wish to spend as much time as possible doing exactly this and an effective home care service can help to achieve this goal (10, 11). Different members of the MDT may be involved in the delivery of home care, in most centres the service is lead by the specialist nurses often with the support of others, especially the physiotherapist and social workers. Assistance with specific drug treatments, home IV antibiotics, or physiotherapy techniques are common examples of homecare provision. A well run homecare service can enhance treatment concordance and help patients to cope with their illness. Remaining at home allows patients to continue with other commitments such as work, education, or childcare. Older adults may be the main carer for other relatives.

Homecare has economic benefits to both the patient and healthcare provider (12) but may not always be appropriate. There is some evidence that hospital IV antibiotics are more effective than home IV antibiotics (13, 14) and the patient's home circumstances may make certain home treatments impractical or unsafe. An inpatient stay may be more appropriate to initiate certain complex medical treatments such as enteral feeding or non-invasive ventilation. It also allows an overall re-assessment of patient management which can be essential when an individual's management is not going as planned.

Psychology and cystic fibrosis

That psychological problems frequently occur in a life limiting, progressive, complex chronic disease like CF cannot be regarded as surprising. We have already touched on some of these issues in earlier sections. Studies of psychological issues in CF remain fairly sparse but their importance is reflected in the growing number of teams taking on dedicated psychologists (15). Adolescents with CF are thought to be approximately three times more likely than healthy controls to experience emotional or behavioural problems (16). Those with more advanced lung disease have been shown to have lower quality of life scores (17) and are at increased risk of depression and relationship problems (18). Chronic diseases are strongly linked to deliberate self-harm and whilst this has not been studied in CF, our patients can be expected to be at increased risk. Some studies have shown the prevalence of clinical depression to be as high as 46% (19). Depression is strongly associated with poor treatment concordance (20) and both poorer lung function and quality of life scores in CF adults (21). Adults are also at increased risk of anxiety disorder (22) and abnormal body image (18), the latter being particularly problematic in adolescents (23). Many patients cope remarkably well with their CF; in fact some studies suggest the prevalence of psychological problems is no higher than in healthy controls (24, 25).

Many CF patients feel isolated from their peers due to rigorous infection control policies. It is now accepted that patients should be isolated from each other to prevent the acquisition of transmissible strains of organisms that may accelerate lung function decline. These organisms are often the most difficult to treat (26). Transmission of the highly virulent organism *Burkholderia cenocepacia* has frequently been described, often from CF centres and summer camps (27, 28) Acquisition of this organism is associated with increased morbidity and mortality (28, 29). The loss of peer group support via camps and direct social contact has had a negative impact on those individuals old enough to remember them. To some extent modern technology has given us tools to fill this void via online chat rooms, instant messaging and social networking sites. We know that many patients continue to socialize outside the hospital environment.

Perhaps the main driver of psychological issues is the conflict generated by attempting to balance an ever increasing treatment burden with the need and desire to live a normal life. A common casualty in this battle is concordance with treatment. Studies in chronic disease consistently show incomplete concordance with medical treatment—typically patients take 50% of the agents prescribed to them (30). Concordance is inversely proportional to the number of treatments given and their complexity (31). Similar results have been observed in CF patients, time-consuming or complex treatments such as nebulized agents and enteral feeding tend to have the lowest concordance (32). Poor concordance is likely to lead to treatment failure and progressive disease. The first step in improving concordance is to acknowledge it as an issue. Clinicians should accept that their patients are unlikely to take everything they are prescribed and tell patients that this is not unusual. By fostering a no-blame atmosphere a more realistic treatment regime can be agreed that the patient may succeed with. Endlessly adding to treatment regimens without asking which are actually being taken will lead to ever decreasing concordance.

Psychological assessment and intervention should not be seen as the exclusive role of the team psychologist. All members of the team can contribute. Good communication skills, active listening, and demonstrating empathy are essential and will lead to earlier detection of psychological problems. An assessment of psychological well-being should be made at annual review and whenever significant problems are identified referral to a psychological therapist or psychiatrist should be made. Cognitive behavioural therapy is widely used in chronic disease groups to treat depression and anxiety disorders and its use in CF is well established (22, 33).

Fertility and pregnancy

CF patients are increasingly becoming parents as their own survival increases. This leads to a range of specific problems. CF adolescents and young adults are often ill-informed about these issues, particularly the dangers that pregnancy may hold for young CF women (34). Adverse outcomes for mother and child are greatest in those with more advanced lung disease (35) whilst pregnancy is well tolerated for those with normal BMI and mild lung disease with no deleterious effect on survival (36).

Pregnancy must be a planned event for CF women with strong emphasis on maximizing pre-conception lung function and BMI. Frank discussions regarding the safety of pregnancy are necessary for those with poorer lung function. CF women have to face the prospect that they may well not live to see their children reach adulthood; 20% die before their child's tenth birthday (36). Supportive care in pregnancy starts with pre-conception genetic counselling and screening of the partner for CF carrier status. Regular monitoring and joint care with obstetrics and fetal medicine are vital. Weight gain is often difficult during pregnancy and enteral feeding may well be necessary. Regular medication should be reviewed for safety and choice of IV agents for respiratory exacerbations may need to be altered.

CF males are almost universally infertile due to congenital absence of the vas deferens (37). Like their female counterparts they are increasingly interested in parenthood, a recent study found 84% wanted to become fathers (38). Whilst this will not have a direct impact on their health they face the same dilemmas linked to their survival. Those who do proceed to fatherhood do so with the help of sperm harvesting and intracytoplasmic sperm injection (ICSI) (39, 40).

Urinary incontinence

The prevalence of urinary incontinence in adult CF women has been reported to be as high as 60% (41), repeated coughing hastening the development of stress incontinence. Incontinence is rarely reported without direct questioning. It can cause significant distress to patients and may lead to inadequate airway clearance via cough avoidance. Pelvic floor exercises are an effective strategy in CF women (42).

Palliation and bereavement

Whilst survival has improved dramatically in recent years, CF remains a life-limiting condition. Patients are acutely aware of their own mortality; most will have known others, perhaps siblings, who have died (43). As with other aspects of CF care successful palliative care is best delivered by the holistic approach of the full MDT. Discussions of end of life issues should be held early. Whilst these discussions will not be easy and may induce patient anxiety, evidence from other specialities suggests they ultimately are helpful (44, 45). Avoidance of these issues ultimately leads to chaotic unsupported deaths and distressing long-term consequences for friends and family. A substantial proportion of those in the terminal phase of their illness will be on the active waiting list for lung transplantation. This inevitably leads to difficulties in the balance and aims of patient care. On the one hand, donor lungs may become available at any moment and the team aims to optimize the patient's respiratory and nutritional status to maximize their chances of successful transplantation. This leads to increasingly intensive and potentially uncomfortable treatment; life-threatening exacerbations, prolonged inpatient stays, non-invasive ventilation, and enteral feeding are usual in this phase of illness. Demand for transplant continues to outstrip donor availability. As a result around 50% of those on the waiting list will die without ever receiving donor lungs (46, 47). These individuals risk losing the chance of a 'good death', if the need for palliation is overlooked in the intense treatment phase leading to transplant. Drugs used for symptom control do not preclude transplant and can be reversed if one becomes available, the balance of treatment and symptom control should be regularly reviewed. Many teams will use the time of initial transplant referral as an opportunity for timely discussion of end of life issues. Assessment of patient insight is followed by open discussion of their wishes on a wide range of issues including: resuscitation; religious/spiritual needs; wills; memory boxes; place of death; family relationships/unfinished business. The use of high-quality communication skills throughout the terminal phase is crucial to its success. The patient must be at the heart of all discussions regarding their care unless they have specifically nominated a proxy amongst their friends and family. Some may choose to document their preferences for end of life care in an advance directive. A recent survey of CF patients in North America found that 30% had done so (48). Exclusion of the patient may avoid difficult discussions but will only lead to a loss of trust with the team and will have a negative impact on their death (49).

All patients in the terminal phase are likely to require symptom control; the vast majority of patients will die from respiratory failure. Breathlessness, anxiety, and fatigue are the commonest symptoms to occur. Pain, nausea, vomiting, and seizures are uncommon (50). Non-medical treatments of breathlessness may be very helpful, e.g. non-invasive ventilation (51) or physiotherapy (52). Drugs to aid symptom control should be used early. The aim should be dose titration to achieve patient comfort without hastening the dying process. Multiple agents are used, a combination of opiates, benzodiazepines, and antiemetics is commonly necessary, often via continuous subcutaneous infusion. Levomepromazine is useful to treat anxiety, terminal agitation, and nausea. Predicting the course of dying is very difficult, particularly its duration. Terminal decline may occur rapidly over hours or take place very gradually over months. This uncertainty along with transplant status means that end of life CF care is very different to that seen in other dying medical patients. Whilst symptom control is similar in both groups it is usual to discontinue therapeutic and long-term medication outside CF practice. One study of paediatric CF patients showed 86% of patients were on opiates for more than a month and 76% remained on IV antibiotics or other acute therapies to within 12 hours of death (53). This means that end of life care pathways used in other patient groups will not be appropriate for CF care. The duration and complexity of end of life care in CF means that 80% of CF patients die in hospital (54).

The loss of a loved one will always be difficult but early, good preparation for death along with excellent medical management will improve the bereavement experience of those close to the patient. Most CF teams will have some sort of bereavement service available to relatives, often this is informal. A member of the team will visit relatives at home; often this is the specialist nurse, social worker, or psychologist. The needs of team members should not be overlooked at this time, many of them will have known the patient for a long time, friendships develop and the patient's loss is often felt deeply. The use of team debriefing for the MDT and ward staff can be helpful in addressing this.

Conclusions

Patients with CF have seen a dramatic improvement in their care over the last 40 years. Survival and quality of life have increased and continue to do so; CF is no longer a disease of childhood. Much of this can be attributed to advances in medical management. Supportive care plays a vital role in CF patient management, providing treatment in its own right as well as enhancing the success of more conventional therapies. Its use is arguably more prominent in CF than any other area of respiratory medicine; other disciplines are likely to benefit from a similar approach.

References

1. UK CF Database, UK CF Trust. *Annual Data Report 2004*. Dundee: UK CF Database, 2006.
2. Riordan JR, Rommens JM, Kerem B, *et al*. Identification of the cystic fibrosis gene: cloning and characterization of complementary DNA. *Science* 1989; **245**:1066–73.
3. Cystic Fibrosis Trust. *UK CF Registry Annual data report, 2008*. London: Cystic Fibrosis Trust, 2008.
4. Standards for the clinical care of children and adults with Cystic Fibrosis in the UK. 2001 *Cystic Fibrosis Trust Clinical Standards and Accreditation Group*. UK CF Trust.
5. Walters S, Britton J, Hodson ME. Hospital care for adults with cystic fibrosis: an overview and comparison between special cystic fibrosis clinics and general clinics using a patient questionnaire. *Thorax* 1994; **49**:300–6.
6. Sharma R, Florea VG, Bolger AP, *et al*. Wasting as an independent predictor of mortality in patients with cystic fibrosis. *Thorax* 2001; **56**:746–50.
7. Pencharz P, Hill R, Archibald E, Levy L, Newth C. Energy needs and nutritional rehabilitation in undernourished adolescents and young adult patients with cystic fibrosis. *J Pediatr Gastroenterol Nutr* 1984; **3**(Suppl 1):S147–53.
8. Steinkamp G, Von Der Hardt H. Improvement of nutritional status and lung function after long-term nocturnal gastrostomy feedings in cystic fibrosis. *J Pediatr* 1994; **124**:244–9.
9. Walker SA, Gozal D. Pulmonary function correlates in the prediction of long-term weight gain in cystic fibrosis patients with gastrostomy tube feedings. *J Pediatr Gastroenterol Nutr* 1998; **27**:53–6.
10. Kuzemko JA. Home treatment of pulmonary infection in cystic fibrosis. *Chest* 1988; **94**:162S–166S.
11. Bramwell E, Harvey H. Care of cystic fibrosis in the community. *Community Nurse* 1998; **3**:16–7.
12. Strandvik B, Hjelte L, Malmborg AS, Widen B. Home intravenous antibiotic treatment of patients with cystic fibrosis. *Acta Paediatr* 1992; **81**:340–4.

13. Thornton J, Elliott RA, Tully MP, Dodd M, Webb AK. Clinical and economic choices in the treatment of respiratory infections in cystic fibrosis: comparing hospital and home care. *J Cyst Fibros* 2005; **4**:239–47.

14. Nazer D, Abdulhamid I, Thomas R, Pendleton S. Home versus hospital intravenous antibiotic therapy for acute pulmonary exacerbations in children with cystic fibrosis. *Pediatr Pulmonol* 2006; **41**:744–9.

15. Kerem E, Conway S, Elborn S, Heijerman H. Standards of care for patients with cystic fibrosis: a European consensus. *J Cyst Fibros* 2005; **4**:7–26.

16. Cadman D, Boyle M, Szatmari P, Offord DR. Chronic illness, disability, and mental and social well-being: findings of the Ontario Child Health Study. *Pediatrics* 1987; **79**:805–13.

17. Gee L, Abbott J, Conway SP, Etherington C, Webb AK. Quality of life in cystic fibrosis: the impact of gender, general health perceptions and disease severity. *J Cyst Fibros* 2003; **2**:206–13.

18. Pfeffer PE, Pfeffer JM, Hodson ME. The psychosocial and psychiatric side of cystic fibrosis in adolescents and adults. *J Cyst Fibros* 2003; **2**:61–8.

19. Burker EJ, Sedway J, Carone S. Psychological and educational factors: better predictors of work status than FEV_1 in adults with cystic fibrosis. *Pediatr Pulmonol* 2004; **38**:413–18.

20. DiMatteo MR, Lepper HS, Croghan TW. Depression is a risk factor for noncompliance with medical treatment: meta-analysis of the effects of anxiety and depression on patient adherence. *Arch Intern Med* 2000; **160**:2101–7.

21. Riekert KA, Bartlett SJ, Boyle MP, Krishnan JA, Rand CS. The association between depression, lung function, and health-related quality of life among adults with cystic fibrosis. *Chest* 2007; **132**:231–7.

22. Oxley H, Webb AK. How a clinical psychologist manages the problems of adults with cystic fibrosis. *J R Soc Med* 2005; **98**(Suppl 45):37–46.

23. Shearer JE, Bryon M. The nature and prevalence of eating disorders and eating disturbance in adolescents with cystic fibrosis. *J R Soc Med* 2004; **97**(Suppl 44):36–42.

24. Blair C, Cull A, Freeman CP. Psychosocial functioning of young adults with cystic fibrosis and their families. *Thorax* 1994; **49**:798–802.

25. Anderson DL, Flume PA, Hardy KK. Psychological functioning of adults with cystic fibrosis. *Chest* 2001; **119**:1079–84.

26. Elborn JS. Difficult bacteria, antibiotic resistance and transmissibility in cystic fibrosis. *Thorax* 2004; **59**:914–5.

27. Jones AM, Dodd ME, Webb AK. Burkholderia cepacia: current clinical issues, environmental controversies and ethical dilemmas. *Eur Respir J* 2001; **17**:295–301.

28. Govan JR, Brown PH, Maddison J, *et al.* Evidence for transmission of Pseudomonas cepacia by social contact in cystic fibrosis. *Lancet* 1993; **342**:15–9.

29. McCloskey M, Mccaughan J, Redmond AO, Elborn JS. Clinical outcome after acquisition of Burkholderia cepacia in patients with cystic fibrosis. *Ir J Med Sci* 2001; **170**:28–31.

30. Sackett D, Snow J. The magnitude of compliance and non-compliance. In Haynes R, Taylor D, Sackett D (eds) *Compliance in healthcare*, pp. 11–22. Baltimore, MA: The Johns Hopkins University Press, 1979.

31. Lask B. Understanding and managing poor adherence in cystic fibrosis. *Pediatr Pulmonol Suppl* 1997; **16**:260–1.

32. Abbott J, Dodd M, Bilton D, Webb AK. Treatment compliance in adults with cystic fibrosis. Thorax 1994; **49**:115–20.

33. Heslop K. Cognitive behavioural therapy in cystic fibrosis. *J R Soc Med* 2006; **99**(Suppl 46):27–9.

34. Sawyer SM, Tully MA, Dovey ME, Colin AA. Reproductive health in males with cystic fibrosis: knowledge, attitudes, and experiences of patients and parents. *Pediatr Pulmonol* 1998; **25**:226–30.

35. Kotloff RM, Fitzsimmons SC, Fiel SB. Fertility and pregnancy in patients with cystic fibrosis. *Clin Chest Med* 1992; **13**:623–35.

36. Goss CH, Rubenfeld GD, Otto K, Aitken ML. The effect of pregnancy on survival in women with cystic fibrosis. *Chest* 2003; **124**:1460–8.

37. Denning CR, Sommers SC, Quigley HJ, Jr. Infertility in male patients with cystic fibrosis. *Pediatrics* 1968; **41**:7–17.

38. Sawyer SM, Farrant B, Cerritelli B, Wilson J. A survey of sexual and reproductive health in men with cystic fibrosis: new challenges for adolescent and adult services. *Thorax* 2005; **60**:326–30.

39. Palermo G, Joris H, Devroey P, Van Steirteghem AC. Pregnancies after intracytoplasmic injection of single spermatozoon into an oocyte. *Lancet* 1992; **340**:17–8.

40. Schlegel PN, Cohen J, Goldstein M, *et al.* Cystic fibrosis gene mutations do not affect sperm function during *in vitro* fertilization with micromanipulation for men with bilateral congenital absence of vas deferens. *Fertil Steril* 1995; **64**:421–6.

41. Cornacchia M, Zenorini A, Perobelli S, Zanolla L, Mastella G, Braggion C. Prevalence of urinary incontinence in women with cystic fibrosis. *BJU Int* 2001; **88**:44–8.

42. McVean RJ, Orr A, Webb AK, *et al.* Treatment of urinary incontinence in cystic fibrosis. *J Cyst Fibros* 2003; **2**:171–6.

43. O'Brien JM, Goodenow C, Espin O. Adolescents' reactions to the death of a peer. *Adolescence* 1991; **26**:431–40.

44. Karasz A, Dyche L, Selwyn P. Physicians' experiences of caring for late-stage HIV patients in the post-HAART era: challenges and adaptations. *Soc Sci Med* 2003; **57**:1609–20.

45. Koenigsmann M, Koehler K, Regner A, Franke A, Frommer J. Facing mortality: a qualitative in-depth interview study on illness perception, lay theories and coping strategies of adult patients with acute leukemia 1 week after diagnosis. *Leuk Res* 2006; **30**:1127–34.

46. De Meester J, Smits JM, Persijn GG, Haverich A. Lung transplant waiting list: differential outcome of type of end-stage lung disease, one year after registration. *J Heart Lung Transplant* 1999; **18**:563–71.

47. Lowton K. 'Double or quits': perceptions and management of organ transplantation by adults with cystic fibrosis. *Soc Sci Med* 2003; **56**:1355–67.

48. Sawicki GS, Dill EJ, Asher D, Sellers DE, Robinson WM. Advance care planning in adults with cystic fibrosis. *J Palliat Med* 2008; **11**:1135–41.

49. Lowton K. Parents and partners: lay carers' perceptions of their role in the treatment and care of adults with cystic fibrosis. *J Adv Nurs* 2002; **39**:174–81.

50. Plonk WM Jr, Arnold RM. Terminal care: the last weeks of life. *J Palliat Med* 2005; **8**:1042–54.

51. Madden BP, Kariyawasam H, Siddiqi AJ, Machin A, Pryor JA, Hodson ME. Noninvasive ventilation in cystic fibrosis patients with acute or chronic respiratory failure. *Eur Respir J* 2002; **19**:310–13.

52. Luce JM, Luce JA. Perspectives on care at the close of life. Management of dyspnea in patients with far-advanced lung disease: "once I lose it, it's kind of hard to catch it… ". *JAMA* 2001; **285**:1331–7.

53. Robinson WM, Ravilly S, Berde C, Wohl ME. End-of-life care in cystic fibrosis. *Pediatrics* 1997; **100**:205–9.

54. Mitchell I, Nakielna E, Tullis E, Adair C. Cystic fibrosis. End-stage care in Canada. *Chest* 2000; **118**:80–4.

Chapter 20

Assessment and management of respiratory symptoms of malignant disease

Jennifer Chard, Peter Hoskin,
and Sam H. Ahmedzai

Supportive care is a major component in the management of malignant diseases that affect the respiratory system. It should be included in the overall management plan for the patient from the very outset. Even in cancers that are potentially curable, the burden of respiratory symptoms and their psychosocial consequences can be significant for the patient and family carers, and supportive care should be instituted alongside the anticancer intervention. It is no longer justified to wait for anticancer treatments with curative intent to be tried and seen to fail before the patient is considered for expert symptom palliation and the family as a whole is offered supportive care. (See Chapter 1, this volume, for a detailed discussion on the timing of supportive care with respect to anticancer therapy.)

Many patients who present with new respiratory or systemic symptoms of lung cancer will need urgent palliation of these problems, even before a definitive histological diagnosis can be made. Indeed, some patients who present late with advanced disease may be too ill for invasive diagnostic investigations, and palliative interventions will be planned on the basis of a working diagnosis of lung cancer, guided on radiological findings and clinical history. However, as will be seen below, it is helpful to pursue the histology if primary lung cancer is suspected, even in quite elderly and frail patients, because the differentiation into small-cell lung cancer (SCLC) or non-small-cell lung cancer (NSCLC) can be a very helpful guide to palliative therapeutic decisions. NSCLC is the commoner of these two main types of lung cancer.

Prevalence of symptoms in cancer

Although this chapter concentrates on supportive care needs of patients with primary thoracic cancers, much of the assessment and therapeutic content applies equally well to patients with extrathoracic primary cancers. Several studies have shown that respiratory symptoms and systemic consequences of malignancy are common to many solid tumours. Using the Memorial Symptom Assessment Scale, Portenoy *et al.* found that dyspnoea, fatigue, and pain were prevalent in most cancer patients, although there are of course variations relating to specific sites (Table 20.1) (1). Thus, dyspnoea affected 28% of patients with colon cancer, 26% of those with breast cancer, and 12% of patients with ovarian cancers.

Hopwood and Stephens (2) reported on symptom prevalence in large numbers of patients with lung cancer who entered the UK Medical Research Council (MRC) clinical trials (Table 20.2). The data on symptoms were derived from the Rotterdam Symptom Checklist (RSCL) (3), a quality-of-life instrument that was widely used in Europe in the mid-1990s. It is worth noting that as these patients were being entered in clinical trials of anticancer treatments, those who were considered too ill for such interventions will have been excluded, so the true picture of symptom and psychosocial burden at presentation may be even worse. In general there was little difference between SCLC and NSCLC, but it is interesting to note that gender differences were detectable using the RSCL (2). Thus, women with early NSCLC reported an average of 16.8 symptoms, whereas men reported an average of 13.8 symptoms. The prevalence of general symptoms was similar but women tended to declare more psychological problems (difference of 20%). In contrast, men reported slightly more physical symptoms, e.g. 12% more haemoptysis, 7% more cough, 3% more dyspnoea, and 2% more chest pain. In early SCLC, these differences were not noted.

There are several published reports on symptom prevalence in patients with advanced lung cancer (4, 5). Once again, it is important to be aware of potential selection bias in these studies, as the criteria for including patients will vary. Many of the patients were

Table 20.1 Prevalence of symptoms in patients attending a cancer hospital

Symptoms	Prevalence (%) by primary site				
	Colon	Prostate	Breast	Ovary	Overall
Shortness of breath	28.3	25.4	25.7	12.0	23.5
Cough	22.2	25.8	37.1	28.0	28.6
Lack of energy	78.3	66.7	80.0	68.0	73.7
Pain	61.7	68.3	60.0	67.3	64.0

Modified with permission from (1). With kind permission from Springer Science+Business Media: Quality of Life Research, Symptom prevalence, characteristics and distress in a cancer population, Volume 3, Number 3, 1994, page 183–189, R. K. Portenoy, H. T. Thaler, A. B. Kornblith et al., Table 2.

Table 20.2 Prevalence (%) of symptoms in patients with early lung cancer. See text for discussion of gender differences in symptoms prevalence

Symptoms	SCLC	NSCLC
Shortness of breath	87	86
Cough	81	87
Haemoptysis	26	36
Lack of energy	88	87
Chest pain	52	50

Modified with permission from (2).

Table 20.3 Prevalence (%) of symptoms in patients with advanced cancer

Symptoms	Primary site						
	Lungs	**Breast**	**Oesophagus**	**Prostate**	**Gynaecological**	**Colorectal**	**Overall**[a]
Dyspnoea	46	24	19	16	11	10	19
Weakness	60	57	64	53	56	68	51
Pain	52	60	44	66	75	64	57

Source: Modified from (4).

[a] Represented mean percentage of all patients in survey (including four other sites).

recruited from palliative care services, and the data will therefore undoubtedly reflect differences between countries (and within countries) regarding how they select patients with advanced disease. Table 20.3 shows prevalence of symptoms in a large international study, conducted on behalf of the World Health Organization (WHO), of patients with advanced cancer who were receiving specialist palliative care (4). Even in hospital-based ambulatory patients, respiratory symptoms were present in a range of non-pulmonary cancer types, e.g. dyspnoea was seen in 25% of ovary and prostate cancer patients, 26% of breast cancer patients, and 29% of colon cancer patients (6). A Japanese hospice study showed that dyspnoea was present in 33% of patients on admission, but this rose to 66% nearer the time of death; prevalence of cough and sputum also rose from 29% to 48% (7).

Causes and assessment of symptoms in cancer

The main symptoms that will be considered in this chapter are dyspnoea, cough, haemoptysis, and pain. The causes of these symptoms are often complex, and the symptoms themselves may come in patterns, which together with clinical findings and evidence from imaging such as chest radiographs and ultrasound, can help to make a working diagnosis. Table 20.4 list the common patterns of symptoms which are seen in patients who have or are suspected of having problems related to cancer or its treatments (7).

Patients with malignant disease often have other reasons for having respiratory and other systemic problems, and it is important to be able to separate the symptoms of comorbidity from those of the cancer. This is particularly relevant with elderly and frail patients, as embarking on a course of management aimed at palliating malignant symptoms can expose them to potentially major side effects, when in fact less harmful treatments may be needed for coexisting chronic or acute conditions. Table 20.5 lists the common comorbid conditions that arise in patients with cancer who complain of respiratory symptoms.

The symptoms caused by these comorbid conditions can easily mimic those that arise directly from malignant disease. Compared with disorders producing chronic airflow limitation, i.e. asthma and chronic obstructive pulmonary disease (COPD), the onset and pattern of breathlessness related to exertion may for some patients be identical to the picture seen in malignant obstruction. Others with asthma or COPD, however, may be able to differentiate the sensations, especially if the new dyspnoea associated with cancer

Table 20.4 Patterns of respiratory symptoms in patients with cancer: symptoms and their anatomical-pathological bases

Anatomical 'site'	Pathological change	Symptom
Pulmonary	Tracheal tumour	Dyspnoea, stridor, cough
	Lung collapse	Dyspnoea, cough
	Airway collapse	Dyspnoea, cough
	Tracheo-oesophageal fistula	Cough, haemoptysis
	Consolidation	Dyspnoea, cough, pleurisy
	Infection	Dyspnoea, cough, pain, haemoptysis
	Lymphangitis carcinomatosa	Dyspnoea, cough
	Thromboembolism	Dyspnoea, cough, pain
	Radiation damage	Dyspnoea, cough
Pleural	Effusion	Dyspnoea
	Thromboembolism	Dyspnoea, pain
	Tumour	Pain, pleurisy
Thoracic cage	Chest wall tumour	Pain, 'Fungating' cancer
	Carcinoma en *cuirasse*	Dyspnoea, pain, 'fungating' cancer
	Diaphragmatic tumour	Dyspnoea, pain, hiccups

Source: Modified from (67).

Table 20.5 Common problems coexisting in patients with cancer (comorbidity)

Problem	Cause
Pain	Arthritis; ischaemia; osteoporosis
Dyspnoea	COPD; heart failure; panic; attacks
Cough	COPD; ACE-inhibitor; neurogenic
Fatigue	Anaemia; nutritional deficit; chronic fatigue syndrome

is not provoked by the usual factors that aggravate their chronic airflow problem. Table 20.6 shows the time course of breathlessness with different causes in such patients.

Other clues which can help to identify dyspnoea caused by cancer come from accompanying symptoms that the patient may report. These include the presence of wheezing, cough, purulent sputum, haemoptysis, chest pain, and oedema (of lower or upper limbs). As can be seen from Table 20.7, even these clues may not be foolproof in making a secure diagnosis and in many cases further investigations will be needed, unless the patient is very ill. The detailed approaches to investigation and assessment of dyspnoea, cough, and pain are discussed elsewhere in this volume (see Chapters 6, 15, 16, and 17).

Table 20.8 lists the minimal useful investigations for dyspnoea, which may help in making a diagnosis before embarking on new therapy. The table also indicates which tests may be helpful in monitoring progress and in estimating prognosis. For example, serial

Table 20.6 Common problems coexisting in patients with cancer (comorbidity)

	Onset acute (h)	Subacute (days or weeks)	Chronic (months)	Recurrent episodes	Nocturnal attacks
Pulmonary					
Asthma	+	+	++	++	++
COPD	+	++			
Infection	+	++			
Pleural				+	
Bronchial obstruction	++	+			
Pulmonary embolism	+	++		+	

Source: Modified from (67).

Key: ++, common: +, occasional.

Table 20.7 Causes of dyspnoea in patients with cancer: associated clinical features

	Wheeze	Purulent sputum	Cough	Haemoptysis	Chest pain	Oedema	
Pulmonary							
Asthma	++	(+)	++				
COPD	++	++	++	(+)		+	(Cor pulmonale legs)
Infection	+	++	(++)	(+)	(+)		
Pleural effusion							
Bronchial obstruction	+	+	++	+	+	(+)	(Superior vena cava obstruction arms/face)
Pulmonary embolism	(+)		+	+	++	+	(Deep vein thrombosis: leg)

Source: Modified from (67).

Key; ++, common; +, occasional; (+), unusual.

lung volumes can be helpful in assessing response to bronchodilator or steroid therapy. Pericardial effusion, detected by cardiac ultrasound, and pulmonary embolism, which is confirmed by ventilation–perfusion scanning, are both poor prognostic findings.

Approaches to symptom management

Once the causes of symptoms have been established, it is possible to make a rational plan for their management. Table 1.2 (see Chapter 1, this volume) presents a generic model for differentiating symptom palliation interventions on the basis of the intention to treat, for both cancer and non-malignant conditions. These categories of treatment intention (prevention/prophylaxis, targeting of primary disease process, manipulation of pathophysiological

Table 20.8 Investigation of dyspnoea in patients with cancer

Recommended	Useful for making diagnosis	Monitoring progress	Determining prognosis
Imaging:			
Chest radiograph	++	+	(+)
CT scan of thorax	++	+	(+)
Ultrasound (to localize pleural or pericardial effusion)	+	(+)	(+)
Ventilation–perfusion lung scan (for pulmonary embolism)	+	(+)	+
Blood:			
Full blood count	++	(+)	
Skin oxygen saturation (SaO$_2$)	++	+	
Pulmonary function:			
Dynamic lung volumes (FEV$_1$, FVC) preferably with bronchodilator	++	+	

Source: Modified from (67).

Key; ++, essential for comprehensive assessment; desirable; (+), optional or limited value.

consequences, and alteration of perception) are exemplified further in the case of cancer-related symptoms in Table 20.9. Thus, where respiratory symptoms are directly related to progressive malignancy, selective use of anticancer treatment (type 2 palliation) is an important component of the management of such patients, even in the setting of advanced incurable disease. Indeed, in the context of lung cancer less than 10% of patients presenting with NSCLC will be suitable for radical (i.e. potentially curative) treatment.

Table 20.9 Classification of palliative intervention in patients with thoracic cancer

Type of palliation	Intention	Examples of intervention
Type 1	Prevention/prophylaxis	Prophylactic cranial irradiation (PCI) to prevent brain metastases in SCLC
Type 2	Direct targeting of the primary disease process	Resection of tumour
		Radiotherapy (RT) for bone destruction
		Chemotherapy for primary SCLC
		RT for primary NSCLC
Type 3	Manipulation of the pathophysiological consequence of the primary disease process	Bisphosphonate for symptoms hypocalcaemia
		Haemostatic treatment for haemoptysis
		Pleural aspiration
Type 4	Alteration of the perception of secondary effects of the symptoms	Analgesia for pain
		Oxygen for breathlessness
		Opioid for cough

Which anticancer treatments are available?

The two principal modalities of treatment available in the management of cancer-related respiratory symptoms are chemotherapy and radiotherapy. Both chemotherapy and radiotherapy have an important role in NSCLC whereas chemotherapy is the treatment of choice for SCLC, as well as breast and colorectal cancer. This partly reflects the relative sensitivities of these tumours to chemotherapy and also the differences in their natural history.

Radiotherapy

Non-small-cell lung cancer

Palliative radiotherapy for NSCLC has been the subject of a series of phase III randomized controlled trials (RCTs) performed by the UK MRC and other collaborative groups in Europe and USA (such as the European Organization for Research and Treatment of Cancer (EORTC) and the South Western Oncology Group (SWOG)) over the last decade or more. These studies have extensively investigated the efficacy of radiotherapy in the management of symptoms from advanced inoperable disease and explored optimal radiation dose schedules. From these results it appears clear that for poorer performance status (PS) patients, symptom control can be achieved either with single doses of 10Gy, or with two treatments given 1 week apart delivering 17Gy in two fractions (8, 9).

One trial suggests that in patients with good PS a more protracted treatment delivering 39Gy in 13 fractions can achieve similar symptom control with a small but statistically significant improvement in survival (10). Similar results have been obtained comparing 20Gy in five fractions with 17Gy in two fractions, again restricted to good prognosis patients although a further study comparing 42.5Gy and 50Gy with 17Gy in two fractions failed to show any advantage for the prolonged fractionation schedule (11). A Cochrane review has concluded that in patients with stage IIIB and IV NSCLC, good PS patients should receive higher dose schedules delivering 20–30Gy in five to ten fractions whilst poor PS patients will achieve good palliation with one or two fractions (12). Estimates of rates of symptom control from these trials are shown in Table 20.10. The issue of deferring treatment in the absence of symptoms has also been explored in a MRC trial in which 230 patients with inoperable NSCLC were randomized to immediate palliative radiotherapy or supportive care and later radiotherapy only if symptoms arose. This study showed that there was no disadvantage in avoiding treatment in the asymptomatic patient (13).

In selected patients radical treatment will be appropriate and offers both the best chance of durable tumour control and also effective symptom palliation. Radical chemoradiotherapy is the standard of care for locally advanced stage IIIB patients with good PS and adequate pulmonary reserve. Radiotherapy is also an option for radical treatment of earlier stage disease that is inoperable. Multiple randomized trials have addressed the role of concurrent chemoradiotherapy in patients with locally advanced disease using platinum-based chemotherapy and thoracic radiotherapy doses in the order of 60–66Gy

Table 20.10 Symptoms response and survival in lung cancer following radiotherapy

	Trial 1[a]		Trial 2[b]		Trial 3[c]	
	17Gy	10Gy	39Gy	17Gy	30Gy	EBRT
Dyspnoea	41%	43%	51%	46%	49%	38%
Cough	48%	56%	36%	48%	45%	65%
Haemoptysis	75%	72%	89%	95%	90%	71%
Fatigue	NS	NS	40%	48%	65%	30%
Chest pain	59%	72%	58%	65%	77%	43%
Median survival (days)	100	122	270	216	287	250

[a] (9): 17Gy in 2 fractions, 10Gy in 1 fraction.

[b] (10): 39Gy in 13 fractions, 17Gy in 2 fractions.

[c] (24):14 30Gy in 8 fractions, 15Gy endobronchial radiotherapy.

NS, not started

in 2-Gy fractions. The optimal chemotherapy regimen is not known (see 'Chemotherapy' section, below); however cisplatin/etoposide and carboplatin/paclitaxel are both common combinations. An individual patient data meta-analysis combined nine trials, with the conclusion that chemoradiotherapy was better than RT alone with a 4% absolute benefit to overall survival at 2 years (14). The optimal way to combine chemotherapy and radiotherapy, whether concurrently or sequentially, is still under debate although there is some evidence that concurrent treatment may be better (15). The role of the targeted agent cetuximab in addition to chemoradiotherapy is the subject of the current phase III RTOG 0617 trial, which is also examining high-dose RT to 74Gy.

The role of altered dose fractionation radiotherapy schedules has also been explored as a means of improving outcomes. In the UK continuous hyperfractionated accelerated radiotherapy (CHART) has been evaluated in a large randomized trial of 563 patients. This schedule treats patients three times a day using fractions of 1.5Gy to a total dose of 54Gy. Radiotherapy is given on consecutive days, including weekends, with the entire course completed in 12 days. The results of the RCT comparing this to standard conventional radiotherapy delivering 60Gy in 6 weeks has shown a consistent improvement in survival, with 30% alive at 2 years compared to 21% and a 5-year survival of 12% compared to 7% (16). This is comparable to the gains seen with chemoradiotherapy.

Technical advances in radiotherapy delivery

The dose of radiotherapy that can be delivered for lung cancer treatment is limited by the tolerances of adjacent normal tissue structures. Conventional external beam radiotherapy treats the cancer with a margin of normal tissue to allow for limitations in delineating the primary tumour and variation in patient set up and organ motion, such as that from respiration. Advances in imaging technology have allowed for more accurate tumour staging and localization and radiotherapy technology such as intensity modulated radiotherapy (IMRT), daily imaging during the course of treatment and respiratory motion compensation mean it is now possible to reduce the margin of normal tissue treated. This may in turn allow for higher doses to be delivered to the primary tumour whilst sparing normal tissue structures with a reduction in side effects, i.e. improving the therapeutic ratio.

Three-dimensional computed tomography (CT)-based radiotherapy planning is recommended for radical treatments in lung cancer. Methods to improve accuracy in contouring gross tumour and involved nodal volumes include the use of intravenous contrast and combining planning CT images with functional imaging such as [18F]-fluorodeoxyglucose positron emission tomography images (FDG-PET), which is commonly performed as a staging investigation in NSCLC. Several methods may be used to account for the motion of tumour with respiration, which may be up to several centimetres. These include four-dimensional respiration correlated planning CT and respiration gated treatments, breath holding techniques, real-time tumour tracking, and abdominal compression.

Stereotactic body radiotherapy (SBRT) is a technique that may be used for smaller lung tumours (<5cm) and limited metastases. It is a highly conformal, precisely targeted form of radiotherapy that delivers treatment in a small number of larger fractions (up to 20Gy). In this treatment accurate tumour delineation, patient positioning and immobilization and tumour motion control are all critical. SBRT is currently the subject of two randomized trials, comparing it with surgery for early stage NSCLC.

Small-cell lung cancer

Radiotherapy is also effective in SCLC; indeed, SCLC is a highly radioresponsive tumour in which rapid regression is often seen. However, systematic trials have not been performed on the role of radiotherapy for palliation of symptoms from SCLC. In general, therefore, an analogy between NSCLC and SCLC is assumed, with similar doses being used for both.

Thoracic radiotherapy in addition to chemotherapy in limited stage disease improves local control rates and adds a modest overall survival benefit of around 5% at 2 years. Early results were conflicting, however a survival benefit was demonstrated in two older meta-analyses (17, 18). The studies included in these meta-analyses used older chemotherapy regimens and sequential treatment, which have been superseded by regimens that allow for concurrent chemoradiotherapy, suggesting the benefit may actually be greater with modern regimens.

Recommended chemoradiotherapy schedules are once daily treatment to doses of 50–60Gy in 2-Gy fractions or hyperfractionated accelerated radiotherapy of 45Gy delivered in 1.5-Gy fractions twice daily. The latter has proven superior to 45Gy delivered in daily fractions, with concurrent cisplatin/etoposide chemotherapy. The overall survival at 5 years in this randomized trial was 26% in the accelerated arm compared with 16% in the standard arm (19). The delivery of radiotherapy is similar to that for NSCLC.

There is a high rate of cerebral metastases in patients with SCLC, as most chemotherapy agents do not penetrate the blood–brain barrier. Prophylactic cranial irradiation (PCI) with doses of 24–36Gy in 2-Gy fractions is an option for patients who have a complete response to initial therapy. PCI has been shown in several randomized trials to significantly reduce the incidence of brain metastases and a meta-analysis of PCI in primarily limited stage disease demonstrated it also confers a survival benefit of 5.4% at 3 years (15.3% vs. 20.7%) (20). PCI also reduces the incidence of brain metastases in locally advanced NSCLC, however no trial has shown a survival benefit for this treatment and it is not currently recommended as standard therapy.

Mesothelioma

There is a limited role for palliative radiotherapy in mesothelioma, usually for localized chest pain. Other symptoms such as pleural effusion, cough, and dyspnoea reflecting diffuse chest-wall disease are not helped by radiotherapy because of the toxicity of delivering radiation to large volumes of the thorax. Palliation has been reported in 60–70% of patients, although this may be maintained for only a few months (21, 22). Retreatment may be effective and no dose–response relationship for palliation has been shown, standard doses being 20–30Gy in five to ten daily fractions over 1–2 weeks.

There are single-institution case series showing long-term survival in highly selected patients with trimodality treatment, including extrapleural pneumonectomy and high-dose postoperative radiotherapy to the chest cavity (23).

Endobronchial therapy

The trials discussed above concerned external beam radiotherapy, but radiation can also be delivered internally to endobronchial tumours using brachytherapy. This is a technique whereby a small radiation source (iridium) is temporarily introduced into the bronchus via a fine-bore catheter (Figure 20.1).

Catheters are placed under direct vision at fibreoptic bronchoscopy and their position verified, following removal of the bronchoscope, by radiography or CT scan (Figure 20.2). The length to be treated is then defined on the film and the brachytherapy source, which is attached to a long wire, is programmed to move in 5-mm steps along the defined length of catheter. It remains at each step position for a few seconds to deliver the radiation dose. This technique is usually performed as a day case procedure, but requires sedation or light general anaesthetic for the catheter insertion.

(a)   (b)

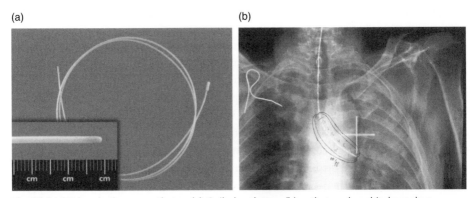

Fig. 20.1 HDR brachytherapy catheter. (a) Coiled catheter; (b) catheter placed in bronchus.

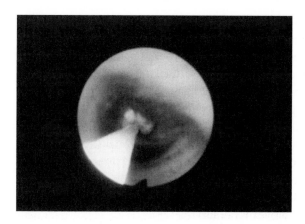

Fig. 20.2 HDR catheter *in situ* following removal of bronchoscope.

The usual dose for a single endobronchial treatment is 7.5–15Gy defined at 1cm from the catheter. Points inside that 1-cm envelope will receive much higher doses, but the dose drops off rapidly with increasing distance from the source, minimizing toxicity to other surrounding structures.

Single-centre studies have shown this to be effective in palliation of endobronchial symptoms. A RCT comparing endobronchial brachytherapy with external beam radiotherapy concluded that fractionated external beam therapy is preferred in patients with good PS (24). External beam radiotherapy gave better and more sustained overall palliation, but it caused greater acute toxicity, in particular dysphagia. As would be expected, there was no survival difference between the two techniques. The relative efficacies for symptom palliation are shown in Table 20.10.

The main acute toxicity with endobronchial brachytherapy is increased cough from the irritant effect of the catheter and radiation reaction. This is typically short-lived and self-limiting over a few days. A late toxicity is the increased possibility of massive haemoptysis in some patients.

The place of endobronchial brachytherapy in the overall management of advanced lung cancer remains unclear. The level I evidence from the RCT suggests that for most patients external beam therapy should be considered initially, and the main role of brachytherapy is in those patients relapsing with chest symptoms after previous external beam treatment.

Chemotherapy

Chemotherapy in advanced NSCLC

There are many modern chemotherapy regimens currently used as first-line treatment in patients with locally advanced or metastatic NSCLC but no single combination regimen that has proven superior (25, 26). Regimens that combine two drugs, typically a platinum compound (cisplatin or carboplatin) with another drug (vinorelbine, paclitaxel, docetaxel, gemcitabine, etoposide, irinotecan, or pemetrexed) are the most common. A meta-analysis has shown carboplatin has a lower response rate compared with cisplatin; however, this did not translate to a significant effect on survival (27). Carboplatin has a more favourable toxicity profile and may be a preferable option over cisplatin in patients treated with palliative intent, particularly those who are elderly or of poor PS. There are also several non-platinum containing regimens available such as gemcitabine plus a taxane. The duration of treatment is generally four to six cycles, guided by objective assessment of response on imaging and treatment toxicity.

The use of two agents compared with single-agent therapy is associated with a higher response rate and modest survival benefits, but at the expense of greater toxicity. A meta-analysis of 65 randomized trials comparing single, two-agent, and three-agent chemotherapy demonstrated an improvement in response rate of 13% versus 26% and in survival at 1 year 30% versus 35% comparing single agents with two drugs but the addition of a third agent did not improve overall survival (28).

Palliative chemotherapy improves survival when given in addition to supportive care. This was best demonstrated in an individual patient data meta-analysis of 16 randomized trials which shows an absolute survival benefit of 9% at 12 months from 20% to 29% for chemotherapy compared with supportive care alone, which translates to an improvement in medial survival of 1.5 months (29).

Analysis of quality of life in patients treated with palliative chemotherapy is somewhat more limited. A subset of patients treated in the European Big Lung Trial were evaluated in regard to quality of life endpoints, with no difference shown between the chemotherapy and supportive care arms (30).

Histology is emerging as a predictive factor for selecting treatment regimens. A phase III study comparing 1725 patients with stage IIIB or IV NSCLC treated with cisplatin/pemetrexed versus cisplatin/gemcitabine chemotherapy demonstrated no difference between the two arms in median survival (10.3 months). However, in planned subset analysis there was a significant survival benefit in the cisplatin/pemetrexed arm for patients with adenocarcinoma and large cell carcinoma compared with squamous cell histology (median 12.6 vs. 10.9 months) (31). The UK National Institute for Health and Clinical Excellence (NICE) guidelines recommend pemetrexed as first-line treatment only for these histological subtypes.

The approach to patients who have progressive disease despite first-line treatment will depend on current symptoms, the site and extent of disease and the initial treatment given, in addition to patient factors. For patients with disseminated disease, second-line chemotherapy or targeted therapy remains an option. Single-agent docetaxel has been shown in one randomized trial to improve median survival (7.5 months vs. 4.6 months) when compared with best supportive care (32). Single-agent pemetrexed used second line shows comparable response rates and median survival to docetaxel in non-squamous histologies, with less neutropenia (33). Both erlotinib and gefitinib (see 'Targeted systemic therapy' section, below) have also been used as second-line treatment.

Elderly and poor performance status patients

A substantial proportion of patients diagnosed with NSCLC are aged over 70 or have comorbid diseases, however first-line chemotherapy should still be considered in these patients.

Age alone should not be a discriminator; with 24% of patients included in the large meta-analysis demonstrating the survival benefit of palliative chemotherapy aged over 70. There was no suggestion that patients in this age group did any worse with chemotherapy than younger patients (28).

Patients with poor PS (ECOG ≥2 or KPS <70) are a heterogeneous group that are often excluded from major trials of chemotherapy in NSCLC. There is, however, evidence from a randomized trial in this population that combination chemotherapy, compared with single agent, provides a higher response rate (38% vs. 16%) but with no statistically significant overall survival benefit (34). It is clear that individualized treatment is required in this patient population, taking into consideration extent of disease, life expectancy, patient preferences, and quality of life.

Adjuvant chemotherapy in resectable disease

Several large randomized trials have demonstrated the benefit of cisplatin-based chemotherapy following complete surgical resection of NSCLC with a meta-analysis of individual patient data from the largest of these trials demonstrating an absolute survival benefit of 5.4% at 5 years, most pronounced in stage II and IIIA disease (35).

Targeted systemic therapy

Targeted systemic therapies are an emerging area in oncology and a method of individualizing treatment based on the molecular features of the cancer. Pathways that may be exploited include: cell signalling, cell proliferation, angiogenesis, or apoptosis. In many tumours there is overexpression of receptors involved in these pathways and by targeting them at a cellular level, the progression of a tumour may be altered. Most targeted therapies are either small-molecule drugs that interact with intracellular targets or monoclonal antibodies that interact with receptors on the cell surface.

Gefitinib and erlotinib are small molecules that inhibit epidermal growth factor receptor (EGFR) tyrosine kinase (TK). They have demonstrated benefit as initial treatment in NSCLC in certain patients and are being further evaluated as an adjunct to first-line chemotherapy. The side effect profile for these oral drugs differs from chemotherapy, with skin rashes and diarrhoea more common.

A phase III trial of 1217 patients from an Asian population who were non-smokers or former light smokers with adenocarcinoma compared first-line carboplatin/paclitaxel chemotherapy with the EGFR TK inhibitor gefitinib. This study demonstrated benefit to gefitinib in a planned subset analysis of patients who had molecular markers performed. In those with EGFR mutations, median survival was improved (9.5 vs. 6.3 months) whilst those without the mutation did better with chemotherapy (36).

As yet no randomized trials have shown a survival benefit to the addition of gefitinib or erlotinib in addition to chemotherapy (37-40). It is possible that with further molecular classification of tumours, a subgroup of patients in whom this treatment is beneficial may emerge, as patient populations in these trials were heterogeneous.

Bevacizumab is a monoclonal antibody that binds to vascular endothelial growth factor (VEGF) receptor. VEGF is thought to play a role in angiogenesis in NSCLC and other tumour types. In patients with non-squamous histology NSCLC bevacizumab has demonstrated modest overall survival benefit when used in addition to carboplatin/paclitaxel chemotherapy (median 10.3 vs. 12.3 months) (41). Progression-free, but not overall survival was improved in a trial of bevacizumab plus cisplatin/gemcitabine (42).

Cetuximab is a monoclonal antibody that binds to EGFR that has also been trialled as an addition to standard chemotherapy doublets. In contrast to gefitinib and erlotinib, cetuximab has demonstrated a small overall survival benefit when added to cisplatin/vinorelbine chemotherapy (median 11.3 vs. 10.1 months) however there was also a significant increase in side effects with this treatment (43).

Small-cell lung cancer

SCLC accounts for approximately 20% of all lung cancers and behaves quite differently to NSCLC, often presenting with rapidly growing, bulky, central tumours. It is highly responsive to chemotherapy, however the results are often short lived.

In patients with limited stage disease chemoradiation is the standard approach using concomitant cisplatin and etoposide with twice daily radiotherapy given between cycles 1 and 2. In patients with extensive stage disease, platinum-based chemotherapy regimens or combinations of cyclophosphamide, adriamycin, and vincristine are used and as with NSCLC no single combination has proven superior. Cisplatin or carboplatin are commonly paired with etoposide but may also be combined with irinotecan, topotecan or epirubicin. No advantage to prolonging treatment beyond three or four cycles has been shown in extensive disease and major symptoms such as cough, dyspnoea and chest pain respond in 60–70% of patients.

Topotecan may be used as a single-agent second-line chemotherapy but with much lower response rates than first-line treatment. In patients who are not candidates for intravenous treatment, oral topotecan has been shown in a randomized trial to prolong survival (26 vs. 14 weeks) and improve symptoms and quality of life when compared with supportive care alone (44).

Mesothelioma

The majority of patients with mesothelioma present with incurable disease. Combination chemotherapy with cisplatin and pemetrexed is considered the standard regimen in good PS patients and has been shown to prolong survival (median 12.1 vs. 9.3 months) compared with placebo (45).

In contrast, a trial in 409 patients comparing chemotherapy using combination mitomycin, vinblastine, and low-dose cisplatin or single-agent vinorelbine with 'active symptom control' using steroids, bronchodilators and analgesics showed no significant benefits to quality of life or overall survival (46). Although this trial used older chemotherapy regimens, it demonstrates that supportive care alone is an appropriate option for some patients.

Radiotherapy or chemotherapy for palliation?

Symptoms of breathless, haemoptysis, cough, and pain due to either NSCLC or SCLC can be effectively palliated in the previously untreated patient with either radiotherapy or chemotherapy. The choice between the two is often difficult and, as shown in

Tables 20.10 and 20.11, response rates are similar. Chemotherapy may be seen as a more debilitating treatment with more associated systemic toxicity, but radiotherapy may also cause acute effects, typically transient dysphagia due to radiation oesophagitis. Chemotherapy may be more effective where symptoms are multiple and due to wide-spread disease, where there is metastatic disease outside the lung, and where other symptoms such as cachexia and anorexia are prominent. Comparison of RCTs suggests that better quality of life will be achieved with chemotherapy than so-called 'best supportive care' alone, not to mention the observed survival advantage.

Radiation therapy is predominantly a locoregional treatment, and where symptoms are due to locoregional tumour progression, e.g. isolated haemoptysis from the bronchus or obstruction secondary to endobronchial tumour growth, then local radiotherapy is effective and simple with toxicity usually limited to a short period of dysphagia. Phase III evidence supports its use in short pragmatic schedules delivering one or two large doses where PS is poor. These doses are close to normal tissue tolerance, however, in particular that of the spinal cord, and in general these treatments cannot be repeated. Brachytherapy localizes the radiation dose within the bronchus and offers an alternative means of retreatment for patients with cough, dyspnoea, or haemoptysis due to recurrent endobronchial tumour.

No direct phase III comparison of chemotherapy versus radiotherapy has been undertaken in the management of symptoms from advanced NSCLC or SCLC. Phase III trials and meta-analyses in NSCLC suggest that chemotherapy has advantages over supportive care alone, although difficulties in the definition and delivery of so-called 'best supportive care' leave these conclusions open to debate. (See Chapter 1 for further discussion of definitions and the proposed composition of a truly comprehensive supportive care programme.)

Both radiotherapy and chemotherapy have been shown to have a small survival advantage, of the order of 3 months. However, this must be viewed in the light of the time taken to undergo a course of treatment and recover from its treatment-related side effects.

Table 20.11 Symptoms response rates (%) with chemotherapy in NSCLC

Symptom	PV+M or I	MIP	MVP	Gemcitabine	
				All	**Mod./severe**
Dyspnoea	78%	46%	59%	26%	51%
Cough	45%	70%	66%	44%	73%
Haemoptysis	91%	92%	–	63%	100%
Anorexia	50%	58%	–	29%	38%
Pain	47%	77%	60%	32%	37%
Malaise	–	–	53%	–	–

PV = cisplatin, vindesine with either M = mitomycin or I = ifosfamide.

MIP = mitomycin, ifosfamide, cisplatin.

MVP (also called CMV) = cisplatin, mitomycin-C and vinblastine

'All' refers to the percentage of patients with symptoms (mild, moderate, and severe) who had relief

'Mod./severe' refers to the percentage of patients with only moderate and severe symptoms who improved.

Modified from Thatcher et al, and Ellis et al—with permission.

A cost-benefit analysis from Canada addressing the role of chemotherapy in NSCLC found a benefit from both cisplatin and vinorelbine and gemcitabine when survival and quality of life were considered against so-called 'best supportive care' alone (47). Whether the survival gains are additive from radiotherapy and chemotherapy has not been tested.

A 'scripted interview' study in the US exploring the views of patients who had had previous cisplatin-based chemotherapy for NSCLC found that although there was considerable individual variation, chemotherapy would be accepted by these patients if there was median survival threshold of 4.5 months for mildly toxic chemotherapy and 9 months for chemotherapy with severe toxicity (48). When considering the effect of chemotherapy on symptoms, 68% would choose chemotherapy if it would substantially reduce symptoms.

Perhaps the most important single factor to take into consideration for planning therapy is PS. Patients with good PS (i.e. ECOG/WHO grade 0 or 1) may gain a survival advantage from protracted radiotherapy (i.e. more than five fractions) or chemotherapy (more than three cycles) whereas patients with poor PS are generally best served by single-fraction palliative radiotherapy, or in SCLC, short (three-cycle) combination chemotherapy.

Treatment choices will also be influenced by previous exposure to treatment. Previous radiation may exclude further exposure if tolerance doses to critical normal tissues are exceeded. This will usually relate to the spinal cord rather than intrathoracic structures. Spinal cord tolerance is generally perceived to be around an equivalent dose of 40–50Gy given in 2-Gy fractions over 4–5 weeks. The palliative schedule of 17Gy in two fractions has been demonstrated to result in fewer episodes of myelitis, with an estimated risk of about 2% across the 1042 patients treated in MRC trials with this schedule (49). Most patients are therefore very close to or at the limits of spinal cord tolerance after palliative radiotherapy, and retreatment after such schedules carries significant hazards.

A different principle applies to re-exposure to chemotherapy relating to drug-resistance. In general re-exposure to a previously administered chemotherapy agent is avoided, on the basis that residual cells progressing after that exposure will be resistant to the original chemotherapy drug. Since in most circumstances there are at least two recognized effective treatment chemotherapy schedules, this limits the need for repeating treatments. The palliative efficacy of second-line chemotherapy has been formally evaluated in NSCLC as described above and in a randomized trial in SCLC an advantage for second-line chemotherapy over 'supportive care' in patients responding to an initial four cycles of treatment was also confirmed (50). There is therefore level I evidence for the use of radiotherapy, first- and second-line chemotherapy in patients with NSCLC and first- and second-line chemotherapy in SCLC.

However, a recent US study has suggested that having conventional anticancer therapies such as chemotherapy in advanced NSCLC may actually be associated with a reduced survival. In a randomized trial of early referral to palliative care (EPC) versus conventional oncological management, patients who had early EPC had not only improved symptoms and psychological health, but also had a mean survival which was longer (11.6 months vs. 8.9 months, P = 0.02) (51). The authors hypothesized that this unexpected finding arose from the observation that EPC patients had evidence of less aggressive care, including fewer chemotherapy treatments near the end of life, compared to standard care patients.

Comprehensive palliation of symptoms

Apart from treatments directed at the cancer itself (type 2 palliation, see Table 20.9) which have been extensively discussed above, management of symptoms can also be considered using the other types of palliative interventions described in Chapter 1, this volume. Examples of these approaches include:

♦ Endobronchial tumour causing obstruction or cough (types 3, 4 palliation).

♦ Lung parenchymal disease which will typically cause breathlessness and may also be associated with cough (types 3, 4 palliation).

♦ Chest wall invasion, predominantly pain (type 4 palliation).

♦ Systemic illness, e.g. fatigue, distant metastases (types 3, 4 palliation).

These are shown in Figure 20.3, along with examples of types 1 and 2 palliation (preventive and direct anticancer intervention).

Breathlessness

Breathlessness due to endobronchial obstruction may be associated with stridor or lung collapse. Initially this may be treated with an endobronchial clearing procedure such as electrocautery, laser therapy (52–54), photodynamic therapy (55), or cryotherapy (56, 57). These are all strictly speaking type 2 palliative interventions, as they work by destruction of the tumour. Airway stenting may also be useful where tumour outside the bronchi is causing external compression.

Airway stenting can give very rapid and dramatic relief of dyspnoea, especially if it is caused by extrinsic compression of bronchi or trachea. Figure 20.4 shows two such examples of extrinsic airways compression arising in mesothelioma and primary lung cancer. Figure 20.5 shows a patient with recurrent NSCLC who was previously treated with external beam radiotherapy, and was successfully palliated with a bronchial stent after complete lung collapse.

For both NSCLC and SCLC, external beam radiotherapy or endobronchial brachytherapy is effective and should be considered. Where breathlessness is due to diffuse parenchymal infiltration or multiple lung metastases or lymphangitis carcinomatosa then chemotherapy is indicated and radiotherapy has no role. Lymphangitis due to primary lung cancer is usually resistant to both types of intervention; however, chemotherapy may be helpful when lymphangitis arises in breast cancer (58).

Where pleural effusion secondary to malignancy is the cause of breathlessness then initial treatment will include drainage and possibly pleurodesis—the methods for these are discussed below. Radiotherapy does not have a significant role in this situation, but chemotherapy may be helpful where recurrent effusions are a problem. One study of 37 patients receiving chemotherapy for malignant pleural effusion using mitomycin C and cisplatin with either 5FU (MCF) or vinblastine (MVP) reported a symptomatic response rate of 78% and objective improvement of the effusion radiologically in 86% (59).

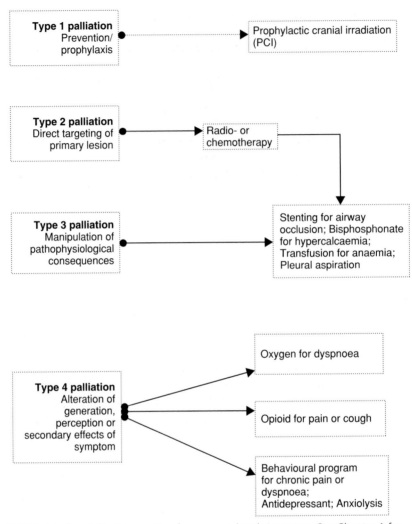

Fig. 20.3 Model of palliative intervention for cancer-related symptoms. See Chapter 1 for explanation.

Where breathlessness is due to diffuse pleural infiltration with multiple deposits of mesothelioma, radiotherapy may be tried if the disease is relatively localized. For more generalized disease, chemotherapy can be considered, but as stated before, the response rate for mesothelioma is very disappointing.

Haemoptysis

Haemoptysis is most commonly due to endobronchial tumour and is more common in NSCLC (60). It is more likely to occur with centrally placed tumours, and with primary lung cancer than with lung metastases.

Patients who have had many years of COPD may well cope with breathlessness if it becomes worse on development of lung cancer; however, the same patients may be very

(a) (b)

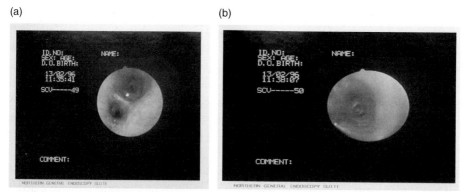

Fig. 20.4 Bronchoscopic appearance of extrinsic compression: (a) Bronchoscopic appearance in a 51-year-old man with extensive left sided pleural mesothelioma. This picture shows narrowing of the left main bronchus due to external compression, arising from mesothelioma infiltration around bronchial roots. (b) Bronchoscopic appearance of left upper lobe bronchus showing marked external compression. Endobronchial biopsies were normal.

(a) (b)

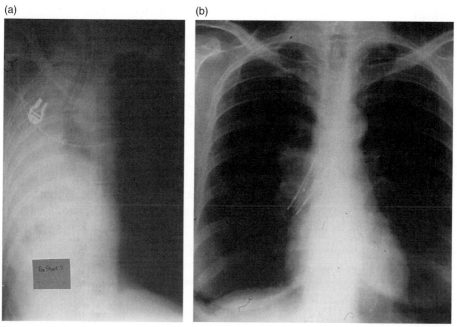

Fig. 20.5 Female patient with recurrent NSCLC treated with endobronchial stent: (a) Complete collapse of right lung. (b) Re-expansion of right lung 1 week after stent placement in right main bronchus.

fearful if haemoptysis develops. They can usually distinguish the fresh blood expectorated from a cancer from the dark staining of sputum associated with an exacerbation of COPD. The bleeding from a cancer may indeed be aggravated by intercurrent infections with increased coughing, and it is helpful to offer the patient antibiotics early on if there are signs of a new respiratory infection developing.

Haemoptysis that is intermittent and mild (often described by the patient as 'specks', 'streaks', or 'small blobs' of blood) may be managed by simple pharmacological means. Two drugs are helpful in this situation. *Tranexamic acid* works by inhibiting the breakdown of fibrin clots, primarily by blocking the binding of plasminogen and plasmin; it can be given orally at a dose of 1g, or IV at 0.5–1g three times daily. Alternatively, *ethamsylate* works not by interfering with coagulation directly, but rather through increasing capillary vascular wall resistance and platelet adhesiveness. This agent is given orally, at a dose of 500mg four times daily. There are no published trials of the use of these agents for haemoptysis.

If haemoptysis is not controlled by these means, or if the patient is unduly at risk of major bleeding, it may be readily controlled with local radiotherapy either given by external beam treatment or endobronchial treatment given in standard palliative doses. Chemotherapy may also be effective, particularly in SCLC (61).

Occasionally haemoptysis may be due to parenchymal lung metastasis. Localized treatment such as radiotherapy is then of less value unless a definite segment of the lung can be identified at bronchoscopy from which haemorrhage is occurring.

Cough

Cough due to malignancy is often a difficult symptom to palliate. Many patients with longstanding lung disease who later develop a primary lung cancer will be familiar with chronic cough which is exacerbated by infective episodes. It is important to allow cancer patients access to antibiotics if infection is definitely the cause of increased cough. The pharmacological management of cough is described fully elsewhere in this volume (see Chapter 15 and 16, this volume). The drug of choice for treating cough in cancer patients is an opioid. Often patients with cancer are already on analgesic doses of opioids: in this situation it does not necessarily help to add another opioid for cough, but it may help to give long-acting forms, especially by night.

When cough is due to endobronchial tumour then palliative external beam radiotherapy, endobronchial brachytherapy, and chemotherapy may all be effective. Overall efficacy rates are similar, as shown in Tables 20.10 and 20.11. It should be recognized that in the short-term cough may be made worse both by external beam radiotherapy and by endobronchial irradiation, which produce localized radiation tracheitis or bronchitis. Patients should therefore be warned of the possibility and they should be offered a short course of opioid linctus, e.g. codeine.

Where cough is due to diffuse parenchymal infiltration, lymphangitis, or multiple pulmonary metastases then chemotherapy may help. Cough may also be due to pleural effusion, and the appropriate therapy for that should be offered (see below).

Pain

Pain is a very common symptom arising in thoracic malignancy. Chapter 18 describes the mechanisms which cause thoracic pain. Up to 60% of patients who have had thoracotomy for curative or attempted resection of tumour may have post-surgical pain, which can extend several intercostal levels above and below the wound (62). The pharmacological

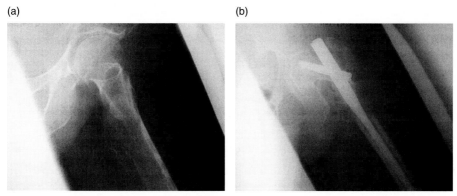

Fig. 20.6 Radiological appearance of left femur affected by metastatic cancer: (a) Multiple lytic lesions in proximal end of femur causing severe pain on weight-bearing and presenting risk of pathological fracture. (b) Prophylactic pining of the proximal end of femur. The patient had reduced pain on mobility and risk of fracture was eliminated.

management of pain is covered in Chapter 18 and in other palliative medicine texts (63). It may be useful to try a combination of NSAID and opioid (codeine, dihydrocodeine, or more potent agents such as morphine, fentanyl, or oxycodone) before considering anti-cancer measures. Even after the latter have been successful, it is likely that the patient will continue to use analgesics, at reduced dose or for usage as required. It is important that patients who have had pain associated with cancer always have access to suitable analgesics at home, should the pain recur or progress. Patients should also be instructed to report worsening pain, which does not respond to their usual regular or as-required medication, sooner rather than later.

Chest pain due to primary lung cancer can be effectively treated, as with other symptoms, by either local radiotherapy using external beam or by chemotherapy; response rates are shown in Tables 20.10 and 20.11. Pleuritic pain due to peripheral lesions may be more difficult to localize and treat, and it may be more appropriate to refer to a pain clinic for local anaesthetic or neurolytic intercostal or paravertebral blockade, rather than for anticancer therapy. Chapter 18 describes these techniques and other invasive approaches for the management of refractory pain.

Patients with lung cancer often develop peripheral metastases which cause local pain. Bone metastases respond well to single fractions of external beam radiotherapy. In some situations, e.g. metastasis to head and neck of femur, very good palliation and restoration of function may be achieved by surgical intervention, e.g. pinning or total hip replacement (see Figure 20.6).

Management of effusions

Pleural effusion frequently arises from primary lung cancer, in the early stages of mesothelioma, and occasionally with metastases affecting the pleura. If it is a presenting feature of a new illness, then it is quite likely that the effusion may be drained for diagnostic purposes. Usually this is done fairly simply using a simple percutaneous needle and syringe with a three-way valve apparatus. If the effusion is large and produces significant dyspnoea at the outset, or if it recurs soon after diagnostic drainage, then a pleural catheter should be considered. It is common now to use a so-called 'pigtail' catheter in the interpleural space, as this adopts a pronounced curvature on removal of the metal guide from the chest wall, which prevents the catheter from falling out (see Figure 20.7) (64). Alternatively, a conventional intercostal drain may be inserted and sutured in well.

A substantial effusion may require 24–48 hours to drain fully. When it is dry, or there is minimal fluid, it may be helpful to instil a sclerosing agent to prevent recurrence. This is not usually necessary until the effusion has recurred two or more times, or if it recurs quickly with a large volume. The purpose of instilling a sclerosing agent is to induce pleural inflammation, which allows the parietal and visceral pleura to adhere, thus preventing further fluid leakage. Various agents have been used, notably talc, but tetracycline (with local anaesthetic to cover for the pain of inflammation) is cheap and reliable (65). Anticancer drugs such as bleomycin do not offer significant advantages for most recurrent malignant pleural effusions.

Pericardial effusions may occur, often developing rapidly, causing patients to be extremely breathless. For rapid relief, they can be drained directly or a catheter may be left *in situ*; see Figure 20.8 for an example of this in a patient with mesothelioma. Pericardial effusion can occur with breast cancer, and may then respond to appropriate chemotherapy. For recurrent pericardial effusion, a permanent 'window' may be placed surgically between the pericardial sac and the interpleural space.

Rarely, a pleural effusion recurs in spite of attempts at chemical pleuradhesis. In this case, it can be helpful to seek the help of a thoracic surgeon to perform a pleurectomy. This can be done under direct vision using a thoracoscope, and allows the surgeon to peel

(a) (b)

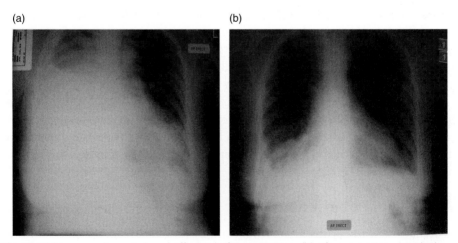

Fig. 20.7 (a) Large malignant pleural effusion before aspiration. (b) After aspiration—residual effusion.

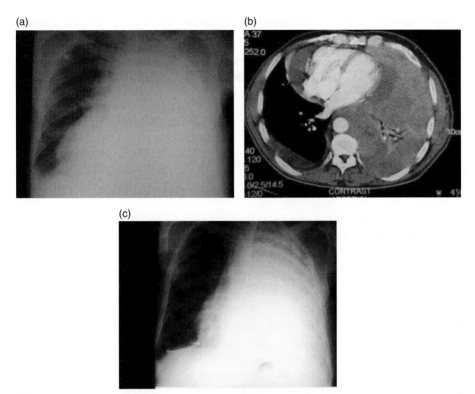

Fig. 20.8 Mesothelioma causing pericardial effusion: (a) A huge left-sided solid mass consisting of mesothelioma, causing mediastinal shift to the right side. Also pericardial effusion which is more clearly demonstrated in (b). The right costophrenic angle is obliterated, indicating a small pleural effusion. (b) CT scan showing complete filling of left hemithorax with mesothelioma. There is a pericardial effusion and also small right pleural effusion. (c) Radiographic appearance after a catheter was placed in the pericardial sac (seen lying at base of right lung). The space between right chest wall and cardiac border was increased indicating loss of pericardial volume. Note that the small pleural effusion has also been drained.

off the affected area of pleura. This technique may be particularly helpful in mesothelioma, but should be reserved for patients with relatively good expected survival (65). In a prospective cohort study of 51 patients with malignant mesothelioma, video-assisted thoracic surgery (VATS) was used to achieve pleurectomy in 17 (34%), but decortication was required for the remainder (using VATS in three and thoracotomy in 31) (66), suggestive that debulking surgery should be reserved for patients who have the epithelial cell type of mesothelioma, and who have not yet suffered significant weight loss.

Key points

- Dyspnoea, cough, haemoptysis, and chest pain are common symptoms in patients with thoracic malignancy.
- For mild symptoms, pharmacological methods are usually helpful.

- Small-cell lung cancer, non-small-cell lung cancer, and metastatic cancers may be palliated by means of radiotherapy; for endobronchial disease, brachytherapy or laser therapy may be helpful.

- Chemotherapy is effective in patients with non-small-cell lung cancer, small-cell lung cancer, breast and colorectal cancer.

- Invasive mechanical procedures including pleural drainage, pleurectomy, and endo-bronchial stenting can give useful palliation of dyspnoea.

References

1. Portenoy RK, Thaler HT, Kornblith AB, *et al.* Symptom prevalence, characteristics and distress in a cancer population. *Qual Life Res* 1994; **3**:183–9.

2. Hopwood P, Stephens RJ. Symptoms at presentation for treatment in patients with cancer; implications for the evaluation of palliative treatment. The Medical Research Council (MRC) Lung Cancer Working Party. *Br J Cancer* 1995; **71**(3):633–6.

3. de Haes JCJM, van Knippenberg FCE, Neijt JP. Measuring psychological and physical distress in cancer patients: structure and application of the Rotterdam Symptom checklist. *Br J Cancer* 1990; **62**:1034–8.

4. Vainio A, Auvinen A. Prevalence of symptoms among patients with advanced cancer: An international collaborative study. *J Pain Symptom Manage* 1996; **12**(1):3–10.

5. Donnelly S, Walsh D. The symptoms of advanced cancer: Identification of clinical and research priorities by assessment of prevalence and severity. *J Palliat Care* 1995; **11**(1):27–32.

6. Cachia E, Ahmedzai SH. Breathlessness in cancer patients. *Eur J Cancer* 2008; **44**:1116–23.

7. Morita T, Tsunoda J, Inoue S, Chichara S. Contributing factors to physical symptoms in terminally ill cancer patients. *J Pain Symptom Manage* 1999; **18**(5):338–46.

8. Medical Research Council Lung Cancer Working Party. Prepared on behalf of the working party and all its collaborators by: N.M. Bleehen, D.J. Girling, D. Machin, and R.J. Stephens. Inoperable non-small-cell lung cancer (NSCLC): a Medical Research Council randomised trial of palliative radiotherapy with two fractions or ten fractions. *Br Jr Cancer* 1991; **63**:265–70.

9. Medical Research Council Lung Cancer Working Party. Prepared on behalf of the working party and all its collaborators by: N.M. Bleehen, D.J. Girling, D.Machin, and R.J. Stephens. A Medical Research Council (MRC) randomised trial of palliative radiotherapy with two fractions or a single fraction in patients with inoperable non-small-cell lung cancer (NSCLC) and poor performance status. *Br J Cancer* 1992; **65**:934–41.

10. Medical Research Council Lung Cancer Working Party. Randomized trial of palliative two-fraction versus more intensive 13-fraction radiotherapy for patients with inoperable non-small cell lung cancer and good performance status. *Clin Oncol* 1996; **8**:167–75.

11. Sundstrom S, Bremnes R, Aasebo U, *et al.* Hypofractionated palliative radiotherapy (17Gy per 2 fractions) in advanced non-small cell lung carcinoma is comparable to standard fractionation for symptom control and survival: a national phase III trial. *J Clin Oncol* 2004; **22**:801–10.

12. Lester JF, Macbeth FR, Toy E, *et al.* Palliative radiotherapy regimens for non-small cell lung cancer. *Cochrane Database Syst Rev* 2006; **4**:CD002143.

13. Falk SJ, Girling DJ, White RJ, *et al.* on behalf of the Medical Research Council Lung Cancer Working Party. Immediate versus delayed palliative thoracic radiotherapy in patients with unresectable locally advanced non-small cell lung cancer and minimal thoracic symptoms: randomised controlled trial. *BMJ* 2002; **325** (7362):465–8.

14. Auperin A, Le Pechoux C, Pignon JP, *et al*, on behalf of the Meta-Analysis of Cisplatin/Carboplatin Based Concomitant Chemotherapy in Non-Small Cell Lung Cancer (MAC3-LC) Group.

Concomitant radio-chemotherapy based on plating compounds in patients with locally advanced non-small cell lung cancer (NSCLC): A meta-analysis of individual data from 1764 patients. *Ann Oncol* 2006; **17**:473–83.

15. Curran WJ, Scott CB, Langer CJ, *et al.* Long-term benefit is observed in a phase III comparison of sequential vs concurrent chemo-radiation for patients with unresectable stage III NSCLC. *Proc Am Soc Clin Oncol* 2003; **22**:621.

16. Saunders MI, Dische S, Barrett A, *et al.* Continuous hyperfractionated accelerated radiotherapy (CHART) versus conventional radiotherapy in non small cell lung cancer: mature data from the randomised multicentre trial. *Radiother Oncol* 1999; **37**:137–48.

17. Pignon JP, Arriagada R, Ihde DC, *et al.* A meta-analysis of thoracic radiotherapy for small-cell lung cancer. *N Engl J Med* 1992; **327**:1618–24.

18. Warde P, Payne D. Does thoracic irradiation improve survival and local control in limited-stage small-cell carcinoma of the lung? A meta-analysis. *J Clin Oncol* 1992; **10**:890–5.

19. Turrisi AT, Kim K, Blum R, *et al.* Twice-daily compared with once-daily thoracic radiotherapy in limited small-cell lung cancer treated concurrently with cisplatin and etoposide. *N Engl J Med* 1999; **340**:265–71.

20. Auperin A, Arriagada R, Pignon JP, *et al.* Prophylactic cranial irradiation for patients with small-cell lung cancer in complete remission. Prophylactic Cranial Irradiation Overview Collaborative Group. *N Engl J Med* 1999; **341**:476–84.

21. Bissett D, Macbeth FR, Cram I. The role of palliative radiotherapy in malignant mesothelioma. *Clin Oncol* 1991; **3**:315–17.

22. Davis SR, Tan L, Ball DL. Radiotherapy in the treatment of malignant mesothelioma of the pleura, with special reference to its use in palliation. *Australas Radiol* 1994; **38**:212–14.

23. Tsao AS, Mehran R, Roth JA. Neoadjuvant and intrapleural therapies for malignant pleural mesothelioma. *Clin Lung Cancer* 2009; **10**:36–41.

24. Stout, R, Barber, P, Burt, P, *et al.* Clinical and quality of life outcomes in the first United Kingdom randomized trial of endobronchial brachytherapy vs external beam radiotherapy in the palliative treatment for inoperable non-small cell lung cancer. *Radiother Oncol* 2000; **56**:323–7.

25. Scagliotti GV, De Marinis F, Rinaldi M, *et al.* Phase III randomized trial comparing three platinum-based doublets in advanced non-small-cell lung cancer. *J Clin Oncol* 2002; **20**:4285–91.

26. Schiller JH, Harrington D, Belani C, *et al.* Comparison of four chemotherapy regimens for advanced non-small cell lung cancer. *N Engl J Med* 2002; **346**:92–8.

27. Ardizzoni A, Boni L, Tiseo M, *et al.* Cisplatin- versus carboplatin-based chemotherapy in first-line treatment of advanced non-small-cell lung cancer: an individual patient data meta-analysis. *J Natl Cancer Inst* 2007; **99**:847–57.

28. Delbaldo C, Michiels S, Syz N, *et al.* Benefits of adding a drug to a single-agent or a 2-agent chemotherapy regimen in advanced non-small-cell lung cancer: a meta-analysis. *JAMA* 2004; **292**:470–84.

29. NSCLC Meta-Analyses Collaborative Group. Chemotherapy in addition to supportive care improves survival in advanced non–small-cell lung cancer: a systematic review and meta-analysis of individual patient data from 16 randomized controlled trials. *JCO* 2008:4617–25.

30. Spiro SG, Rudd RM, Souhami RL, *et al.* Chemotherapy versus supportive care in advanced non-small cell lung cancer: improved survival without detriment to quality of life. *Thorax* 2004; **59**:828–36.

31. Scagliotti GV, Parikh P, von Pawel J, *et al.* Phase III study comparing cisplatin plus gemcitabine with cisplatin plus pemetrexed in chemotherapy-naive patients with advanced-stage non-small-cell lung cancer. *J Clin Oncol* 2008; **26**:3543–51.

32. Shepherd FA, Dancey J, Ramlau R, *et al.* Prospective randomized trial of docetaxel versus best supportive care in patients with non-small-cell lung cancer previously treated with platinum-based chemotherapy. *J Clin Oncol* 2000; **18**:2095–103.

33. Hanna N, Shepherd FA, Fossella FV, *et al.* Randomized phase III trial of pemetrexed versus docetaxel in patients with non-small-cell lung cancer previously treated with chemotherapy. *J Clin Oncol* 2004; **22**:1589–97.

34. Lilenbaum R, Villaflor VM, Langer C, *et al.* Single-agent versus combination chemotherapy in patients with advanced non-small cell lung cancer and a performance status of 2: prognostic factors and treatment selection based on two large randomized clinical trials. *J Thorac Oncol* 2009; **4**:869–74.

35. Pignon JP, Tribodet H, Scagliotti GV, *et al.* Lung adjuvant cisplatin evaluation: A pooled analysis by the LACE collaborative group. *J Clin Oncol* 2008; **26**:3552–9.

36. Mok TS, Wu YL, Thongprasert S, *et al.* Gefitinib or carboplatin-paclitaxel in pulmonary adenocarcinoma. *N Engl J Med* 2009; **361**:947–57.

37. Herbst RS, Prager D, Hermann R, *et al.* TRIBUTE: a phase III trial of erlotinib hydrochloride (OSI-774) combined with carboplatin and paclitaxel chemotherapy in advanced non-small-cell lung cancer. *J Clin Oncol* 2005; **23**:5892–9.

38. Gatzemeier U, Pluzanska A, Szczesna A, *et al.* Phase III study of erlotinib in combination with cisplatin and gemcitabine in advanced non-small-cell lung cancer: the Tarceva Lung Cancer Investigation Trial. *J Clin Oncol* 2007; **25**:1545–52.

39. Giaccone G, Herbst RS, Manegold C, *et al.* Gefitinib in combination with gemcitabine and cisplatin in advanced non-small-cell lung cancer: a phase III trial—INTACT 1. *J Clin Oncol* 2004; **22**:777–84.

40. Herbst RS, Giaccone G, Schiller JH, *et al.* Gefitinib in combination with paclitaxel and carboplatin in advanced non-small-cell lung cancer: A Phase III Trial—INTACT 2. *J Clin Oncol* 2004; **22**:785–94.

41. Sandler A, Gray R, Perry MC, *et al.* Paclitaxel-carboplatin alone or with bevacizumab for non-small-cell lung cancer. *N Engl J Med* 2006; **355**:2542–50.

42. Reck M, von Pawel J, Zatloukal P, *et al.* Phase III trial of cisplatin plus gemcitabine with either placebo or bevacizumab as first-line therapy for nonsquamous non-small-cell lung cancer: AVAiL. *J Clin Oncol* 2009; **27**:1227–31.

43. Pirker R, Pereira JR, Szczesna A, *et al.* Cetuximab plus chemotherapy in patients with advanced non-small-cell lung cancer (FLEX): an open-label randomised phase III trial. *Lancet* 2009; **373**:1525–31.

44. O'Brien ME, Ciuleanu TE, Tsekov H, *et al.* Phase III trial comparing supportive care alone with supportive care with oral topotecan in patients with relapsed small-cell lung cancer. *J Clin Oncol* 2006; **24**:5441–7.

45. Vogelzang, NJ, Rusthoven, JJ, Symanowski, J, *et al.* Phase III study of pemetrexed in combination with cisplatin versus cisplatin alone in patients with malignant pleural mesothelioma. *J Clin Oncol* 2003; **21**:2636–44.

46. Muers MF, Stephens, RJ, Fisher, P, *et al.* Active symptom control with or without chemotherapy in the treatment of patients with malignant pleural mesothelioma (MS01): a multicentre randomised trial. *Lancet* 2008; **371**:1685–94.

47. Berthelot JM, Will BP, Evans WK, *et al.* Decision framework for chemotherapeutic interventions for metastatic non-small-cell lung cancer. *J Natl Cancer Inst* 2000; **92**: 1321–9.

48. Silvestri G, Pritchard R, Welch G, *et al.* Preferences for chemotherapy in patients with advanced non small cell lung cancer: descriptive study based on scripted interviews. *BMJ* 1998; **317**:771–5.

49. Macbeth FR, Wheldon, TE, Girling DJ, *et al.* Radiation myelopathy: estimates of risk in 1048 patients in three randomized trials of palliative radiotherapy for non small cell lung cancer. *Clin Oncol* 1996; **8**:176–81.

50. Spiro SG, Souhami RL, Geddes DM, *et al.* Duration of chemotherapy in small cell lung cancer: a Cancer Research Campaign trial. *Br J Cancer* 1989; **59**:578–83.

51. Temel JS, Greer JA, Muzikansky A, *et al.* Early palliative care for patients with metastatic non–small-cell lung cancer. *N Engl J Med* 2010; **363**:733–42.

52. George PJ, Garrett CP, Nixon C, *et al.* Laser treatment for tracheobronchial tumours: local or general anaesthesia? *Thorax* 1987; **42**:656–60.

53. Tobias JS, Brown SG. Palliation of malignant obstruction–use of lasers and radiotherapy in combination. *Eur J Cancer* 1991; **27**:1352–5.

54. George PJM, Clarke G, Tolfree S, Garrett CPO, Hetzel MR. Changes in regional ventilation and perfusion of the lung after endoscopic laser treatment. *Thorax* 1990; **45**:248.

55. Lam S. Photodynamic therapy of lung cancer. *Thorax* 1993; **48**:469.

56. Walsh DA, Maiwand MO, Nath AR, *et al.* Bronchoscopic cryotherapy for advanced bronchial carcinoma. *Thorax* 1990; **45**:509–13.

57. Walsh DA, Nath, AR, Maiwand M. Authors' reply. *Thorax* 1990; **45**:150.

58. Isaacs, C. Lymphatic spread of breast cancer. In: J.R. Harris, M.E. Lippman, M. Morrow, and S. Hellman, (ed.) *Diseases of the breast*, pp. 827–33. Philadelphia, PA: Lippincott-Raven, 1996.

59. Bonnefoi H, Smith IE. How should cancer presenting as a malignant pleural effusion be managed? *Br J Cancer* 1996; **74**:832–5.

60. Salajka F. Occurrence of haemoptysis in patients with newly diagnosed lung malignancy. *Schweiz Med Wochenschr* 1999; **129**(41):1487–91.

61. James LE, Gower, NH, Rudd, RM, *et al.* A randomised trial of low dose high frequency chemotherapy as palliative treatment of poor prognosis small cell lung cancer: a Cancer Research Campaign trial. *Br J Cancer* 1996; **73**:1563–8.

62. Wildgaard K, Ravn J, Kehlet HC. Chronic post-thoracotomy pain: a critical review of pathogenic mechanisms and strategies for prevention. *Eur J Cardio-Thoracic Surg* 2009; **36**:170–80.

63. Twycross, R, Wilcock, A. *Palliative care formulary PCF3*. Abingdon: Radcliffe Medical Press, 2007.

64. Saffran L, Ost DE, Fein AM, Schiff MJ. Outpatient pleurodesis of malignant pleural effusions using a small-bore pigtail catheter. *Chest* 2000; **118**:417–21.

65. Neragi-Miandoab S. Surgical and other invasive approaches to recurrent pleural effusion with malignant etiology. *Support Care Cancer* 2008; **16**(12):1323–65.

66. Martin-Ucar AE, Edwards JG, Rengajaran A, Muller S, Waller DA. Palliative surgical debulking in malignant mesothelioma. Predictors of survival and symptom control. *Eur J Cardiothorac Surg* 2001; **20**(6):1117–21.

67. Ahmedzai S. Palliation of respiratory symptoms. In Doyle D, Hanks GWC, MacDonald N (eds) *Oxford Textbook of Palliative Medicine*, pp. 583–616. 2nd edn Oxford: Oxford University Press, 1998.

Chapter 21

Comprehensive supportive care for chronic pulmonary infections

Gary T. Buckholz and Charles F. von Gunten

Background

Chronic respiratory infections are a major healthcare issue around the world associated with significant morbidity and mortality. Treatment of these infections often entails prolonged antimicrobial regimens which have toxicities and may or may not be successful. Sometimes therapies are used with the goal of control rather than cure. Tuberculosis (TB) and other chronic pulmonary infections associated with HIV infection will be a focus of this chapter. Tuberculosis and HIV (in addition to malaria) are considered the primary diseases of poverty and occur all over the world. Other pulmonary diseases which predispose to frequent or chronic infections such as cystic fibrosis and chronic obstructive pulmonary disease (COPD) will be reviewed as well. In fact, there is a deleterious and synergistic interaction between TB, HIV, tobacco smoking, and COPD in a large proportion of the world's population (1). Our aim is to describe optimal supportive and palliative care of the symptoms encountered with chronic respiratory infections broadly. Symptoms frequently encountered in this patient population include: dyspnoea or breathlessness, secretions, persistent cough, and haemoptysis.

Comprehensive supportive care of respiratory symptoms should be systematic, evidence-based, individualized, regularly monitored, and iteratively updated. Optimal management of symptoms frequently encountered with chronic respiratory infections involves the combination of potentially restorative therapies such as antimicrobials as well as global therapies. Historically acute and chronic pulmonary infections have been viewed as an 'either/or' plan of care (cure versus comfort). It has been challenging for healthcare providers to overcome this 'false dichotomy' (2).

Figure 21.1, adapted from Ferris et al. (3), shows an integrative focus of care including both the use of antimicrobials which may be restorative and/or help control symptoms and global therapies which specifically control symptoms rather than modifying the infection. Upon diagnosis, symptom burden is often high; while many times antimicrobials may be the best palliative treatment; these medications generally take time to work. Therefore, upon diagnosis, specific attention should be given to the use of global therapies that are available in many healthcare settings. If antimicrobials are helpful or successful, the need for global therapies may decrease over time with overall better symptom control. However, if an infection becomes chronic, either 'controlled' with antimicrobials

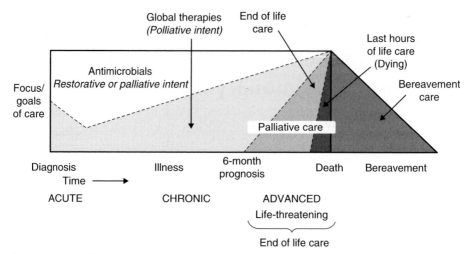

Fig. 21.1 Comprehensive supportive care for chronic pulmonary infections. Adapted from (3) with permission from Elsevier.

or refractory to antimicrobials, the need for global therapies may increase over time while antimicrobials may become less helpful over time. Near the end of life, optimal management may still include antimicrobials if there are continued benefits of symptom control by decreasing or controlling microbial load. As illness progresses, management must include global therapies to decrease symptom burden as well as specialized care-planning for the patient and family to prepare for death. An interdisciplinary team model is needed throughout the care planning as psychosocial and spiritual issues for the patient and family are expected.

Whenever possible the focus of care should balance the use of potentially restorative therapies, global therapies, and end of life care planning when appropriate, over time. This balance requires clinician knowledge of locally available and affordable therapies and healthcare systems. This knowledge must be applied in the context of the patient's individual situation and goals. It is important to assess whether a patient's goals are realistic and make specific recommendations for the plan of care.

Patients' goals have the potential to conflict with public health policies, however this is rare. For example, antimicrobial therapy of active pulmonary TB is mandated in many countries.

Chronic pulmonary infections—associated restorative therapies

Pulmonary tuberculosis

Over time, TB has been a significant problem experienced across the world. However, this problem has shifted dramatically to developing countries where there are significant social (such as overcrowding) and economic factors. Nearly one-third of the world's population is thought to be infected with latent *Mycobacterium tuberculosis* (4). The World Health Organization (WHO) estimates that 9.4 million new cases of TB occurred in 2008. Asia (the South-East and Western Pacific regions) accounts for 55% of the global cases and the African region for 30%. Many of the countries with the highest estimated TB incidence are in Africa. This phenomenon is linked to high rates of co-infection with HIV. Among the total new cases of TB, 15% were HIV positive. Tuberculosis prevalence is associated with dramatic morbidity and mortality as almost 1.8 million people died from TB in 2008 and approximately 28% of these deaths were among HIV-positive people (5).

If latent TB becomes active, approximately 75% of the cases are pulmonary. Spread from the lungs to other sites is more common in immunocompromised individuals. Those with the primary stage of disease are often asymptomatic or may have flu-like symptoms. Those who develop miliary TB or post-primary pulmonary TB have significant change in the architecture of the lungs which may lead to respiratory failure and subsequent challenging respiratory symptoms. In spite of the prevalence of this disease there is scant data on respiratory symptoms experienced from a population-based perspective. A prospective questionnaire study in one area of the US showed that of patients with pulmonary disease, 52% experienced persistent cough and approximately 24% experienced haemoptysis. Other respiratory symptoms such as dyspnoea were not measured (6).

If an individual has sputum-positive fully sensitive TB, restorative treatment generally requires a combination of antimicrobials for at least 6 months. This prolonged, complex treatment regimen is drastically different than treatment for most acute pulmonary infections. For the first 2 months, this usually means four different antimicrobials (rifampicin, isoniazid, pyrazinamide, and ethambutol) and the subsequent 4 months require two antimicrobials (usually rifampicin and isoniazid). Individuals are generally considered non-infectious after 2 weeks of starting treatment.

Restorative therapies with combinations of antimicrobials have great potential for success and complete recovery, however the duration of treatment and other social factors, such as isolation or use of masks sometimes used during treatment, can make adherence challenging. In order to improve public health, many countries have developed directly observed therapy (DOT) programmes where a healthcare provider directly monitors the patient's use of restorative medications.

Unfortunately, multidrug resistant TB (MDR-TB) is becoming more of a problem. This means that the organism is resistant to the two most effective drugs, rifampicin and isoniazid. For an individual this can change the likelihood of cure from higher than 97% to approximately 50%. The global burden of MDR-TB is estimated to be 511,000 incident cases. The median prevalence of MDR-TB in new TB cases is 1.6%, ranging from 0% in eight countries with low TB prevalence to 19.4% in Moldova and 22.3% in Baku, Azerbaijan (7). A successful outcome requires good laboratory services to determine antibiotic sensitivity and a very prolonged treatment regimen. This often entails continued use of antimicrobials for 2 years after negative cultures. It also may take many months of treatment before being considered non-infectious.

HIV-related pulmonary infection

Significant progress has been achieved in prevention of new HIV infections and overall mortality is on the decline. However, in spite of AIDS-related mortality peaking in 2004, the number of people living with HIV continues to grow due to infected individuals living longer with HIV combined with individuals still becoming newly infected. The WHO provides statistics from 2008 which indicate 2.7 million people were newly infected with HIV worldwide in 2008 and 33.4 million people live with HIV/AIDS worldwide. While mortality has peaked, AIDS-related illness remains one of the leading causes of death globally. The toll remains astounding—two million people died from HIV/AIDS in 2008. While Sub-Saharan Africa remains the most heavily affected region, accounting for 71% of all new HIV infections, the prevalence is increasing in some areas of the world such as Eastern Europe and Central Asia. Additionally there is a resurgence of the epidemic among men who have sex with men (8).

Optimal treatment of HIV involves a combination of antiretroviral medications. These combinations of antiviral medication are also known as highly active antiretroviral therapy, or HAART. HAART is the reason people are living longer with HIV; however, it only suppresses the virus rather than curing the illness. Life-long therapy has changed the trajectory of this illness to one of chronic disease rather than terminal illness. This change is not always seen in developing parts of the world where these drugs may not be widely available or too expensive. Opportunistic infections are common once an individual's CD4 count is less than 200 cells/microlitre. Therefore monitoring of CD4 count and prophylaxis, if indicated, is important for prevention of opportunistic infections and subsequent symptoms.

Respiratory symptoms are a common complaint among individuals with HIV and the frequency of these complaints often increases as CD4 counts decrease. Studies on the prevalence of respiratory symptoms show complaints of dyspnoea occurring in 15–48% of patients, cough in 19–60%, and phlegm production in 42%. Among HIV-infected individuals, current or past cigarette smoking was the most important predictor for respiratory symptom burden (2, 9, 10).

A person with HIV/AIDS may experience respiratory symptom burden from opportunistic infections, neoplasms, general debility, multiorgan disease, and/or non-HIV-related respiratory conditions. Pulmonary opportunistic infections are the most likely cause of respiratory symptoms and can be bacterial, mycobacterial, fungal, viral, and/or parasitic. Common HIV-associated opportunistic pneumonias are listed in Table 21.1 according to CD4 count (11). Pulmonary TB is an AIDS-defining illness and these individuals are much more likely to present with disseminated or lymph node-positive TB and to be sputum negative.

The principles of antibiotic and potentially restorative treatment for all of the HIV-related pulmonary infections are similar to a general patient population with a couple of important distinctions. Clinicians treating persons with both HIV and TB need to be aware of drug interactions between the rifamycins and both protease inhibitors and non-nucleoside reverse transcriptase inhibitors.

Table 21.1 Common HIV-associated opportunistic pneumonias

CD4 cell count	Organism
Any	Bacterial pneumonia (especially *Streptococcus pneumoniae* and *Hemophilus* species)
	Tuberculosis (TB)
<200 cells/µL	*Pneumocystis* pneumonia (PCP)
	Cryptococcus neoformans pneumonia
	Bacterial pneumonia accompanied by bacteraemia or septicaemia
	Extrapulmonary or disseminated TB
<100 cells/µL	Bacterial pneumonia due to *Pseudomonas aeruginosa*
	Toxoplasma gondii pneumonia
<50 cells/µL	*Coccidioides immitis*, usually accompanied by disseminated disease
	Histoplasma capsulatum, usually accompanied by disseminated disease
	Cytomegalovirus, usually accompanied by disseminated disease
	Mycobacterium avium complex, usually accompanied by disseminated disease
HIV risk factors: injection drug use: increased incidence of bacterial pneumonia and TB	
Habits: cigarette smoking: increased incidence of bacterial pneumonia	
Prior opportunistic infections: increased incidence of recurrence	
Use of opportunistic infection prophylaxis: decreased incidence of opportunistic pneumonia	
Sustained combination antiretroviral therapy: decreased incidence of opportunistic pneumonia	

For bacterial pneumonia, HIV-infected patients should receive a beta-lactam plus macrolide due to the increased risk of drug-resistant *Streptococcus pneumoniae* with macrolide monotherapy (12).

Continuation or initiation of HAART may also improve treatment response for pulmonary infections. In a trial of 642 patients, initiation of antiretroviral therapy during tuberculosis therapy significantly improved survival (13).

COPD-related pulmonary infection

COPD is a common lung disease that interferes with breathing by causing inflammation and damage to the airways subsequently blocking air flow from the lungs. The primary cause of COPD is through inhaled tobacco smoke from direct tobacco use or second-hand smoke. Additionally, indoor air pollution especially from fuel used for indoor heating and cooking is a significant problem in resource-poor countries. An estimated 210 million people have COPD worldwide and approximately 3 million people died from COPD in 2005. The most common symptoms experienced are breathlessness, abnormal sputum production, and chronic cough (14). While individuals with COPD generally experience acute exacerbations, the exacerbations are often during times of pulmonary infection and the symptoms experienced are the same as those experienced by patients with chronic pulmonary infections. Additionally much of the evidence-base for treating these symptoms from a global perspective is in the COPD patient population.

Restorative therapies for treatment of COPD exacerbations generally include bronchodilators, a brief course of corticosteroids, and oxygen if the patient is hypoxemic. Antibiotics to treat bronchitis are often part of this approach. Several meta-analyses support the concept that patients with increased dyspnoea, increased sputum volume, and increased sputum purulence will benefit from antimicrobial therapy. However, even though there are well-established guidelines regarding the use of antibiotics during exacerbation, antibiotics may be overused. In one study, there was no statistically significant relationship between the presence of an established indication for antibiotic administration and the use of antibiotics, with roughly 75% of patients in all groups receiving therapy. A significant fraction of patients received combination therapy that was more appropriate for the management of pneumonia than for acute exacerbation (15).

Over time some patients with COPD develop chronic bronchitis or bronchiectasis. With these conditions, chronic sputum production is common and does not usually require antibiotic therapy. However when symptoms are chronically severe enough to interfere with daily activities, it is reasonable to consider suppressive antibiotic therapy.

Clinically, pneumonia should be considered if symptoms include worsening cough and dyspnoea in addition to fever and/or chest discomfort. A chest radiograph should help confirm the diagnosis. Establishing the exact aetiology, however, is often challenging and sputum diagnostics are not always helpful. Although pneumococcal pneumonia remains common, Gram-negative organisms may be the major pathogens in individuals who have recently been hospitalized, who have been treated with antibiotics previously, or who live in a nursing facility. Therefore, broad-spectrum antibiotics should be utilized. Antibiotic coverage should account for possible atypical pneumonias such as *Legionella*, *Chlamydia pneumoniae*, *Moraxella catarrhalis*, and *Mycoplasma pneumoniae*. Erythromycin, if tolerated, is a cost-effective antibiotic over newer macrolides to cover for atypical pneumonia. Patients with underlying COPD are also more susceptible to atypical mycobacterial disease.

Cystic fibrosis-related pulmonary infection

Cystic fibrosis (CF) is the most common life-limiting autosomal recessive inherited disease affecting Caucasians. Modern medicine has transformed it from a fatal diagnosis in infancy to a chronic disease of children and young adults. Chronic lung disease results from clogging of the airways from mucous build-up and subsequent inflammation. Changes in the lung architecture over time result in bronchiectasis, pulmonary hypertension, and heart failure with secretions, recurrent pulmonary infections, and hypoxia being major life-limiting problems. Common organisms such as *Staphylococcus aureus* and *Hemophilus infuenzae* become overgrown and cause frequent pneumonia. Over time the changing architecture of the lungs predisposes to *Pseudomonas aeruginosa*. The median age at death is currently 36.8 years, most commonly due to respiratory failure (16). Most individuals have a gradual, progressive decline in their health allowing for a thoughtful, planned approach.

Respiratory symptoms are common in these individuals with dyspnoea experienced by up to 100% of patients, difficulty expectorating sputum in 69%, persistent cough in 80%, haemoptysis in 6–9%, and massive haemoptysis experienced by 4% of patients (18–20). The ranges reflect different studies and different degrees of illness progression. Patients dying from end-stage CF have a high level of complex symptoms.

Restorative therapies with palliative and life-prolonging intent focus on managing secretions, suppressing pulmonary infections (often with chronic use of systemic and inhaled antibiotics), treating acute pulmonary infections, and managing hypoxia with oxygen and/or invasive or non-invasive ventilation. In studies looking at an integrated model of providing palliative care for patients with CF, 85–100% of patients received intravenous anti-pseudomonas antibiotics during their terminal phase of their illness for 'mixed therapeutic and palliative intent'. Many clinicians utilize ventilatory support for these patients near the end of life as well (18, 21).

Symptoms—associated global therapies

Global therapies are ones that do not restore previous function or reverse underlying pathology. These therapies are used in conjunction with restorative therapies. As chronic infection potentially advances and restorative therapies are less helpful, the focus of care may shift toward global therapies in conjunction with end of life care. The term global is also appropriate in that many of these therapies are inexpensive and in many healthcare settings readily available. There are many non-pharmacological therapies to consider as well.

Much of the research targeting global therapies for respiratory symptoms are in the COPD patient population. Some research is from cancer or congestive heart failure (CHF) populations. It is likely that these data can be extrapolated usefully to those suffering from chronic pulmonary infections.

Dyspnoea

Dyspnoea is a subjective sensation defined as an uncomfortable awareness or sensation of breathing. The term is used interchangeably in the medical literature with shortness of breath and breathlessness. It is a very common symptom described by patients with chronic pulmonary infections. The pathophysiology of dyspnoea is complex and incompletely understood. The cerebral cortex integrates the various sensory (chemoreceptors, mechanoreceptors, and vagal afferents) and motor inputs along with cognitive and emotional factors. The symptom of dyspnoea results when the integration of these factors equals the inability to meet the perceived demand.

The differential diagnosis of dyspnoea is extensive and underlying causes should be addressed whenever possible while being consistent with the patient's goals of care. Similar to pain, there is an inter-relationship between the experience of dyspnoea and how one feels about the experience. This can result in a vicious cycle of anxiety and increased dyspnoea with subsequent panic. Cortical limbic and paralimbic areas as well as frontoparietal attention networks of the brain are activated during breathlessness (17, 18).

It is likely that these areas of the brain are involved in perception as well as modulation of dyspnoea. Therefore, a mind–body approach is warranted. From a global perspective, symptomatic management is aimed at decreasing the patient's sense of effort of breathing.

There are many pharmacological and non-pharmacological interventions that can potentially change physiological factors as well as emotional and cognitive factors to ameliorate the symptom of dyspnoea. Additionally, case management (i.e. hospice or home health) and pulmonary rehabilitation programmes may integrate many of these therapies and have been effective at reducing the symptom of dyspnoea in certain populations (19, 20).

Non-pharmacological therapies

Non-pharmacological therapies to treat the symptom of dyspnoea are abundant. These therapies may be considered first line for mild to moderate dyspnoea as many have a low risk profile and allow for an integrative approach while avoiding polypharmacy. Table 21.2 (21) summarizes potentially useful non-pharmacological therapies. Generally the evidence-base for these therapies is weak; however, there is strong evidence for the use of walking aids in debilitated patients to assist in both energy conservation and lean forward position. The lean forward position allows the rib cage to form a barrel shape providing better efficiency of the diaphragm thereby permitting the lungs to expand better and decrease the use of accessory muscles.

Non-invasive positive pressure ventilation (NIPPV) is an alternative to invasive ventilation for dyspnoea relief, but can act as a bridge to invasive ventilation. NIPPV has a role for select patients in ameliorating dyspnoea, but given the potential bridging aspect to chronic, invasive ventilation it should be considered carefully in the context of the overall trajectory of the: chronic illness; possible disease progression if the patient is not responding to restorative therapies; and the patient's goals of care.

Table 21.2 Non-pharmacological therapies for dyspnoea

Physiological factors	Emotional and cognitive factors
Muscle strengthening (i.e. exercise, neuromuscular electrical stimulation, respiratory muscle training)	Counselling and support
Chest wall vibration	Open environment
Sit up or lean forward position	Relaxation (i.e. guided imagery, progressive muscle relaxation)
Energy conservation (i.e. walking aids)	Distraction (i.e. music)
Breathing training (i.e. pursed lips, diaphragmatic breathing)	Psychotherapy
Cool air	
Moving air (i.e. fan, forced air via nasal cannula)	
Acupuncture/acupressure	
Nutritional supplementation	
Ventilation	

For patients with COPD, lung volume reduction surgery is superior to medical therapy alone for patients with predominately upper lobe disease and low exercise capacity. In these patients, surgery may improve dyspnoea and survival (22). Surgery is once again playing a role in the management of TB for those patients who have MDR-TB. The focus of pulmonary resection in this population has been with focus of disease eradication and survival rather than symptom control. Not surprisingly, the symptom of dyspnoea may worsen with this intervention (23).

Pharmacological therapies

For severe dyspnoea, a combined approach using both non-pharmacological and pharmacological therapies has the best chance for success. There are several medications to consider when treating dyspnoea. Currently opioids are the class of medications with the most evidence to support their use in various patient populations (24–26). The mechanism of action is not well understood, but the areas of the brain activated during feelings of dyspnoea are similar to ones activated during perception of pain. Therefore, opioids may change the perception of dyspnoea in a similar manner to their alteration of the perception of pain (27). Furthermore, there are many opioid receptors throughout the tracheobronchial tree, however their role in relief of dyspnoea remains unclear and there is no convincing evidence of benefit with nebulized opioids (24). Thus, the mechanism is most likely central and systemic administration is currently preferable.

Given reports of respiratory depression with opioids there is considerable fear among prescribers when contemplating opioids for dyspnoea. However, the chronic dosing of regular, low-dose opioids has been established as safe for the symptomatic relief of dyspnoea (28). Clinicians must be well versed in appropriate dosing and titration strategies to steer clear from serious adverse effects. Generally, the opioid titration strategies are the same as those used for pain and often relatively low doses accomplish good control. For those suffering from prolonged or constant dyspnoea, a regimen with extended release opioids should be considered and has been established as effective in a randomized, double-blind, placebo-controlled cross-over trial (29). Morphine has been the opioid most utilized and studied to treat this symptom however other opioids appear to be effective.

Oxygen is often used to treat dyspnoea. Hypoxia alone is a relatively weak stimulus for the symptom of dyspnoea. Often hypoxia does not correlate with increased severity of dyspnoea and those who are feeling breathless often have normal oxygen saturation. Compressed air via nasal cannula is just as effective as oxygen in treating the symptom of dyspnoea (30). It is postulated that nasal cold receptors in the nose arising from the V2 distribution of the trigeminal nerve give sensory input to affect respiration and decrease breathlessness. Moving cold air across the face has been shown to be effective in small studies (31, 32). If a patient is hypoxic, oxygen should be utilized and may help decrease feelings of breathlessness. If a patient is not hypoxic, techniques which get cool air moving across the face may be just as effective as oxygen in reducing the symptom. Patients will often report that keeping their room cool with moving air via open window or fan is helpful. These techniques should be utilized as first line in outpatient settings where providing oxygen can be quite expensive.

Historically, benzodiazepines have often been used to treat the symptom of dyspnoea along with the subsequent experience of anxiety. A 2010 Cochrane review analysed seven studies (with meta-analysis of six) including 200 total participants with COPD and advanced cancer. It revealed no evidence for beneficial effect of benzodiazepines specific to breathlessness in that patient population (33). Although further study is needed, benzodiazepines should be considered third-line therapy. Other medications used to treat anxiety such as buspirone or selective serotonin reuptake inhibitors have insufficient evidence to support routine use specifically for dyspnoea.

There are several other pharmacological therapies which may play a role in treating dyspnoea. These therapies require further investigation, but warrant being mentioned. Nebulized furosemide may have beneficial effects on breathlessness independent of diuresis. It appears to have a mild bronchodilator effect (28). Low-dose chlorpromazine and possibly other phenothiazines may play a role in management of dyspnoea; however the mechanism of action is unclear (34, 35). Heliox is a gas mixture of helium and oxygen which may decrease airway resistance and decrease work of breathing. It may be useful in reducing lung hyperinflation and for management of obstruction of large airways such as trachea or main bronchi (40, 41). It is best administered by mask rather than nasal cannula to minimize entrainment of room air, and is generally used on a short-term and in-patient basis because of its high cost.

Secretions

One of the symptomatic challenges in chronic pulmonary infections is the control of secretions. Their presence worsens the sense of shortness of breath and cough. Those listening hear a distressing chest rattle. Airway mucus hypersecretion is now recognized as a key pathophysiological feature in many patients. For supine patients, non-pharmacological interventions such as re-positioning, oropharyngeal suctioning, and decreasing parenteral fluids, if present, can be considered. However suctioning can be traumatic for the patient and some pharmacological interventions are more effective when started early with lower initial rattle intensity (42). Conventional therapies include anticholinergics, corticosteroids, and mucolytics. Novel pharmacotherapeutic targets are being investigated (43). A princial choice is whether to try to liquify or to dry the secretions.

Liquify secretions

A variety of approaches have been advocated to liquify secretions in order that they may be better expectorated. Nebulized saline enhances mucociliary clearance and stimulates mucociliary transport. Hypertonic saline has been postulated to break ionic bonds within mucus gel and hence lower viscosity and elasticity. Patients with cystic fibrosis have better cough clearance with increasing concentrations of nebulized hypertonic saline.

Guaifenesin is a ubiquitous expectorant found in many cough preparations. The data supporting its effectiveness, however, is sparse and weak. In a recent Cochrane review, two trials compared guaifenesin with placebo, one indicated significant benefit whereas the other did not (36). One trial found that a mucolytic reduced cough frequency and symptom scores. Two studies examined antihistamine–decongestant combinations and found conflicting results. Three studies compared other combinations of drugs with placebo and indicated some benefit in reducing cough symptoms.

Mucolytic medications depolymerize the mucin network reducing viscosity and aiding cough clearance. N-acetylcysteine and carbocysteine hydrolyse the disulfide bonds that link mucin monomers within sputum. For patients with cystic fibrosis, DNAase reduces the size of DNA molecules within the mucus, thereby reducing sputum viscosity. Inhaled indomethacin has been advocated to improve sputum viscosity and relieve symptoms in patients with chronic bronchitis and bronchiectasis.

Dry secretions

Antimuscarinic anticholinergic agents dry secretions by competitively inhibiting the muscarinic effects of acetylcholine. In other words, these agents functionally block the parasympathetic division of the nervous system (parasympatholytics) and fall either into tertiary amines or quaternary ammonium compounds. Tertiary amines readily cross the blood–brain barrier and can have significant adverse clinical effects, while quaternary ammonium compounds do not readily penetrate the CNS. All antimuscarinics have variable effects on the parasympathetic nervous system, from inhibitory effects on secretions in salivary, bronchial and sweat glands, to heart rate and ocular effects, inhibition of bladder detrusor activity and gastrointestinal smooth muscle activity, as well as gastric secretion.

Atropine (a racemic mixture of dextro- and levo-hyoscyamine) is the prototype antimuscarinic drug—and is also useful for remembering the side effects of tertiary amines (xerostomia, blurred vision, cycloplegia, mydriasis, photophobia, anhidrosis, urinary retention, tachycardia, palpitations, constipation, and mental confusion/delirium). For purposes of symptom control in drying secretions, it is one of these 'side effects', the antisecretory effect, that is desired. Other tertiary amine-antimuscarinics are hyoscyamine (Levsin©) and scopolamine (Transderm-Scop©). Belladonna leaf extract contains a mixture of atropine (d-l-hyoscyamine) and scopolamine, and is also used clinically; combination preparations containing atropine, scopolamine, hyoscyamine and phenobarbital (Donnatal©, for example) are also available. The quaternary ammonium compounds that are clinically useful are ipratropium and glycopyrrolate.

A novel approach expands the use of octreotide for the management of secretions (37). Octreotide is an analogue of the naturally occurring polypeptide hormone somatostatin (34, 38, 39). Somatostatin's effects are widespread in the human body, but its short half-life ($t_{1/2}$ = 3–5min) makes it difficult to use clinically. Octreotide has a significantly longer half-life of approximately two hours. The net effect of octreotide is generally inhibitory. It causes inhibition of the glandular secretion of GH, TSH, ACTH and prolactin; as well as decreasing the release of gastrin, CCK, insulin, glucagon, gastric acid and pancreatic enzymes.

Octreotide is generally well tolerated with the most common side effect being dry mouth amenable to ice chips and moist troches. Long-term therapy has been shown to lead to biliary sludging with actual stone formation (15–20%). Additionally, octreotide can cause nausea, abdominal pain and diarrhoea (4–7%), but anecdotal reports in MBO show improvement in these symptoms. Due to its effects on insulin and glucagon, octreotide has been reported to cause a mild hyperglycaemia.

Cough

Cough is a reflex defence mechanism to remove either inhaled foreign material, or excess secretions. The reflex begins with either mechanical or chemical stimulation of irritant receptors. A cough response is generated in the medulla oblongata. An effective cough, resulting in relief of the inciting irritation, depends upon the speed of air, the tenacity of the secretions, and a functioning mucociliary transport system (40). Consequently, in the setting of chronic pulmonary infections, where there is a chronic inflammatory response, there may be chronic cough.

Symptomatic management involves stopping medications that may be causing or exacerbating the cough. Many medications have anticholinergic side effects, and may be causing the mucus to be excessively dry and difficult to expel. Angiotensin converting enzyme (ACE) inhibitors can cause a dry cough; the effect is not related to dose and may take up to 4 weeks to resolve after discontinuing the ACE inhibitor.

Antihistamines may be effective if there is an allergic component to mucus production. However, for chronic infections, it is likely that the anticholinergic effects of many antihistamines lead to improvement of symptoms. In a recent Cochrane review, three trials found antihistamines were no more effective than placebo in relieving cough symptoms (36).

Corticosteroids may have a diffuse benefit on the underlying inflammatory response. While some are concerned about their use in the setting of chronic infections, in combination with the antimicrobial, they may help with intractable cough. They may be given systemically, or, in an attempt to limit systemic effects, in aerosolized form.

All of the agonist opioids have antitussive effects. While marketing efforts highlight one over another (e.g. codeine) there is little evidence to support this. Recent data suggests dextromethorphan, commonly marketed as an antitussive, is no more effective than placebo (41). Benzonatate is chemically related to the anesthetic procaine and is thought to act peripherally by anesthetizing stretch receptors. While weak in its own right, combined with an opioid, benzonatate 100mg three times daily may improve observed effectiveness.

Haemoptysis

In most chronic infections, haemoptysis is mild; scattered flecks of blood in the sputum. However, what is mild to the clinician may be the cause of paralysing anxiety in a patient or family member. Reassurance and explanation of the cause are helpful for most. Empathic listening to the fears of the patient and family may help to resolve any conflicts.

However, with some infections, notably TB, bleeding may be more serious, and may even be the ultimate cause of death.

Treatments to enhance clotting such as tranexamic acid may be considered (42). Case reports and small clinical trials give conflicting data on efficacy and safety. Therefore, further study is warranted and treatments to enhance clotting should only be considered in patients who experience severe distress secondary to haemoptysis. Specific contraindications include a history of thromboembolic events or haematuria.

If there is significant bleeding, meaning that the sight of the blood is distressing to the patient and family, minimize its visual impact by using dark towels, dark sheets, dark cloths, and dark basin. Even a small amount of blood on a white background looks like exsanguination. In selected patients, preparation for anxiolysis even to the point of sedation may be needed. Any benzodiazepine will work (e.g. lorazepam starting at 0.5mg three or four times daily). However, if urgent sedation is anticipated, midazolam 5mg in a prefilled syringe for intravenous or subcutaneous administration may be kept at the bedside.

Withdrawal of therapies—special considerations
Withdrawal of restorative therapies

In the course of treatment, interventions to cure or restore function may no longer be effective or desired. In chronic pulmonary infection, this may mean a variety of treatments including antimicrobials, as well as treatments such as mechanical ventilation. One reason for this may be that the treatment-associated burden seems to outweigh its benefit.

Patients are open to such discussions. Studies show that between 85% and 95% of patients want to have honest discussions with their healthcare providers regarding life-threatening diseases (43). Yet, healthcare providers do not adequately meet this need. Studies have shown that doctors and nurses underestimate patients' concerns, do not elicit the goals and values of seriously ill patients or include them in treatment decisions, and generally fail to address their patients' emotional concerns (44–46).

The three chief reasons that doctors do poorly in communicating honestly with patients and families are as follows:

1. Medical education does not devote much time or attention to the development of good communication skills, and medical students see few role models (47).

2. The culture of medicine in the Western world focuses on organ systems rather than on whole-patient care.

3. The physicians' own attitudes and underlying emotions regarding death and dying also interfere with adequate goals-of-care discussions (48).

The importance of good communication has been well recognized in the field of palliative medicine. Major educational initiatives such as Education for Physicians on End-of-life Care (EPEC) and End-of-Life Nursing Education Consortium (ELNEC) devote significant time on skills training in this area. Communication is a learnable skill that, like many other skills, requires ongoing practice. Brief educational interventions are likely not sufficient to change physician behaviour (49). Intensive communication skills training, however, has been shown in a randomized trial to improve physician communication skills in practice (50).

As a guide for inexperienced clinicians, a six-step communication protocol for the delivery of bad news can be useful. The model uses the general principle of shared decision-making. Shared decision-making is a process that puts great emphasis on patient autonomy while acknowledging the physician's responsibility to make treatment recommendations that are based both on the patient's stated overall goals of care and the physician's medical expertise.

When conveying medical information, it is generally recommended that the information be given in small pieces. The physician should use words that the patient can understand and should pause frequently to check for the patient's responses. The higher the emotional impact of the given information on the patient, the less likely the patient is to hear what is being said (51). It may therefore be necessary to repeat the information at a later time. The use of written information, summary letters, or voice recordings improves patient recall and understanding (52). Using an informational video after a verbal goals-of-care discussion significantly altered patients' decision towards end of life care in a study of 50 cancer patients, increasing patients' choice for comfort care from 22% to 91% (53).

Stone and colleagues suggested always preparing and having difficult conversations at three levels: facts, emotions, and identity issues involved (54).

An example of this triad regarding goals-of-care discussions would be to spend some time discussing the different clinical options, then looking for and validating the patient's emotional responses such as fear, worry, and sadness. Last, but not least, the physician would reflect on what the discussed options would mean for the patient's and healthcare provider's identity. Examples of identity issues that influence goals-of-care discussions are as follows: 'I have always been a fighter and now you're asking me to give up?' or 'I am not someone who just gives up on a patient'.

Six-step protocol

A stepwise approach to goals-of-care discussions helps to remind the clinician to include all major components of the discussion.

Step 1: prepare and establish an appropriate setting for the discussion

Assess the patient's or family member's readiness to have this conversation, and to address cultural or personal priorities regarding medical decision making in general. Ask whether your patient would want to have this discussion with you, if someone else should be present, or if your patient would prefer to defer the conversation to someone else such as a family member or designated medical decision-maker. A recent study from Australia comparing awareness of treatment goals in patients and their caregivers shows significant discrepancy in nearly half of them, suggesting that we should attempt to include surrogates in as much of these conversations as possible (55). You can elicit these preferences using the following sentences:

> 'Some patients like all the information, others like me to speak with someone else in the family. I wonder what is true for you?'
> 'Tell me how you like to receive medical information.'
> 'Is there anyone else you would like to have present for our discussion?'

When you enter the actual goals-of-care discussion, do it with a clear understanding of the purpose of the meeting and be prepared to discuss information that the patient and family will need to learn. An example could be the outcomes of different treatment options such as antibiotics, cardiopulmonary resuscitation survival data, and common treatment side effects. In general, patients are more interested in outcomes ('Life is not worth living if I won't be able to speak') than in the details of interventions ('That means that we would have to put a tube down your throat that is about as thick as your finger') (56).

In addition to medical information, it can be helpful before entering the discussion to reflect on expected emotional responses and possible identity issues that may arise for the patient. This approach allows you to gain more insight into the patient's and family's perspective and to feel prepared, especially when their perspective seems 'unrealistic'.

Arrange to have the meeting itself in a private and comfortable place where everyone participating can sit at eye level. The atmosphere should be unhurried and undisturbed. After general introductions, the purpose of the meeting should be made clear. You can introduce the subject by phrases such as the following:

> 'I'd like to talk to you about your overall goals of care.'
> 'I'd like to review where we are and make plans for the future.'
> 'I'd like to discuss something today that I discuss with all my patients.'

Be prepared for the possibility that setting up a meeting and asking for a support person to be there may be taken by some patients to be sign that they are about to get very bad news. There will be patients who do not want to wait for a more formal meeting in order to get information as the waiting may lead them to assume the very worst. The more routinely you have such meetings, and the degree to which you really mean you do this routinely, will lead to a demeanour that won't connote you are saving up really, really bad news. It may help to acknowledge this by saying:

> 'Many patients are concerned that we are saving up really bad news by arranging such a meeting, is that true for you?'

You can then use this opportunity to contrast the purpose of a goals-of-care meeting with a bad news meeting at this time.

Step 2: ask the patient and family what they understand

Start out with an open-ended question to elicit what the patient understands about his or her current health situation. This is an important question and one that many clinicians skip. If the doctor is doing all the talking, the rest of the conversation is unlikely to go well. You could start with phrases such as the following:

> 'What do you understand about your current health situation?'
> 'Tell me how you see your health.'
> 'What do you understand from what the doctors have told you?'

Starting with these questions not only helps to establish trust and set the tone for patient-centred decision-making, it also helps to address misconceptions and conflicting or missing information and allows you a quick glimpse into the patient's emotional response to his or her current health state such as fear, anger, or acceptance. More time may be needed to clarify the current situation before the patient is able to address future medical decisions.

Step 3: find out what they expect will happen

For patients who have a good understanding of the status of their disease, the third step is to ask them to consider their future. Examples of how you could start are as follows:

> 'What do you expect in the future?'
> 'Have you ever thought about how you want things to be if you were much more ill?'
> 'What are you hoping for?'

This step allows you to listen while the patient has the opportunity to contemplate and verbalize his or her goals, hopes, and fears. This step creates an opportunity for you to clarify what is likely or unlikely to happen. You may need to ask follow-up questions to understand the patient's vision of the future as well as his or her values and priorities more clearly. If there is a significant discontinuity between what you expect and what the patient expects from the future, this is the time to discover it.

Step 4: discuss overall goals and specific options

Now that you have set the stage for a joint understanding of the patient's present and future, you can discuss overall goals of care and specific options. Allowing the patient to reflect on goals that may still be realistic despite reduced functional abilities and a limited life expectancy can be a very effective tool to maintain realistic hope and build trust. Your insight into the patient's values and priorities should then structure the conversation of medical options and should guide your expert opinion. Use language that the patient can understand, and give information in small pieces. As discussed earlier, you should focus the discussion on treatment outcomes rather than on details of medical interventions (56, 57). Stop frequently to check for emotional reactions and to clarify misunderstandings.

It is often helpful to summarize the patient's stated overall goals and priorities as an introduction to the specific options. Following the principle of shared decision-making, after the discussion of the available options, you should make clear recommendations that are based both on the patient's stated overall goals of care and on your medical expertise. For example:

> 'You have told me that being at home with your family is your number one priority and that the frequent trips to the hospital have become very bothersome for you. You do have three options at this point (…). Getting more service at home seems to be the option that best helps you to realize your goals.'
>
> 'If I heard you correctly, your first priority is to live to participate in your granddaughter's wedding in June. Taking that into account, it may be best to continue therapy but try to treat your infection with a different regimen.'
>
> 'I heard you say that you are particularly concerned about being a burden to your children. Your family could get extra support from the nurse, chaplain, and a social worker who would come to see you at the house.'
>
> 'It is clear you want to pursue all options to extend your life as long as possible. That includes being cared for in an intensive care setting with maximal support. However, if you are unable to

communicate, and there is no reasonable chance of recovery, you want life support to be stopped.'

A recent Canadian analysis of expert opinion regarding 'code status' discussions suggests that clinicians may initiate them at any point during an illness or even when a patient is in good health. The discussion should be framed as an overall goals discussion. It should distinguish between life sustaining therapies (LST) and cardiopulmonary resuscitation (CPR), describe a cardiac arrest, CPR, LST, and palliative care, explain outcomes of cardiac arrest, offer a prognosis and make clear recommendations (58).

A study looking at US patient and caregiver preferences regarding end of life care conversations shows that these discussions should include different treatment options, future symptoms, the terminal phase, and, separately, preference for place of death. Fears about dying should be addressed, and myths dispelled. The needs of patients and caregivers differed significantly when discussing dying: while patients emphasized the importance of reassurance that pain would be controlled, and their dignity maintained, caregivers often wanted more detail about the terminal phase and practical information about how to look after a very sick person. Both wanted reassurance that their healthcare professionals would be available (59).

Step 5: respond to emotions

Patients, families, and healthcare providers may experience profound emotions in response to an exploration of goals of care. It should not be surprising that patients, when considering the end of their life, may cry. Parents of children with life-threatening diseases are especially likely to be emotional and need extra support from the healthcare team. In contrast to common worries in the healthcare community, however, emotional responses tend to be brief. Respond empathetically. The most profound initial response a physician can make may be silence and offering a facial tissue. Consider using open statements such as the following:

'I can see this makes you sad.'
'Tell me more about how you are feeling.'
'People in your situation often get angry. I wonder what you are feeling right now.'
'I notice you are silent.'
'Many people experience strong emotions. I wonder whether that is true for you.'

A common barrier to this step is the physician's fear to precipitate overwhelming emotional outbursts that they may not be able to handle. Therefore, conversations between physicians and their patients remain in the cognitive realm where emotions are not addressed (60). The best way to overcome this barrier is to learn how to respond to patient emotions empathically and to learn to be comfortable with silence. Most patients are embarrassed by being emotional and keep their discussions brief. This is because most patients have adequate coping skills and resilience, and appreciate the presence of a doctor while they work through the experience and their emotions. As with most aspects of being a physician, a sense of competence then leads to a willingness to engage in the challenge.

Step 6: establish and implement the plan

The last step of the goals-of-care discussion protocol involves the establishment and implementation of a plan on which that the patient, family members, and physician have agreed. You should verbalize a plan that is clear and well understood by everyone involved. Consider using language such as the following:

> 'You said that it is most important for you to continue to live independently for as long as possible. Because you are doing so well right now and need your current breathing machine only at night, we will continue what we are doing. However, when your breathing becomes worse, you do not want to be placed on a continuous breathing machine. We will then focus on keeping you comfortable with medicines to making sure that you do not feel short of breath.'

> 'The different regimens we have used to fight your infection are not working. There is no other antimicrobial therapy that is known to be effective. We discussed your options at this point including getting a second opinion from one of my pulmonary colleagues or asking a home care programme to get involved in your care. In light of what you told me about your worries about being a burden to your family, you thought that hospice or palliative care may be the best option at this point because you would get extra help at home from the team members that come to see you at your house. I am going to call the home care team today and arrange for them to call you in the morning so they can see you and explain more about what they offer. We can talk more after you see them.'

It is often helpful to ask patients or family members to summarize the plan and underlying reasoning in their own words to ensure understanding. Especially for emotionally overwhelmed patients, good continuity of care is important. Ensuring this continuity, for example by arranging for follow-up appointments, speaking to the referring physician, or writing the appropriate orders, is part of the physician's responsibility. You may want to conclude your conversation with information that gives hope such as a promise of ongoing care.

Psychosocial aspects

In addition to issues faced by all patients with chronic or advancing illness, individuals with chronic pulmonary infections have unique aspects of their care that require additional exploration by an interdisciplinary team. Some of these infections require respiratory isolation. Management of pulmonary TB requires respiratory isolation until sputum cultures are negative. CF patients are sometimes isolated from other CF patients to avoid transmission of specific microbes. This can create challenges for generating a healthy support system. Respiratory isolation with masks can cause feelings of isolation in the extreme as there is always a barrier to human contact and human expression as well as fears of transmission to loved ones. Fears or other emotional responses must be addressed and misconceptions require further patient, family, and often healthcare provider education.

Summary

Comprehensive management of chronic pulmonary infections and supportive care of subsequent respiratory symptoms requires combining restorative and global therapies provided by skilled interdisciplinary team members. The care plan must consider the context of the individual's illness and his or her goals of care. If restorative therapies are not available or not helpful in achieving physical improvement or patient-centred goals, the focus of care may shift to global symptom-oriented therapies including non-pharmacological and pharmacological interventions. Clinicians need high-level communication skills in discussing withdrawal of therapies such as antimicrobials and mechanical ventilation when appropriate. For some pulmonary infections, such as those encountered by patients with CF, therapies traditionally thought to be restorative may continue to have palliative intent even if cure is not possible late into the disease trajectory.

While many of the global therapies are available in most countries and more people die from non-malignant pulmonary diseases and complications of these illnesses such as infection, this patient population accesses global therapies and support systems much less often when compared to cancer patients (61). Proper utilization of these therapies and support systems must increase to provide the best care for patients and their families.

References

1. van Zyl Smit RN, Pai M, Yew WW, *et al.* Global lung health: the colliding epidemics of tuberculosis, tobacco smoking, HIV and COPD. *Eur Respir J* 2010; **35**(1):27–33.

2. Selwyn PA, Forstein M. Overcoming the false dichotomy of curative vs palliative care for late-stage HIV/AIDS: 'let me live the way I want to live, until I can't'. *JAMA* 2003; **290**(6):806–14.

3. Ferris FD, Balfour HM, Bowen K, *et al.* A model to guide patient and family care: based on nationally accepted principles and norms of practice. *J Pain Symptom Manage* 2002; **24**(2):106–23.

4. Jasmer RM, Nahid P, Hopewell PC. Clinical practice. Latent tuberculosis infection. *N Engl J Med* 2002; **347**(23):1860–6.

5. WHO. *Global Tuberculosis Control. A Short Update to the 2009 Report.* Geneva: WHO. Available from: http://www.who.int/ (accessed 23 April 2010).

6. Miller LG, Asch SM, Yu EI, Knowles L, Gelberg L, Davidson P. A population-based survey of tuberculosis symptoms: how atypical are atypical presentations? *Clin Infect Dis* 2000; **30**(2):293–9.

7. Migliori GB, D'Arcy Richardson M, Sotgiu G, Lange C. Multidrug-resistant and extensively drug-resistant tuberculosis in the West. Europe and United States: epidemiology, surveillance, and control. *Clin Chest Med* 2009; **30**(4):637–65, vii.

8. WHO. *Towards Universal Access. Scaling up priority HIV/AIDS interventions in the health sector. Progress Report 2009.* Geneva: WHO. Available from: http://www.who.int/ (accessed 23 April 2010).

9. George MP, Kannass M, Huang L, Sciurba FC, Morris A. Respiratory symptoms and airway obstruction in HIV-infected subjects in the HAART era. *PLoS One* 2009; **4**(7):e6328.

10. Diaz PT, Wewers MD, Pacht E, Drake J, Nagaraja HN, Clanton TL. Respiratory symptoms among HIV-seropositive individuals. *Chest* 2003; **123**(6):1977–82.

11. Huang L, Crothers K. HIV-associated opportunistic pneumonias. *Respirology* 2009; **14**(4):474–85.

12. Guidelines for prevention and treatment of opportunistic infections in HIV-infected adults and adolescents. *MMWR* 2009; **58**(RR-4):34.

13. Abdool Karim SS, Naidoo K, Grobler A, *et al.* Timing of initiation of antiretroviral drugs during tuberculosis therapy. *N Engl J Med* 2010; **362**(8):697–706.

14. WHO. *Quick COPD Facts.* Geneva: WHO. Available from: http://www.who.int/ (accessed 23 April 2010).

15. Farkas JD, Manning HL. Guidelines versus clinical practice in antimicrobial therapy for COPD. *Lung*; **188**(2):173–8.

16. Yankaskas JR, Marshall BC, Sufian B, Simon RH, Rodman D. Cystic fibrosis adult care: consensus conference report. *Chest* 2004; **125**(1 Suppl):1S–39S.

17. Evans KC, Banzett RB, Adams L, McKay L, Frackowiak RS, Corfield DR. BOLD fMRI identifies limbic, paralimbic, and cerebellar activation during air hunger. *J Neurophysiol* 2002; **88**(3): 1500–11.

18. Peiffer C, Poline JB, Thivard L, Aubier M, Samson Y. Neural substrates for the perception of acutely induced dyspnea. *Am J Respir Crit Care Med* 2001; **163**(4):951–7.

19. Rabow MW, Dibble SL, Pantilat SZ, McPhee SJ. The comprehensive care team: a controlled trial of outpatient palliative medicine consultation. *Arch Intern Med* 2004; **164**(1):83–91.

20. Lacasse Y, Goldstein R, Lasserson TJ, Martin S. Pulmonary rehabilitation for chronic obstructive pulmonary disease. *Cochrane Database Syst Rev* 2006; **4**:CD003793.

21. Buckholz GT, von Gunten CF. Nonpharmacological management of dyspnea. *Curr Opin Support Palliat Care* 2009; **3**(2):98–102.

22. Shah AA, D'Amico TA. Lung volume reduction surgery for the management of refractory dyspnea in chronic obstructive pulmonary disease. *Curr Opin Support Palliat Care* 2009; **3**(2):107–11.

23. Pomerantz BJ, Cleveland JC, Jr, Olson HK, Pomerantz M. Pulmonary resection for multi-drug resistant tuberculosis. *J Thorac Cardiovasc Surg* 2001; **121**(3):448–53.

24. Jennings AL, Davies AN, Higgins JP, Gibbs JS, Broadley KE. A systematic review of the use of opioids in the management of dyspnoea. *Thorax* 2002; **57**(11):939–44.

25. Ben-Aharon I, Gafter-Gvili A, Paul M, Leibovici L, Stemmer SM. Interventions for alleviating cancer-related dyspnea: a systematic review. *J Clin Oncol* 2008; **26**(14):2396–404.

26. Currow DC, Plummer J, Frith P, Abernethy AP. Can we predict which patients with refractory dyspnea will respond to opioids? *J Palliat Med* 2007; **10**(5):1031–6.

27. Thomas JR, von Gunten CF. Clinical management of dyspnoea. *Lancet Oncol* 2002; **3**(4):223–8.

28. Currow DC, Ward AM, Abernethy AP. Advances in the pharmacological management of breathlessness. *Curr Opin Support Palliat Care* 2009; **3**(2):103–6.

29. Abernethy AP, Currow DC, Frith P, Fazekas BS, McHugh A, Bui C. Randomised, double blind, placebo controlled crossover trial of sustained release morphine for the management of refractory dyspnoea. *BMJ* 2003; **327**(7414):523–8.

30. Bruera E, Sweeney C, Willey J, *et al.* A randomized controlled trial of supplemental oxygen versus air in cancer patients with dyspnea. *Palliat Med* 2003; **17**(8):659–63.

31. Schwartzstein RM, Lahive K, Pope A, Weinberger SE, Weiss JW. Cold facial stimulation reduces breathlessness induced in normal subjects. *Am Rev Respir Dis* 1987; **136**(1):58–61.

32. Burgess KR, Whitelaw WA. Effects of nasal cold receptors on pattern of breathing. *J Appl Physiol* 1988; **64**(1):371–6.

33. Simon ST, Higginson IJ, Booth S, Harding R, Bausewein C. Benzodiazepines for the relief of breathlessness in advanced malignant and non-malignant diseases in adults. *Cochrane Database Syst Rev* 2010; **1**:CD007354.

34. O'Neill PA, Morton PB, Stark RD. Chlorpromazine—a specific effect on breathlessness? *Br J Clin Pharmacol* 1985; **19**(6):793–7.

35. McIver B, Walsh D, Nelson K. The use of chlorpromazine for symptom control in dying cancer patients. *J Pain Symptom Manage* 1994; **9**(5):341–5.

36. Smith SM, Schroeder K, Fahey T. Over-the-counter medications for acute cough in children and adults in ambulatory settings. *Cochrane Database Syst Rev* 2008; **1**:CD001831.

37. Hudson E, Lester JF, Attanoos RL, Linnane SJ, Byrne A. Successful treatment of bronchorrhea with octreotide in a patient with adenocarcinoma of the lung. *J Pain Symptom Manage* 2006; **32**(3):200–2.

38. Lamberts SW, van der Lely AJ, de Herder WW, Hofland LJ. Octreotide. *N Engl J Med* 1996; **334**(4):246–54.

39. Fallon M. The physiology of somatostatin and its synthetic analog, octreotide. *Eur J Palliat Care* 1996; **1**(1):20–2.

40. Thomas T WR, Booth S. Other respiratory symptoms (cough, hiccup and secretions). In Bruera E, Higginson IJ, Ripamonti C, von Gunten, C (eds) *Textbook of Palliative Medicine*, pp. 663–72. London: Hodder Arnold, 2006.

41. Lee PCL, Jawad MS, Eccles R. Antitussive efficacy of dextromethorphan in cough associated with acute upper respiratory tract infection. *J Pharm Pharmacol* 2000; **52**(9):1137–42.

42. Marsden S. Other infectious disease: malaria, rabies, tuberculosis. In: Bruera E, Higginson IJ, Ripamonti C, von Gunten C (eds) *Textbook of Palliative Medicine*, PP. 944–54. London: Hodder Arnold, 2006.

43. Jenkins V, Fallowfield L, Saul J. Information needs of patients with cancer: results from a large study in UK cancer centres. *Br J Cancer* 2001; **84**(1):48–51.

44. Goldberg R, Guadagnoli E, Silliman RA, Glicksman A. Cancer patients' concerns: congruence between patients and primary care physicians. *J Cancer Educ* 1990; **5**(3):193–9.

45. Tulsky JA, Fischer GS, Rose MR, Arnold RM. Opening the black box: how do physicians communicate about advance directives? *Ann Intern Med.* 1998; **129**(6):441–9.

46. Maguire P, Faulkner A, Booth K, Elliott C, Hillier V. Helping cancer patients disclose their concerns. *Eur J Cancer* 1996; **32A**(1):78–81.

47. Billings JA, Block S. Palliative care in undergraduate medical education. Status report and future directions. *JAMA.* 1997; **278**(9):733–8.

48. The AM, Hak T, Koeter G, van Der Wal G. Collusion in doctor-patient communication about imminent death: an ethnographic study. *BMJ* 2000; **321**(7273):1376–81.

49. Shorr AF, Niven AS, Katz DE, Parker JM, Eliasson AH. Regulatory and educational initiatives fail to promote discussions regarding end-of-life care. *J Pain Symptom Manage* 2000; **19**(3):168–73.

50. Fallowfield L, Jenkins V, Farewell V, Saul J, Duffy A, Eves R. Efficacy of a Cancer Research UK communication skills training model for oncologists: a randomised controlled trial. *Lancet* 2002; **359**(9307):650–6.

51. Eden OB, Black I, MacKinlay GA, Emery AE. Communication with parents of children with cancer. *Palliat Med* 1994; **8**(2):105–14.

52. Rodin G, Zimmermann C, Mayer C, *et al.* Clinician-patient communication: evidence-based recommendations to guide practice in cancer. *Curr Oncol* 2009; **16**(6):42–9.

53. El-Jawahri A, Podgurski LM, Eichler AF, *et al.* Use of video to facilitate end-of-life discussions with patients with cancer: a randomized controlled trial. *J Clin Oncol* 2010; **28**(2):305–10.

54. Stone D, Patton B, Heen S. *Difficult Conversations. How to Discuss What Matters Most.* New York: Penguin Books, 2000.

55. Burns CM, Broom DH, Smith WT, Dear K, Craft PS. Fluctuating awareness of treatment goals among patients and their caregivers: a longitudinal study of a dynamic process. *Support Care Cancer* 2007; **15**(2):187–96.

56. Pfeifer MP, Sidorov JE, Smith AC, Boero JF, Evans AT, Settle MB. The discussion of end-of-life medical care by primary care patients and physicians: a multicenter study using structured qualitative interviews. The EOL Study Group. *J Gen Intern Med* 1994; **9**(2):82–8.

57. Frankl D, Oye RK, Bellamy PE. Attitudes of hospitalized patients toward life support: a survey of 200 medical inpatients. *Am J Med* 1989; **86**(6):645–8.

58. Downar J, Hawryluck L. What should we say when discussing 'code status' and life support with a patient? A Delphi analysis. *J Palliat Med* 2010; **13**(2):185–95.

59. Clayton JM, Butow PN, Arnold RM, Tattersall MH. Discussing end-of-life issues with terminally ill cancer patients and their carers: a qualitative study. *Support Care Cancer* 2005; **13**(8):589–99.

60. Levinson W, Gorawara-Bhat R, Lamb J. A study of patient clues and physician responses in primary care and surgical settings. *JAMA* 2000; **284**(8):1021–7.

61. Shuttleworth A. Palliative care for people with end-stage non-malignant lung disease. *Nurs Times* 2005; **101**(6):48–9.

Index

abdominal muscles 38
  compression 222
Abernethy, A.P. 129, 130, 133, 136
accelerometers 147
accessory muscles 38
acinus 43
active cycle of breathing (ACBT) 275
active, progressive (definition of term) 12
activities of daily living (ADLs) 170
activity monitors 147
activity pacing 149
activity planning 150
acupuncture/acupressure 173–4
acute respiratory distress syndrome (ARDS) 209
Adams, S.G. 167
adriamycin 332
advance care planning 206–7, 211
advance directives 30–1, 207, 315
affective component 85–6
afferent receptors/signals 44, 73, 75, 78–9
Africa 349
age factors 8, 235
AIDS see HIV/AIDS
air travel and oxygen therapy 139–40
airflow:
  obstruction 84
  see also diffuse airflow obstruction; oxygen
airway
  cells 51
  lining fluid (ALF) 50–1
  obstruction 71, 72, 74, 78
  proteins 51
  resistance 45–6, 47
  stenting 335
alcohol intake reduction 246–7
allergies 247, 261
allodynia 290, 293
alprazolam 116
alvelolar-material oxygen gradient 48
alveolar cell carcinoma and expectoration 272
alveoli 41–2, 48
American College of Chest Physicians 114
  Position Statement 165
American College of Sports Medicine 155
American Thoracic Society definition of
  dyspnoea 91
anabolic steroids 223
analgesics/analgesia 291–2, 294, 295, 339
  adjuvant 294
  modern classification 295
  see also WHO analgesic ladder
anatomy and physiology 37–52
  accessory muscles 38
  airway resistance 45–6, 47

breathing during exercise 49
breathing regulation 49
bronchial circulation 42
diaphragm 37, 38
innervation 44
integration 44–5
intercostal muscles 38
lower airways 39–42
lung defence mechanisms 50–1
lung inflammation 51–2
lymph 42, 43
obesity 49–50
pleura, pleural space and pleural fluid 38
pulmonary gas exchange 46–8
pulmonary vessels 42, 44
upper airways 39
angiotensin-converting enzyme (ACE)
  inhibitors 358
  associated cough 260–1
anorexia and malignant disease 333
antibiotics 262, 263, 266, 337, 338
  chronic obstructive pulmonary disease-related
    infection 352
  cystic fibrosis-related infection 310, 312, 315, 353
  HIV-related infection 350
anticholinergics 275, 357
antidepressants 22, 117–19, 227
  tricyclic 117–19, 205
antiemetics 315
antihistamines 262, 357, 358
antimicrobials 347–8, 352
  see also antibiotics
antitussive therapies 264–5
anxiety 94–5
  buspirone 117
  and complementary exercises 172
  cystic fibrosis 313, 314
  diffuse airflow obstruction 205
  dyspnoea 163
  hyperventilation syndrome 235, 244
  and music therapy 173
  neuromuscular and skeletal disorders 222
  non-pharmacological strategies 174–5
  obstructive sleep apnoea 227
  occupational therapy and environmental
    modifications 149, 150–1
  pharmacological treatment 356
  psychotropic medications 115
  pulmonary rehabilitation 166
  6-minute walking test (6MWT) 353
Argyropoulou, P. 117
arterial blood gas (ABG) analysis 124
arterial pH 79–80
arterioles 42

asbestosis 209
Asia 349
  Central 350
  South East 262
Assist UK 153
assisted dying and euthanasia 33–4
Association for Palliative Medicine of Great Britain
    and Ireland 12
asthma 47
  acupuncture/acupressure 174
  and affective dimension of dyspnoea 164
  clinical investigations 94
  cough variant 259–60, 261
  and expectoration 272
  and hyperventilation syndrome (HVS) 235, 242–3,
    244, 247
  self-management programmes 166
  visual analogue scales 96
Asthma Bother Profile 54, 55, 56
Asthma Quality of Life Questionnaire 54, 55
atropine 275, 357
Australia 111, 133, 360
autogenic drainage 275
autogenic training 151
Azerbaijan 349

baclofen 263
Baku 349
basal metabolic rate (BMR) 190
baseline dyspnoea index/transitional
    dyspnoea index (BDI/TDI) 93–4, 98, 99–100, 132,
    201
behavioural observation scores 283
Belgium 33
belladonna leaf extract 357
Ben-Aharon, I. 131
benzodiazepines 86, 115–16, 206, 315, 356, 359
benzonatate 358
bereavement 314–16
  counselling/services 31–2, 316
beta agonists/blockers 244, 274
beta-lactam 351
bevacizumab 331–2
bisphosphonates 297
bleomycin 266
blood sugar levels, fluctuating 247
blood tests 93
body mass index 157, 200, 311
Booth, S. 130
Borg score 130, 132, 136
  see also modified Borg
Bowler, S.D. 243
brachytherapy 328–9, 333, 335, 338
branched chain amino acids (BCAA) 189
breath-hold test 241
Breathe Easy 152
breathing:
  active cycle of breathing (ACBT) 275
  deep breathing manoeuvres 220
  diaphragm 220, 245
  and exercise 49, 246
  frog 220–1, 222

and hyperventilation syndrome (HVS) 237–8
  intermittent positive pressure breathing
    (PPPB) 222
  mouth 239
  nose 238, 245
  pursed lip 170, 203, 220
  quiet 245
  rate 246
  regulation 49
  retraining 170, 203–4, 244
    factors preventing 247
  and talking 246
  techniques in neuromuscular and skeletal
    diseases 220–1
  upper chest 238, 239
  while sitting and standing 246
Breathing Problems Questionnaire 55, 57
breathlessness see dyspnoea
breathlessness clinics, hospital-based 24
Brief Pain Inventory 283
British Lung Foundation 152
British Thoracic Society guidelines 140, 198
bronchi 40, 48
bronchial circulation 42
bronchial epithelium 50
bronchiectasis 198–9, 261, 262, 352
  and expectoration 272, 357
  and hyperventilation syndrome (HVS) 244
bronchioles 40–1, 42, 48
bronchiolitis 197
bronchitis 197, 352, 357
  chronic 172, 261, 262, 273, 274, 275, 352
  eosinophilic 259–60, 261, 272
bronchoconstriction 83–4
bronchodilators 274, 352
Bruera, E. 94, 130
bupivacaine 82
buprenorphine 299, 303
bupropion 204
Burdon, J. 97
burn-out 32–3
buspirone 117, 356
Buteyko breathing techniques 243
Buteyko, K. 242–3

C-fibres 78, 81, 83–4, 254
cachexia see nutrition and cachexia
caffeine 235, 246–7
calcium channels 293
Calicut model 9
Campbell, M.L. 97
Canada 9–10, 133, 333–4, 363
Canadian Occupational Performance
    Measure (COPM) 147–8
cancer see malignant disease
Cangiano, C. 189
cannabinoids 188
capnographs 241
capsaicin 254, 255, 259, 264–5, 293
carbocysteine 357
carbon dioxide measurement 241
  see also $PaCO_2$; PCO_2

carboplatin 329–30
/paclitaxel 326, 331, 332
cardiopulmonary resuscitation 27
Care and Repair schemes 152
carer, role of 151–2
carers, needs of in end of life care 31–2
Carers UK 151–2
Central and Eastern Europe 9, 350
central nervous system areas
responding to breathlessness 113
central sleep apnoea 216, 219
cetuximab 326, 332
Chaitow, L. 247
charities 3
chemoradiotherapy 325–6, 327, 332
chemoreceptors 72, 73, 79–80
chemotherapy 265–6, 326, 330, 335–6, 338–40
in advanced non-small cell lung cancer
(NSCLC) 329–31
late effects 29
for palliation 332–4
in resectable disease 331
chest wall:
disorders and oxygen therapy 134
muscles, weakness of 217–18
receptors 84
vibrators 84
Chevallier, J. 275
Cheyne-Stokes respiration 216
Childhood Asthma Questionnaires 55–6, 57
children:
and cough 266–7
Harrison's sulcus 37
neuromuscular disorders 222
China 163
chlorpromazine 356
Christie, M.J. 55
Chronic Care Model (CCM) 166–7
chronic obstructive pulmonary disease
(COPD) 46, 47, 71, 80
acupuncture/acupressure 174
and affective dimension of dyspnoea 164
antidepressants 118
benzodiazepines 115, 116
breathing retraining 170
buspirone 117
cachexia 190–1
clinical investigations 93–4
clinical prognostic indicators 207
cognitive-behavioural therapy (CBT) 174–5
and complementary exercises 172–3
complications 199
dietary support 204
diffuse airflow obstruction 197, 199, 203
disease-modifying treatments 201
energy conservation 149, 170
exercise tolerance 156
and expectoration 272
fatigue 148
furosemide 82–3, 119, 356
and hyperventilation syndrome (HVS) 243–4
illness trajectory 165

inspiratory muscle training 170
long-term oxygen therapy (LTOT) 127–9, 205
lower airway receptors 81–3
modified Borg dyspnoea scale (MBS) 97
neuromuscular stimulation 171
non-invasive positive pressure ventilation
(NIPPV) 171
nutritional status 157
opioids 112–14
oxygen therapy 131, 132, 133, 134, 135
psychological support 205
pulmonary rehabilitation 154
relaxation exercises 172
self-management programmes 166–8
stages 200
surgical options 206
chronic pulmonary infections:
supportive care 347–65
chronic obstructive pulmonary-related 351–2
cystic fibrosis-related 352–3
global therapies 353–9
cough 358
dry secretions 357–8
dyspnoea (breathlessness) 353–4
haemoptysis 358–9
non-pharmacological therapies 354–5
pharmacological therapies 355–6
secretions 356–7
HIV-related 350–1
psychosocial aspects 364
pulmonary tuberculosis 348–9
restorative therapies, withdrawal of 359–60
six-step protocol 360–4
Chronic Respiratory Disease
Questionnaire (CRDQ) 54, 56, 102–3, 132, 167
Chronos, N. 80
cisplatin 329, 331, 334, 335
/etoposide 326
/gemcitabine 330, 332
/pemetrexed 330
/vinorelbine 332
citalopram 118
clorazepate 116
codeine 117, 263, 264, 294, 298, 338, 339
cognitive behavioural therapy (CBT) 165, 174–5,
205, 314
cognitive impairment 283
communication skills 315
training 359–60
communication/language difficulties 283
comorbidity 18
complementary exercises 172–3
complementary therapies 28, 245, 310, 314
compressed air via nasal cannula 355
computed tomography pulmonary angiogram
(CTPA) 286
congenital abnormalities 266
congestive heart failure and self-management
programmes 167
continuous hyperfractionated accelerated
radiotherapy (CHART) 326
continuous positive airway pressure (CPAP) 226–7

coping capacity 94
corollary discharge 75–6, 77, 80
corticosteroids 260, 262, 266, 352, 358
cost-benefit analysis 62
cost-effectiveness analysis 62, 65–6, 67
cost-minimization analysis 62
cost-utility analysis 62–8
   clinical question definition and identification of all
      relevant comparisons 63
   cost and effects 65–7
   health outcomes 64
   resource use 64–5
   uncertainty 67–8
   viewpoint and time-horizon of analysis 63–4
cough:
   antitussives 264–5
   assistance machines 221–2
   chronic obstructive pulmonary disease-
      related 351, 352
   cystic fibrosis-related 353
   global therapies 358
   HIV-related 350
   malignant disease-associated 320–3, 326, 329,
      332–3
   palliation 338
   peak cough expiratory flow rate (PCEF) 222
   tuberculosis-associated 349
   see also cough physiology and pathophysiology
cough physiology and pathophysiology 253–67
   acute cough 253, 255, 257–8
   angiotensin-converting enzyme inhibitor-
      associated 256, 260–1
   children 266–7
   chronic cough 253, 254, 257, 261
   corticosteroid-responsive cough 257
   cough centre 254
   cough reflex 253–5
   cough variant asthma/eosinophilic
      bronchitis 259–60
   frequency determination 255
   gastro-oesophageal reflux 261, 262
   in health and disease 255
   malignancy and palliative care 265–6
   non-eosinophilic cough 257
   patient evaluation 255–9
   post viral cough 261
   rhinitis/upper airway cough 261–2
   treatment of chronic cough 263–5
   upper airway cough 261–2
   voluntary cough suppression 264
Council of Healthcare Ministers of the European
    Union 14
counselling interventions 63
creatine 223
cryptogenic organizing pneumonia (COP) 266
cultural factors 31, 32
cyanosis, central 216
cyclophosphamide 332
cystic fibrosis 51
   and cough 266
   diffuse airflow obstruction 199
   and expectoration 272, 273, 274, 275

   medications for secretions 356, 357
   oxygen therapy 134
   psychosocial aspects 364
   -related pulmonary infection 352–3
   see also supportive care in cystic fibrosis
cytokines 51

Da Costa, J.M. 233
daily activity monitoring 146–7
Dean, N.C. 132
decision-making, shared 360
deconditioning 78, 80, 243, 246
definitions of palliative care 10–14
delegation 150
depression 117–18
   and complementary exercises 172
   cystic fibrosis 313, 314
   diffuse airflow obstruction 205
   dyspnoea 163
   hyperventilation syndrome 235
   neuromuscular and skeletal disorders 222
   non-pharmacological strategies 174–5
   obstructive sleep apnoea 227 occupational
      therapy and
   environmental modifications 149
   pulmonary rehabilitation 166
dextromethorphan 263, 264, 358
diabetes 244, 309
diamorphine 264, 300
diaphragm 37, 38, 218
   breathing 220, 245
   hyperventilation syndrome 237–8, 247
diazepam 115, 117, 225–6
diet *see* nutrition
dietician 311
diffuse airflow obstruction and
   'restrictive' lung disease 197–211
   advance care planning 206–7, 211
   advance directives 207
   assessment of severity 199–200, 209–10
   chronic diffuse airflow
      obstruction 197–9
   dietary support 204
   drugs for severe breathlessness 206, 211
   general measures 210
   lung transplantation 211
   medicolegal issues 211
   non-obstructive/restrictive lung disease 208–9
   oxygen therapy 205, 210
   posture, breathing technique training and
      respiratory muscle training 203–4
   psychological support 205
   pulmonary rehabilitation 202–3, 210
   self-management 204
   smoking cessation 204
   supportive care needs assessment 201–2
   supportive care in non-obstructive lung
      disease 210
   supportive care role 200–1
   surgical options 206
   treatment 209–10
diffuse parenchymal lung diseases (DPLD) 208

diffuse pleural thickening 208
diffusing capacity for carbon monoxide (DLCO) 48
dihydrocodeine 115, 339
directly observed therapy (DOT) programmes 349
Disabled Facilities Grant 152
Disabled Living Centres 153
Disabled Living Foundation 153
disease management (DM) programme 167–8
disease-directed therapies 20–2
disease-specific scales 54–7
DNAase 273, 357
docetaxel 329, 330
double effect principle 34, 303
drug-resistance 334
drugs *see* pharmacological treatment
Duchenne muscular dystrophy 215, 216, 221, 222, 224
Dudgeon, D.J. 96
dynamic hyperinflation 84
dysaesthesias 290
dyspnoea (breathlessness):
  anchored to activities 97–101
  chronic 111–12
  chronic obstructive pulmonary disease-related
      infection 351, 352
  cystic fibrosis-related infection 353
  definitions and prevalence 111–12
  drug treatment 211
  global therapies 353–4
  HIV-related infection 350
  malignant disease 319–20, 321, 322, 323, 324, 326, 332, 333
  multidimensional assessment 91–104
    choice of instrument 103
    clinical investigations 93–4
    medical history 92
    physical examination 92–3
    psychological factors 94–5
    qualitative dimensions 95
    quality of life instruments 101–3
    unidimensional scales 95–9
  non-pharmacological strategies 163–75
    acupuncture/acupressure 173–4
    affective dimension 164
    anxiety and depression 174–5
    assessment 165
    breathing retraining 170
    chronic obstructive pulmonary disease
        (COPD) 168–9
    cognitive-behavioural perspective 165
    complementary exercises 172–3
    end of life phase 175
    energy conservation 169–70
    exercise training 166
    fresh air and fans 171
    illness trajectories 165
    inspiratory muscle training (IMT) 170
    intensity and distress, factors related to 164–5
    multidimensional symptom, dyspnoea
        as 163–4
    music therapy 173
    neuromuscular stimulation (NMES) 171
  non-invasive positive pressure ventilation
      (NIPPV) 170–1
    patient education 169
    pulmonary rehabilitation 165–6
    relaxation exercises 171–2
    self-management programmes 166–8
    symptom perception phases 164
    symptom prevalence and comorbidities 163
  and obstructive sleep apnoea 215–17, 218, 219, 220
  occupational therapy 145
  oxygen and airflow 126–7, 128–9
  palliation 335–6
  physiology and pathophysiology 71–86
    advanced disease 86
    affective dimension 85–6
    afferent receptors 78–9
    chemoreceptors 79–80
    corollary discharge 75–6
    descriptors associated with increased ventilatory
        muscle work 76–7
    efferent-reafferent dissociation 77–8
    mechanoreceptors 80–4
    multiple origins 72–3
    qualitative descriptions 73–5
  pulmonary rehabilitation 154
  refractory 123
  see also baseline dyspnoea
      index/transitional dyspnoea
      index
Dyspnoea Self-Management Programme
    (DSMP) 167
dystrophia myotonica 215, 216

early disease detection 18
Eaton, T.C. 133
economic evaluation *see* cost-utility analysis
Education for Physicians on End-of-life Care
    (EPEC) 359
efferent-reafferent dissociation 73, 75, 77–8, 79, 80, 81
effort, sense of 76
effusions, management of 339–41
Efthimiou, J. 191
eicosapentaenoic acid (EPA) 188–9
Eimer, M. 116
electrocardiogram (ECG) 286
emphysema 197, 220
end of dose failure 291
end of life care 8–9, 29–33
  family and other carers, needs of 31–2
  healthcare professionals, needs of 32–3
  non-pharmacological strategies 175
  oxygen and airflow 136–7
  pain management 302–3
  physical symptom management 30
  psychological aspects of management 30–1
  social aspects of patients' and families' lives 31
  spiritual and cultural aspects of care 31
End-of-Life Nursing Education Consortium
    (ELNEC) 359
endobronchial therapy 328–9, 335, 338
endurance shuttle walking test (ESWT) 156, 157

energy conservation 149–50, 169–70, 219–20
enteral nutrition 187, 311, 312
environmental modifications 152–4
epirubicin 332
Epler, G.R. 94
EQ-5D 64
equipment provision 152–4
erectile dysfunction 227
erlotinib 330, 331
erythromycin 352
ethambutol 349
ethamsylate 338
etoposide 326, 329, 332
EuroPall project 14
Europe 25, 28, 158, 197, 320, 325
European Big Lung Trial 330
European Organization for Research and Treatment
    of Cancer QLQ-C30 56, 284
European Organization for Research and Treatment
    of Cancer QLQ-LC13 284–5
European School of Oncology 14
European Union 14
euthanasia 33–4
exacerbation rate 272–3
excessive daytime sleepiness and cognitive
    defects 226–7
exercise programmes 157–8, 166
  and anxiety and depression 174–5
  and breathing 246
  cardiovascular/aerobic 157, 221
  cycle-based 157
  diffuse airflow obstruction 203
  endurance shuttle walking test (ESWT) 156, 157
  endurance training 203
  field-based exercise test 155–6
  home-based 158, 166, 173
  hyperventilation syndrome 243
  incremental shuttle walking test (ISWT) 155–6, 157
  lower- and upper-extremity 165–6
  neuromuscular and skeletal diseases 221
  progressive exercise testing 94
  relaxation exercises 151, 171–2
  resistance training 157–8, 203
  respiratory muscle training 203–4, 221
  rowing 157
  shuttle walking test 94
  6-minute walking test (6MWT) 131, 155–6, 173, 174
  stepping 156, 157
  strength training 166
  treadmill exercise 173
  walking/walking tests 94, 157, 158, 223
exercise testing 94, 95
exercise tolerance 155–6
expectoration 50, 350, 351
  care pathway 276
  chronic obstructive pulmonary disease-related
    infection 352
  cystic fibrosis-related infection 353
  pathophysiology, measurement and therapy 271–6
    anticholinergics 275
    beta agonists 274
    measurement 272–3

mucokinetic agents 274
mucolytic agents 273
pathophysiology 271–2
physiotherapy with autogenic drainage 275
secretagogues 273–4
therapy 271
water and saline 274
expiration 45
  forced 47
  maximal expiratory pressure (PEmax) 93
  peak cough expiratory flow rate (PCEF) 222
  positive end expiratory pressure (PEEP) 82, 84
  see also forced expiratory volume
expiratory reserve volume 50
extended dominance 66

face mask 223
'faces' pain scale 283
family and other carers, needs of in end of life
    care 31–2
family support 18
far-advanced disease (definition of term) 12
fat-free mass (FFM) 190
fatigue/malaise 148, 185–6 malignant disease 319,
    320, 322, 326, 333
fear of impending loss and future helplessness 31
fentanyl 294, 296, 299, 303, 339
Ferreira, J.M. 191
Ferris, F.D. 347
fertility/pregnancy and cystic fibrosis 314
fibrosing alveolitis 42, 46
fibrosis 197
Filshie, J. 173
financial advice and support from the state 32
fire risk and oxygen therapy 137
5FU (MCF) 335
focus of care is quality of life (definition
    of term) 13
forced expiratory volume (1-second)(FEV1) 46–7,
    71, 94
  diffuse airflow obstruction 197–8, 200
  furosemide 82–3, 119, 356
  Sickness Impact Profile 101
forced vital capacity (FVC) 94, 119
forward leaning posture with shoulder girdle
    support 203–4, 354
Foster, S. 210
Foundations 152
fractionated external beam therapy 329
French, D.J. 55
fresh air and fans 171, 355
Friedreich's ataxia 215
frog breathing 220–1, 222
functional capacity utilization 146
functional electrical stimulation of abdominal
    muscles 222
functional magnetic resonance imaging (fMRI) 286
functional performance 146
functional reserve 146
functional residual capacity (FRC) 45–6, 50
functional status scales 146–7
furosemide 82–3, 119, 356

Galbraith, S. 130
Garrod, R. 132
gastro-oesophageal reflux disease 244, 262
gefitinib 330, 331
gemcitabine 329, 330, 332, 334
gender factors 8, 235
    cough 255, 260, 263, 267
    malignant disease 320
generic model 6–7
generic scales 57–8
genetic screening programmes 18, 20
Germany 28
ghrelin 187–8
Gift, A.G. 92
Global Initiative on Obstructive Lung Disease 114
global therapies 347–8
    see also chronic pulmonary infections
glutamate 293
glutamine-enriched solutions 189–90
glycopyrrolate 357
Gold Standards Framework 206–7
Gorecka, D.K. 127–8
guaifenesin 273–4, 356
Guyatt, G.H. 56, 96, 102

haemoptysis 358–9
    cystic fibrosis-related infection 353
    malignant disease 320, 321, 323, 326, 329, 332, 333
    palliation 336–8
    tuberculosis 349
Harrison's sulcus 37
health outcomes, measurement and valuation of 64
health-related quality of life (HRQL) 64
healthcare professionals, needs of in end of life care 32–3
heart failure and oxygen therapy 134
helium/oxygen (Heliox) 203, 356
Henoch, I. 94
Hering-Breuer reflex 44
highly active antiretroviral therapy (HAART) 350–1
HIV/AIDS 185, 347, 349, 350–1
holistic approach 28, 245, 310, 314
Holloway, E. 244
home care services and cystic fibrosis 312
home-based exercise programmes 158, 166, 173
Hopwood, P. 320
hospice movement 8–9, 10, 26
Hospital Anxiety and Depression Scale (HADS) 94–5, 149, 242
hospital-based breathlessness clinics 24
hospital-based pain clinics 24
hydromorphone 114
∃-hydroxy—methylbutyrate (HMB) 190
Hyland, M.E. 55, 56
hyoscine 266, 275
hyoscyamine (Levsin©) 357
hyperalgesia 290, 291, 293
hypercalcaemia 5–6
hypercapnia/hypercarbia 71–2, 73, 78, 127
    acute 79, 80
    chronic 80
    and obstructive sleep apnoea 216, 219, 221, 223
    and oxygen therapy 137

hyperinflation 71, 72, 76, 78
    dynamic 79
hyperventilation syndrome (HVS) 233–48
    acute 234
    and asthma 242–3
    breathing, efficient 237–8
    breathing and exercise 246
    breathing rate 246
    breathing while sitting and standing 246
    and bronchiectasis 244
    causes 235
    chronic 234–5
    and chronic obstructive pulmonary disease (COPD) 243–4
    diagnosis 239–42
        breath-hold test 241
        carbon dioxide measurement 241
        Hospital Anxiety and Depression scale 242
        provocation test 241
        recording symptoms 240–1
    diaphragm breathing 245
    factors preventing breathing retraining 247
    lifestyle changes 246–7
    management 244–5
    minute ventilation 239
    mouth breathing 239
    musculoskeletal rehabilitation 247
    nose breathing 245
    prevalence 235
    quiet breathing 245
    symptoms 235–7
    talking and breathing 246
    terminology and history 233–4
    upper chest breathing 238
hypocapnia 234, 242
hypocarbia 233, 239
hypopnoea 216, 219
hypoventilation 125
hypoxaemia 71–2, 73, 83–4, 126–7
    acute 80, 125
    antidepressants 118
    chronic 125, 127, 128, 205
    chronic obstructive pulmonary disease-related infection 352
    mild 80, 127
    moderate 80, 128
    oxygen therapy 131, 134, 135
hypoxia 216, 219, 355

iatrogenic peripheral neuropathy 293
idiographic scales 58
incremental analysis 66
incremental cost-effectivness ratio (ICER) 66–7
incremental costs 65–6
incremental health outcomes 65
incremental shuttle walking test (ISWT) 155–6, 157
independence, declining 148
India 8–9
indomethacin 357
infertility 314

information:
  centres 24
  resources 22
  services 28
inhaled foreign body 256, 266
innervation (lungs) 44
inspiration 45
  maximal inspiratory pressure (PImax) 93–4
  peak inspiratory pressure 156
inspiratory muscle training (IMT) 156, 170
integration (lungs) 44–5
integrative step 18–19
intercostal drain 340
intercostal muscles 38, 237–8
interdisciplinary team model 348
intermittent positive pressure breathing (PPPB) 222
International Association for the Study of Pain 14
internet-based dyspnoea self-management
    programme (eDSMP) 168
interstitial lung disease 134, 208, 266
interstitium 41
interventional (anaesthetic) procedures for pain
    management 301–2
ipratropium 357
  bromide 262, 274
irinotecan 329, 332
isokinetic dynamometer 156
ISOLDE study 273
isometric strength (Nm) 156
isoniazid 349

Japan 262, 321
Jobs, K. 173
Jones, P.W. 57
Juniper, E.F. 55, 57
juxtapulmonary (J) receptors 44, 83

Kapella, M.C. 148
Karagener's syndrome 51
∀-ketoisocaproate 190
Klastersky, J. 17
kyphoplasty 297

Lacasse, Y. 118
'language of dyspnoea' 126
larynx 39
Leicester Cough Questionnaire 259
Leidy, N.K. 146
leucine 189, 190
levomepromazine 315
lidocaine 83, 263
life-maintaining therapies 21
life-prolonging treatments 21
lifestyle factors 235, 245, 246–7
Light, R.W. 117
lignocaine 233, 264
Likert scales 96
Liss, H.W. 130
Living with Asthma Questionnaire 56–7
living wills 30–1
lobules 42, 43, 48
local anaesthesia 301

long-term oxygen therapy (LTOT) 124, 127–9,
    134–5, 137, 139, 200, 205
lorazepam 359
lower airways 39–42
  receptors 81–4
lung:
  defence mechanisms 50–1
  disease and acupuncture/acupressure 173
  function tests 93
  inflammation 51–2
  transplantation 211, 315
  volume reduction surgery 206, 355
  volume subdivisions 45
lymph 42, 43
lymphoedema clinic 24

Maa, S.H. 174
McDonald C.F. 132
MacDonald, N. 4, 15
McGavin, C.R. 98
McGill Pain Questionnaire 283, 284
McGill Quality of Life Questionnaire 58, 130
MacMillan Durham Cachexia pack 204
macrolides 351
magnetic resonance imaging (MRI) 286
Mahler, D.A. 93–4, 98
malignant disease and respiratory symptoms 319–42
  acupuncture/acupressure 173, 174
  adjuvant chemotherapy in resectable disease 331
  and affective dimension of dyspnoea 164
  approaches to symptom management 323–4
  benzodiazepines 116
  cachexia syndrome 185
  causes and assessment of symptoms 321–3
  chemotherapy 332–4
  cough 264, 265–6, 338
  dyspnoea (breathlessness) 335–6
  dyspnoea scale (CDS) 100–1
  effusions, management of 339–41
  haemoptysis 336–8
  opioids 113–14
  oxygen therapy 131, 134
  pain 338–9
  prevalence of symptoms 319–21
  radiotherapy 326–9, 332–4
  reading numbers aloud test 98
  self-management programmes 167
  survivors and supportive care 28–9
  systemic therapy, targeted 331–2
  visual analogue scales 96
  see also non-small cell lung cancer; small-cell lung
    cancer
Man, G.C. 116
maximal expiratory pressure (PEmax) 93
maximal inspiratory pressure (PImax) 93–4
maximal voluntary ventilation (MVV) 94
mechanoreceptors 72, 80–4
Medical Outcomes Study Short Form (SF-36) 101,
    102, 285
Medical Research Council (MRC) 325
  breathlessness scale 98
  clinical trials 320

dyspnoea grades 3-5 155
   long-term oxygen therapy study 127–8
   scale 98, 201–2
medicine, changing aims of 3–7
medicolegal issues 211
medroxyprogesterone (MPA) 187
megestrol acetate (MEGACE) 187, 189
melanocortin antagonists 188
Memorial Symptom Assessment Scale 319
menopause and cough 255, 257
Mental Capacity Act (2005) 207
mepivicaine 263
metabolic alkalosis 219
metaboreceptors 80
methadone 296–7
midazolam 116, 359
Miller, S. 275
mindfulness meditation 172–3
minimal important difference (MID) 131
minute ventilation 239
Missoula-VITAS quality of life index 58
Mitchell-Heggs, P. 115
mitomycin 332, 335
modafinil 226–7
models of palliative care 9–15
modified Borg dyspnoea scale (MBS) 96, 97, 174
Moldova 349
Molken, M.R. 103
mood disorders/disturbance 172, 227
Moore, R.P. 132, 133
Mor, V. 96
morphine 206
   chronic pulmonary infections 355
   cough 264
   malignant disease 339
   pain 294, 298
   respiratory symptoms 112–14, 116, 117
motivation, loss of 148
motor cortex 76, 77
motor neuron disease 222, 224
mouth breathing 239
movement detectors 147
mucokinetic agents 274
mucolytic agents 266, 273
multidimensional assessment *see* dyspnoea
   (breathlessness): multidimensional assessment
multidisciplinary team and cystic fibrosis 310, 312,
   314
muscle wasting *see* cachexia syndrome
musculoskeletal rehabilitation for hyperventilation
   syndrome 247
music therapy 173
myasthenia gravis 221
myofibrillar protein 192
myotonic dystrophy 220

N-acetylcysteine 273, 357
naloxone 112–13
nasal mask 223–4
National Hospice Study 96
National Institute for Health and Clinical
   Excellence 62

cancer technology appraisals 63
   guidelines on chemotherapy 330
   quality of life 64, 67
National Reference costs 65
Navigante, A.H. 115–16
negative pressure ventilation system 224–5
Netherlands 33
neural respiratory drive 77
neuromuscular electrical stimulation (NMES) 171, 203
neuromuscular and skeletal diseases 215–26
   breathing techniques 220–1
   chest wall muscles, weakness of 217–18
   clinical features 215–17
   cough assistance 221–2
   energy conservation and physiotherapy 219–20
   exercise training 221
   nutrition 222–3
   oxygen therapy 134, 223
   psychotherapy 222
   respiratory drive abnormalities 219
   sedative drugs 225–6
   sleep 219
   upper airway muscles 218
   ventilatory support 223–5
neutrophils 52
new concept of care, necessity for 16–17
New Zealand 133
NHS End of Life Care Strategy 206
nicotine replacement therapies 204
Nijmegen questionnaire 240, 242
Nocturnal Oxygen Therapy Trial (NOTT) 127–8
non-governmental organizations 3
non-invasive positive pressure ventilation
   (NIPPV) 81–2, 84, 170–1, 223–5, 354
   cystic fibrosis 312, 353
non-nucleoside reverse transcriptase inhibitors 350
non-obstructive/restrictive lung disease 46, 94, 208–9
non-small cell lung cancer (NSCLC) 319–20, 324–5,
   331–7
   chemotherapy 329–31
   radiotherapy 325–6
non-steroidal anti-inflammatory drugs
   (NSAIDs) 339
nortriptyline 118
nose 39
   breathing 238, 245
numeric rating scale (NRS) 96, 130, 136, 174, 282
nutrition 157
   diet 204, 247
   enteral 187, 311, 312
   neuromuscular and skeletal diseases 222–3
   total parenteral nutrition 187, 189, 192
   see also nutrition and cachexia
nutrition and cachexia 185–92
   definition of cachexia syndrome 185–6
   malignant (cancer) cachexia 186–90
      food intake enhancement 187–8
      nutraceuticals 188–90
      nutritional support 186–7
   non-malignant cachexia related to respiratory
      system 190–2
   nutritional support and exercise combined 191–2

obesity 49–50
obstructive sleep apnoea 215–17, 218, 219, 220, 226–7
occupational therapy 145–60
  anxiety and depression 149, 150–1
  carer, role of 151–2
  daily activity monitoring, objective 147
  dyspnoea (breathlessness) 145
  energy conservation 149–50
  environmental modifications 152–4
  fatigue 148
  functional status scales 146–7
  independence, declining 148
  self-esteem and motivation, loss of 148
  sexual dysfunction 151
  see also pulmonary rehabilitation
octreotide 357–8
O'Donnell, D.E. 95, 97, 130, 132
omega-3-polyunsaturated fatty acids (PUFA) 188–9
opioids 112–15
  anti-social addictive behaviour 27
  clinical use 113–15
  cough 266, 358
  cystic fibrosis 315
  dyspnoea (breathlessness) 355
  malignant disease 338–9
  mechanisms of action 112–13
  neuromuscular and skeletal diseases 225–6
  pain 291, 296, 298–300, 303
  palliation and supportive care 27
  physical dependence 27
  receptors 293
  restrictive lung disease 206, 211
  strong 294
  weak 294
  see also hyperalgesia
opportunistic infections/pneumonias 350–1
opportunity cost 61
orthopnoea 216
oxidative injury, risk of 137–8
oxycodone 339
oxygen 123–41, 352
  air travel 139–40
  ambulatory 124, 134
  concentrator 138
  -conserving devices 138–9
  cost diagram (OCD) 98, 99
  cylinders 138
  cystic fibrosis-related infection 353
  definitions 123–4
  demand oxygen pulsing devices 138–9
  diffuse airflow obstruction and 'restrictive' lung disease 205, 210
  domiciliary 124, 134
  dyspnoea (breathlessness) 126–7, 128–9, 355
  dyspnoeic patient at rest 129–31, 136
  dyspnoeic patient exercising 131–3, 136
  end of life care 136–7
  /energy/vitality cost 149
  hazards 137–8
  humidified 266
  levels, measurement of 124–5

neuromuscular and skeletal diseases 223
  palliative 124
  PaO_2 85
  patient preference and education 135
  proposed guidelines for use 133–5
  psychological addiction 138
  saturation 93, 174
  SpO_2 value 124–5
  see also long-term oxygen therapy

paclitaxel 326, 329, 331, 332
$PaCO_2$ 48, 49, 76, 79, 124, 125
pain:
  assessment 281–7
    checklist for seniors with limited ability to communicate (PACSLAC) 283
    evaluation 281–2
    history 282
    investigations 286
    multidimensional 283
    pain diary 285
    physical examination 285–6
    quality of life 283–5
    in research 286
    tools 282–3
    utility of assessment tools 285
  bone 297
  breakthrough 290–1, 293, 296
  burning in chest 73
  chronic 293, 296
  diffuse 290
  incident 290–1
  localized 290
  long-term post-surgical 29
  malignant disease 290, 319–23, 326, 332–3
  management 26
  matrix 293, 286
  mechanisms and management 289–304
    analgesics 295
    anatomical basis of thoracic pain 289
    biological basis 291–4
    bisphosphonates 297
    end of life 302–3
    future developments in pain control 303–4
    interventional (anaesthetic) procedures 301–2
    non-pharmacological therapies 302
    opioids 298–300
    rational approach to pharmacological management 294–7
    surgical techniques 297
    types of pain 289–91
  neuropathic 289–90, 281, 283
  nociceptive 289–90, 281
  palliation 338–9
  pleuritic 289
  post-mastectomy 290
  post-thoracotomy 290
  pressure-like 73
  pyramid model/approach 296, 297
  radicular 290
  severity 282
  sharp 73

signals: transduction, transmission and
 inhibition 292
 somatic 289–90, 281
 speed of onset 282
 thoracic 291, 301
 visceral 289–90, 281
pain clinics, hospital-based 24
palliative care:
 and cough 265–6
 in cystic fibrosis 314–16
palliative sedation 303
palpation 285–6
pamidronate 297
panbronchiolitis, diffuse 262–3
panic 353
PaO$_2$ 124–5
parasympathetic vagal nerves 44
paroxetine 118
Payment by Results (PbR) tariff 65
PCO$_2$ 85
peak cough expiratory flow rate (PCEF) 222
peak inspiratory pressure 156
Pediatric Asthma Caregiver's Quality of Life
 Questionnaire 57
Pediatric Quality of Life Questionnaire 57
pemetrexed 329, 330, 332
percutaneous cervical cordotomy 302
performance status (PS) 325, 331, 332, 333, 334
peripheral muscle proteolysis 189
peripheral receptors 78
pertussis infection 257, 266
pH 124
pharmacological treatment 63, 111–19
 chronic pulmonary infections 355–6
 dyspnoea 111–12, 206, 211
 furosemide, inhaled 82–3, 119, 356
 opioids 112–15
 pain 294–7
 psychotropics 115–19
pharynx 39
phenobarbital (Donnatal©) 357
phenothiazines 117–19
phosphodiesterase inhibitors 227
physiology see anatomy and physiology
physiotherapy 219–20, 264, 266, 275, 311, 312
'pigtail' catheter 340
platypnoea 216
pleura, pleural space and pleural fluid 38
pleurectomy 340–1
pneumoconiosis 208–9
pneumonectomy 209
pneumonia 266, 350–1, 352
poliomyelitis 225
Portenoy, P.K. 319–20
positive end expiratory pressure (PEEP) 82, 84
positron emission tomography (PET) 286
post-pneumonectomy supportive care 208
postgraduate membership of Royal College of
 Physicians or General Practice 15
potassium channels 293
Poznan declaration 9
prednisolone 260

pressure work 76
pressure-dependent airway narrowing 47
probabilistic sensitivity analysis (PSA) 67–8
prochlorperazine 117
progesterone 247
prognosis is limited (definition of term) 12–13
progressive massive fibrosis 209
progressive muscle relaxation (PMR) 151, 173
promethazine 117
prophylactic cranial irradiation (PCI) 327–8
proprioceptive neuromuscular facilitation (PNF) 220
protease inhibitors 350
protriptyline 118–19
provocation test 241
psychological addiction to oxygen therapy 138
psychological aspects of management in end of life
 care 30–1
psychological factors 302
 cystic fibrosis 312–14
 and dyspnoea (breathlessness) 94–5
psychological support:
 diffuse airflow obstruction and 'restrictive' lung
  disease 205
 and hyperventilation syndrome 244
psychological well-being measures 157
psychosocial factors 164, 166, 364
psychotherapy 205, 222
psychotropics 115–19
 benzodiazepines 115–16
 buspirone 117
 phenothiazines 117–19
pulmonary alveolar macrophages (PAMs) 41–2, 51
pulmonary arteries 44
pulmonary fibrosis 208
pulmonary function tests 93–4, 95
Pulmonary Functional Status and Dyspnoea
 Questionnaire (PFSDQ) 100, 174
Pulmonary Functional Status Instrument (PFSI) 118
Pulmonary Functional Status Scale (PFSS) 100
pulmonary gas exchange 46–8
pulmonary hypertension 197
 and oxygen therapy 134
pulmonary infections see chronic pulmonary
 infections
pulmonary receptors 78
pulmonary rehabilitation 4–5, 28, 86, 154–9, 165–6
 anxiety and depression 174
 chronic respiratory disease questionnaire 102
 diffuse airflow obstruction and 'restrictive' lung
  disease 202–3, 210
 educational programme 158
 exercise programme 157–8
 exercise tolerance 155–6
 health-related quality of life and psychological
  well-being measures 157
 hyperventilation syndrome 243, 246
 nutritional status 157
 patient selection 155
 pulmonary functional status scale 100
 strength 156
 structured 165
pulmonary vascular disease 208, 209

pulmonary vessels 42, 44
pulse oximetry 124
pursed lip breathing 170, 203, 220
pyrazinamide 349

quality domains for patients and families 175
quality of life 53–9, 67
   and complementary exercises 172
   definitions 53
   disease-specific scales 54–7
   and expectoration 272–3
   generic scales 57–8
   health-related 64
   idiographic scales 58
   implications for treatment selection and patient
      management 59
   instruments 101–3, 157
   malignant disease 330, 333
   oxygen therapy 129, 133
   and pain 283–5
quality-adjusted life year (QALY) 64
quaternary ammonium compounds 275, 357
quiet breathing 245

radiological investigations 93, 286
radiotherapy 265–6, 336
   continuous hyperfractionated accelerated
      (CHART) 326
   external beam 335, 338, 339
   non-small cell lung cancer (NSCLC) 325–6
   for palliation 332–4
   stereotactic body (SBRT) 327
   technical advances 326–9
   three-dimensional computed
      tomography-based 327
   see also chemoradiotherapy
Rajagopal, M.R. 8–9
rapidly adapting irritant receptors (RARs) 44, 254
Ravasco, P. 186–7
Read, J.A. 189
'reading numbers aloud' test 98–9
reafferent signals 77
reductive step 18–19
rehabilitation *see* pulmonary rehabilitation
relaxation exercises 151, 171–2
reservoir cannulae 139
residual volume (RV) 45–7
resistance training 157–8, 203
resource use, measurement and valuation of 64–5
respiratory alkalosis 234
respiratory depression 114–15
respiratory distress observation scale (RDOS) 97
respiratory drive abnormalities 219
respiratory failure, acute 171
respiratory isolation 364
respiratory muscle strength 156
respiratory muscle training programmes 203–4, 221
respiratory syncytial virus (RSV) 266
restorative therapies, withdrawal of for chronic
     pulmonary infections 359–60
restrictive pulmonary disease 46, 94
   see also diffuse airflow obstruction

Reuben, D.B. 96
rhDNase 273
rhinitis/upper airway cough 261–2
Rice, K.L. 117, 167
rifampicin 349
rifamycins 350
ritual for a breathing crisis 175
Rooyacker, J.M. 132
Rotterdam Symptom Checklist (RSCL) 320
rowing 157
Royal College of Physicians guidelines for oxygen
     use 133–5, 205

S-carboxymethylcysteine 273
St George Respiratory Questionnaire (SGRQ) 54,
     57, 103, 157, 201, 273
   saline:
      hypertonic 274, 356
      isotonic 274
      nebulized 356
sarcoidosis 199
Saunders, C. 10
scalene muscles 38
Scandinavian countries 28, 297
Schedule for the Evaluation of Individual Quality of
     Life (SEIQoL) 58
Schols, A.M. 191
sclerosing agent 340
scoliosis 215, 217, 218, 219, 224
scopolamine (Transderm-Scop©) 357
Scottish Intercollegiate Guidelines Network (SIGN)
     guidelines on asthma 198
secretagogues 273–4
secretions 356–8
   see also expectoration
sedative drugs 34, 225–6
segment (lung) 48
selective serotonin reuptake inhibitors (SSRIs)
     117–18, 205, 356, 357
self-esteem, loss of 148
self-management programmes 166–8, 174, 204
sensory component 85
sensory cortex 77
sensory nerves 292–3
sertraline 118
sexual dysfunction 151
SF-36 *see* Medical Outcomes Study Short Form
Sheffield model of supportive care 18–22, 26, 28, 29
shortness of breath questionnaire (SOBQ) 100
shuttle walking test 94
Sickness Impact Profile (SIP) 101–2
sighing 239
sildenafil 227
silicosis 209
Silver Lining Questionnaire 58
Simon, P.M. 74
Singh, N.P. 117
Singh, V.P. 173
six-step protocol 360–4
6-minute walking test (6MWT) 131, 155–6, 173, 174
skeletal diseases *see* neuromuscular and skeletal
     diseases

sleep apnoea:
  central 19, 216
  obstructive 215–17, 219, 220, 226–7
slowly-adapting stretch receptors (SAR) 44, 254
small-cell lung cancer (SCLC) 319–20, 325, 332–5, 338
  chemotherapy 332
  radiotherapy 327–8
smoking 235, 347
  chronic obstructive pulmonary disease-related
      infection 351
  and cough 262
  diffuse airflow obstruction and 'restrictive' lung
      disease 197–8, 200, 204
  HIV-related infection 350
  non-obstructive lung disease 210
  and oxygen therapy 136
social aspects of patients' and families' lives in end of
    life care 31
social issues 302
social worker 311–12
social-environmental influences 164–5
sodium channels 293, 301
specialist medical team 310
specialist nurses 302, 311, 312
specialized palliative care 14, 15
speech, excessive and hyperventilation 235
speech therapy intervention 264
spinal cord injuries 81, 221, 222
spinal cord tolerance 334
spiritual/religious issues 31, 302
spirometry 93
SpO$_2$ value 124–5
sputum see expectoration
State-Trait Anxiety Inventory Scale (STAI) 117, 174
Steiner, M.C. 191
step tests 156, 157
Stephens, R.J. 320
steroids:
  anabolic 223
  see also corticosteroids
stimulant intake reduction 235, 246–7
Stone, D. 360
strength training 166
stress management 172, 235, 245
stretch receptors 73–4, 78, 81, 254
Strigo, I.A. 286
Stulbarg, M.S. 102
Sub-Saharan Africa 350
sulphydryl moieties 273
supportive care:
  best 63, 333–4
  chronic cough 264
  diffuse airflow obstruction and 'restrictive' lung
      disease 200–2
  malignant disease 330
  non-obstructive lung disease 210
  therapies 20
  see also chronic pulmonary infections: supportive
      care
supportive care in cystic fibrosis 309–16
  fertility and pregnancy 314
  home care services 312

medical management 310
  palliation and bereavement 314–16
  psychological aspects 312–14
  social worker 311–12
  specialist dietician 311
  specialist medical team 310
  specialist nurse 311
  specialist physiotherapist 311
  urinary incontinence 314
supportive care network:
  Group A 23–5
  Group B 23–5
  Group C 23–6
supportive care and palliation 3–34
  assisted dying and euthanasia 33–4
  cancer survivors 28–9
  composition 23–6
  end of life care 8–9, 29–33
  implementation 17–21
  medicine, changing aims of 3–7
  models of palliative care 9–15
  needs at earlier stages of illness 27–8
  new concept of care, necessity for 16–17
  relationship between 26–7
  specialty, palliative medicine as 15
  symptom perception, factors determining 7–8
Suresh, K. 8–9
surgical interventions 339
surgical options 206
surgical techniques 297
Swinburn, C.R. 130
sympathetic nerves 44
symptom perception, factors determining 7–8
systemic therapy, targeted 331–2

tai chi 172–3
talc 340
talking and breathing 246
Tanaka, K. 94
taxane 330
Tayek, J.A. 189
team debriefing 316
terminal care see end of life care
tertiary amines 357
tertiary ammonium compounds 275
tetracycline 340
Thomas, H.M. 210
Thomas, M. 242–3, 244
thoracic compression 222
thoracoplasty 215
Thornby, M.A. 173
tidal volume 239
Tomíska, M. 187
topotecan 332
total lung capacity (TLC) 45–6, 49–50
total parenteral nutrition 187, 189, 192
tracheostomy ventilation 224–5
tramadol 298
tranexamic acid 338, 358–9
transcutaneous electrical nerve stimulation
    (TENS) 173–4
transfer coefficient for carbon monoxide (TLCO) 48

transient receptor potential vanilloid-1
(TRPV-1) 254
treadmill exercise 173
treatment concordance 313
treatment, previous exposure to 334
treatment selection and quality of life 59
tricyclic antidepressants 117–19, 205
tryptophan 189
tuberculosis (TB) 199, 224, 347, 348–9, 355
haemoptysis 358
multidrug resistant (MDR-TB) 349, 355
psychosocial aspects 364
type 1 palliation:
prevention/prophylaxis 6, 16
type 1 receptors (rapidly adapting) 44, 254
type 1 respiratory failure 125
type 2 palliation: direct targeting of primary disease
process 6, 16
type 2 respiratory failure 125
type 3 palliation: manipulation of pathophysiological
consequences of primary disease process 6, 16,
21, 26
type 4 palliation: alteration of perception or
secondary effects of symptom 6, 16, 22, 26
type II receptors (slowly adapting) 44, 254
type III receptors (J receptors) 44, 83

uncertainty, analysis of impact of 67–8
unidimensional scales 95–9
United States
assisted dying and euthanasia 33
chronic obstructive pulmonary disease
(COPD) 197
cystic fibrosis 315
end of life care preferences 363
malignant disease 325, 334
opioids 297
palliation and supportive care 19, 28, 202
tuberculosis 349
University of California, San Diego shortness of
breath questionnaire (SOBQ) 100
upper airway 39
muscles 218
receptors 81
urinary incontinence and cystic fibrosis 314
Uronis, H.E. 131

valid daily activities 146–7
Van Norren, K. 189
varenicline 204

Velloso, M. 148
ventilatory support 44–5, 46, 222, 223–5
compressed air via nasal cannula 355
continuous positive airway pressure 226–7
intermittent positive pressure breathing
(PPPB) 222
non-invasive positive pressure ventilation 81–2,
84, 170–1, 223–5, 312, 353, 354
see also oxygen
venules 44
verbal rating scale 282
Vermeeren, M.A. 191
vertebroplasty 297
vinblastine 332, 335
vincristine 332
vinorelbine 329, 332, 334
visual analogue scales (VAS) 95–6, 97, 113, 130, 136,
172, 283
visual imagery 151
vital capacity 45, 47, 49
forced 94, 119
volume work 76
volunteers and palliative care principles 3

walking 157, 158
aids 354
tests 94, 223
Washington DC Consensus Group 185
water used in expectoration 274
Wells, C.K. 93–4, 98
West, R. 244
Wijkstra, P.J. 102–3
Wilcock, A. 95
Wilson, D.O. 190
Wood, P. 233
Woodcock, A.A. 117
World Health Organization 3, 14
analgesic ladder 294, 295, 296, 301, 303
Cancer pain relief and palliative care 10–11, 12
HIV infection 350
malignant disease 321
quality of life definition 54
resource model for organizing cancer services 11,
19–20
tuberculosis 349

yawning 239
yoga 172–3

zoledronic acid 297